Case-Based Neurology

Case-Based Neurology

Anuradha Singh, MD
Neurology Attending
Assistant Professor
Department of Neurology
New York University Langone Medical Center
New York, New York

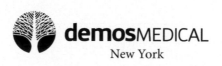

demosMEDICAL

New York

Visit our website at www.demosmed.com

ISBN: 978-1-9338-6425-9
E-book ISBN: 978-1-9352-8192-4

Acquisitions Editor: Beth Barry
Compositor: Newgen Imaging

Medicine is an ever-changing science. Research and clinical experience are continually expanding our knowledge, in particular our understanding of proper treatment and drug therapy. The authors, editors, and publisher have made every effort to ensure that all information in this book is in accordance with the state of knowledge at the time of production of the book. Nevertheless, the authors, editors, and publisher are not responsible for errors or omissions or for any consequences from application of the information in this book and make no warranty, express or implied, with respect to the contents of the publication. Every reader should examine carefully the package inserts accompanying each drug and should carefully check whether the dosage schedules mentioned therein or the contraindications stated by the manufacturer differ from the statements made in this book. Such examination is particularly important with drugs that are either rarely used or have been newly released on the market.

Library of Congress Cataloging-in-Publication Data

Singh, Anuradha.
  Case-based neurology / Anuradha Singh.
    p. ; cm.
  Includes bibliographical references and index.
  ISBN 978-1-933864-25-9 (alk. paper) — ISBN 978-1-935281-92-4 (e-book)
  I. Title.
  [DNLM: 1. Nervous System Diseases—diagnosis—Case Reports. 2. Nervous
System Diseases—therapy—Case Reports. WL 141]
  616.8—dc23   2011040244

Special discounts on bulk quantities of Demos Medical Publishing books are available to corporations, professional associations, pharmaceutical companies, healthcare organizations, and other qualifying groups. For details, please contact:
Special Sales Department
Demos Medical Publishing
11 West 42nd Street, 15th Floor
New York, NY 10036
Phone: 800-532-8663 or 212-683-0072
Fax: 212-941-7842
E-mail: rsantana@demosmedpub.com

Printed in the United States of America by Hamilton Printing.
11 12 13 14 / 5 4 3 2 1

Contents

Contents

Contributors

Lauren E. Abrey, MD
Attending Physician
Department of Neurology
Memorial Sloan-Kettering Cancer Center
New York, NY

Phillip Paul Amodeo, MD
Neurologist/Clinical Neurophysiologist
Department of Neurology
Shore Neurology, P.A.
Tom's River, NJ

Sonia Anand, MD
Neurology Resident
Department of Neurology
New York University Langone Medical Center
New York, NY

Deepti Anbarasan, MD
Resident Physician
Department of Neurology and Psychiatry
New York University School of Medicine
New York, NY

Ramesh P. Babu, MBBS, Mch(Neurosurgery), MD
Associate Clinical Professor
Neurosurgery Department
New York University Langone Medical Center
New York, NY

Michael Boffa, MD
Resident Physician
Department of Neurology
Rush University Medical Center
Chicago, IL

Robert J. Bollo, MD
Assistant Professor
Department of Neurology
Baylor College of Medicine
Houston, TX

Ritvij Bowry, MD
Neurology Resident
Department of Neurology
New York University School of Medicine and Medical Center
New York, NY

Rachel Brandstadter, BS
Mount Sinai Hospital
New York, NY

Marjorie E. Bunch, BS, MD
Instructor
Department of Neurology
Beth Israel Deaconess Medical Center
Boston, MA

Chad Carlson, MD
Assistant Professor
Department of Neurology
New York University Langone Medical Center
New York, NY

Adrian T. Chan, MD
Neurology Attending, Movement Disorder
Department of Neurology
WellSpan Neuroscience and Pain Center
York, PA

Yaniv Chen, MDCM
Neurologist
Department of Neurology
New York University Langone Medical Center
New York, NY

Mary Lynn Chu, MD
Co-Director
Department of Neurology
Neuromuscular Disease Center
Rusk Institute of Rehabilitation Medicine and
    Medical Director, Center for Children
Hospital for Joint Diseases
New York University Langone Medical Center
New York, NY

Christina Coyle, MD, MS
Director of Tropical Medicine Clinic
Jacobi Medical Center
Assistant Dean for Faculty Development
Albert Einstein College of Medicine
Bronx, NY

Contributors

Sara C. Crystal, MD
Assistant Professor
Department of Neurology
New York University Langone Medical Center
New York, NY

Philippe Douyon, MD
Resident
Department of Neurology
New York University Langone Medical Center
New York, NY

John Engler, MD
Neurosurgery Housestaff
Department of Neurosurgery
New York University Langone Medical Center
New York, NY

Mohammad Fouladvand, MD
Associate Professor
Neurology and Ophthalmology Department
New York University Langone Medical Center
New York, NY

Benjamin Ge
Department of Radiology
Hospital of the University of Pennsylvania
Philadelphia, PA

Rebecca Wolf Gilbert, MD, PhD
Clinical Assistant Professor of Neurology
Department of Neurology
New York University Langone Medical Center
New York, NY

Samuel A. Goldlust, MD
Co-Chief, Brain and Spine Institute
John Theurer Cancer Center
Hackensack, NJ

Varendra Gosein, MD
Department of Psychiatry
New York University School of Medicine
New York, NY

Jerome J. Graber, MD, MPH
Director of Adult Neuro-Oncology
Assistant Professor of Neurology and Oncology
Montefiore Medical Center of the Albert Einstein
    College of Medicine
Bronx, NY

Jonathan H. Howard, MD
Clinical Instructor
Departments of Neurology and Psychiatry
New York University
New York, NY

Thomas J. Kaley, MD
Assistant Attending Physician
Department of Neurology
Memorial Sloan-Kettering Cancer Center
New York, NY

Maya Katz, MD
Clinical Fellow
Department of Neurology
University of California
San Francisco, CA

Muznay Naveed Khawaja
Fourth-year medical student
Pakistan

Minjee Kim, MD
Resident
Harvard University Residency Program
Neurology Department
Masscchusetts General Hospital and Brigham and
    Women's Hospital
Boston, MA

Jason L. Kiner, MD
Neurohospitalist
Department of Neurology
Baptist Health System, Neuroscience Consultants
Miami, FL

Kiril Kiprovski, MD
Assistant Professor
Department of Neurology
Hospital for Joint Diseases
New York University Langone Medical Center
New York, NY

Arielle Kurzweil, MD
Resident
Department of Neurology
New York University School of Medicine
New York, NY

Geneviève Legault, MD
Fellow, Pediatric Neuro-oncology
Department of Pediatrics
New York University Langone Medical Center
New York, NY

Brijesh Malkani, MD
Resident
Department of Neurology
New York University Langone Medical Center
New York, NY

Lara V. Marcuse, MD
Assistant Professor, Co-Director of the Mount
    Sinai Epilepsy Center
Mount Sinai Medical Center
New York, NY

Mitchell G. Miglis, MD
Fellow in Autonomic Neurophysiology
Department of Neurology
Beth Israel Deaconess Medical Center
Harvard University School of Medicine
Boston, MA

Sarah S. Milla, MD
Assistant Professor
Department of Radiology
New York University Langone Medical Center
New York, NY

Betty Mintz, MD
Department of Neurology
Mount Sinai School of Medicine
New York, NY

Matthew Morrison, BS
Department of Medical Education
Mount Sinai School of Medicine
New York, NY

Vincci Ngan, MD
Chief Resident
Department of Neurology
New York University School of Medicine
New York, NY

Irina Ok
Research Assistant
New York Sleep Institute
City University of New York
New York, NY

Rachael Oxman, BA
Medical Student
Mount Sinai School of Medicine
New York, NY

Kimberly Parker Monzor, BSN, MA, ANP BC, GNP BC
Nurse Practitioner
Department of Epilepsy
New York University Langone Medical Center
New York, NY

Addie Peretz, MD
Department of Internal Medicine
Georgetown University Hospital
Washington, DC

Jai S. Perumal, MD
Assistant Professor
Department of Neurology
Weill Cornell Medical College
New York, NY

Maria Philip, MD
Resident
Department of Neurology
New York University School of Medicine
New York, NY

Rikki Racela, MD
Department of Neurology
New York University School of Medicine
New York, NY

Shahzad Raza, MD
Department of Neuro-Oncology
New York University School of Medicine and Doctor,
    Department of Internal Medicine
Brookdale University Hospital & Medical Center
New York, NY

Alcibiades J. Rodriguez, MD
Assistant Professor
Department of Neurology
New York University School of Medicine and
    Medical Director
New York Sleep Institute
New York, NY

Martin J. Sadowski, MD, PhD
Assistant Professor
Department of Neurology, Psychiatry, and Pharmacology
New York University School of Medicine
New York, NY

Contributors

Daniel Sahlein, BA, MD
Fellow
Department of Radiology
New York University Langone Medical Center
New York, NY

David Schick, MD
Department of Neurology
Albert Einstein College of Medicine/Montefiore Medical
    Center
New York, NY

Sana S. Shah, BA, MD
Department of Internal Medicine
Emory University School of Medicine
Atlanta, GA

Susan C. Shin, BS, MD
Department of Neurology
Mount Sinai Medical Center
New York, NY

Anuradha Singh, MD
Neurology Attending, Assistant Professor
Department of Neurology
New York University Langone Medical Center
New York, NY

Maria Stefanidou, MD, MSc
Epilepsy Fellow
Comprehensive Epilepsy Center
New York University
New York, NY

Ashish Vyas, MBBS, MD
Resident
Department of Neurology
New York University Hospital
New York, NY

Kristin M. Waldron, MD
General Neurologist
New York University School of Medicine
New York, NY

Qingliang Wang, MD, PhD
Attending Stroke Neurologist and Interventional
    Neuroradiology Fellow
Department of Neurology and Radiology
Mount Sinai Medical Center
New York, NY

Winfred Poayi Wu, MD
Neurology Associates of Norwalk
Norwalk, CT

Niushen Zhang, MD
Department of Neurology
Stanford University
Stanford, CA

The accumulation of first-hand experience with patients is the surest path to a successful career in medicine. As Sir William Osler brilliantly stated, "He who studies medicine without books sails an unchartered sea, but he who studies medicine without patients does not go to sea at all." The most able clinicians build upon their experiences with individual patients to formulate their approach to diagnosis and treatment for their next patient. Osler, whose early career was devoted to neurology, established the idea of residency training so that today doctors in training make up most of the hospital medical staff of the major academic medical centers. Within these settings, bedside teaching and clinical case conferences focusing on actual patients have become the most important component in medical education. When faced with perplexing new patients, we hark back to our experience with prior patients in whom we recognize similarities.

Dr. Singh, the editor of this wonderful compendium, and the many trainees, former trainees, and faculty she has invited as contributors have compiled a stellar collection of actual patient experiences representing the broad panoply that is clinical neurology. While the patient encounters described in this collection may be considered typical of the diseases they represent, we must remain aware of differences that can occur from case to case of the same disorder.

The diversity of patients described mirrors the enormous variety of patients seen daily at the New York University Langone Medical Center. Bellevue Hospital, one of the oldest city hospitals in the nation and the major teaching hospital of NYU, attracts patients originating from every part of the world and from a wide diversity of cultural and socioeconomic backgrounds. Its tradition in neurology extends back to William Hammond, MD, a Surgeon General of the United States during the Civil War. Dr. Hammond, formerly a military surgeon, came to Bellevue Hospital in 1864 and made a specialty of diseases of the nervous system, publishing in 1871 the first textbook of neurology in the United States. Many outstanding neurologists succeeded him, building a tradition of clinical excellence that has been passed on to the young practitioners who within this text share some of their favorite patient experiences.

Just as Osler, a giant of American medicine, was firmly grounded in neurology, so too have other influential physicians found the study of neurology to be a strong influence on their careers. Lewis Thomas, MD, well known to readers of the *New England Journal of Medicine* for his regular column titled "Notes of a Biology Watcher" (1971–1981), completed a neurology residency and later served as chairman of the pathology department at the NYU Medical School, then as chairman of the NYU Department of Medicine, and subsequently as dean of the NYU School of Medicine. Indeed, it was Dr. Thomas who encouraged me while I was a Bellevue Hospital Resident in Medicine to study neurology. It was a choice that I have cherished, opening doors to a career that has been witness to so many advances in science.

Every practitioner of medicine and related health sciences will enjoy reading these first-hand case reports and studying the accompanying figures, tables, and suggested readings. Many depend upon a multidisciplinary approach so common in the complex highly technical world in which we practice. I look forward to more presentations in this format by our next generation of trainees.

Edwin H. Kolodny, MD
Bernard A. and Charlotte Marden Professor of Neurology
New York University School of Medicine

How do we learn neurology? Localization in neurology seems to be a daunting challenge for many medical students and residents. Neurology is often perceived to be the most exigent branch in medicine. Neurologists need to master the complex neuroanatomical pathways for precise localization. Still, localizing a lesion is creative and I feel, at times, it can be an exciting journey of discovery akin to solving a complex mathematical problem.

What motivated me to write this book? I have always enjoyed lectures and grand rounds where speakers present challenging cases and give clinical pearls because I can translate that knowledge to improve my clinical acumen. During my fellowship year, I felt thrilled and honored when one of my mentors, Dr. David Younger, asked me to write a chapter in his textbook titled *Motor Disorders*. Later when I thought of writing a case-based neurology book, I wanted to give motivated trainees the same chance and invited medical students, neurology residents, and attendings with special expertise in the field to write up interesting cases and help me shape this project.

This book is a collective effort,and I sincerely hope that our readers enjoy and learn by reading it. The authors have retained a uniform case format despite variances in their approach to clinical problems and the discussion of differential diagnoses. There are abundant illustrations, as well as useful information in tables that can be quickly accessed and appreciated. If it is true that a picture is worth a thousand words, a visual of a good clinical case will be retained and absorbed in a way that traditional text readings cannot do.

Case-Based Neurology is organized by chief complaint; each case includes an introduction, physical examination, case questions, laboratory testing, imaging findings, diagnosis, and discussion, including differential diagnosis and treatment. The back of the book provides a topic list for readers who want to review cases by disease pathology or subject. All major areas of neurology and both typical and atypical presentations of a disease are included. We have covered important topics such as critical care, multiple sclerosis, epilepsy, movement disorders, stroke, neurodegenerative diseases, spinal cord pathologies, neuro-oncology, muscular dystrophy, peripheral nervous system disorders, neuro-immunology and neuro-infectious diseases. Cases are illustrated with high-quality images, and diagnosis and clinical management is emphasized. For each case, controversies in management are discussed to highlight differences in treatment philosophy and further hone clinical skills.

Although not exhaustive, suggested readings are included at the end of each chapter. As readers go through the cases, they may realize how the same chief complaints can still lead to totally different diagnoses emphasizing the role of careful history taking, physical examination and appropriate diagnostic studies. While it is beyond the scope of this book to include all cases in depth, we have included a good overview of a wide range of common neurological conditions.

Acknowledgments

I would like to express my gratitude to all the neurology residents, medical students, fellows, attendings, and mentors who made this work possible. My deepest thanks go out to Dr. Edwin H. Kolodny who agreed to write the foreword of this book.

Many thanks to Beth Barry and Lindsay Claire at Demos Medical Publishing and Ashita Shah at Newgen Imaging for their patience and tolerance. They are the ones who have encouraged and pushed me to finish this work in a timely fashion.

Last but not least, I want to thank my parents, siblings, and lovely daughters (Parul and Pallavi) for their unwavering support.

3-T	3-Tesla
5-HT	5-Hydroxytryptamine
AA	Anaplastic astrocytoma
A & O	Alert and oriented
A1	First segment of the anterior cerebral artery
A2	Second segment of the anterior cerebral artery
AA	Anaplastic astrocytoma
AAN	American Academy of Neurology
AASM	American Academy of Sleep Medicine
Ab	Antibody
ABC	Airway, breathing, and circulation
ACA	Anterior cerebral artery
ACE	Angiotensin converting enzyme
Ach	Acetylcholine
ACTH	Adrenocorticotropic hormone
AD	Alzheimer's disease
ADC	Apparent diffusion coefficient
ADEM	Acute disseminated encephalomyelitis
ADHD	Attention deficit hyperactivity disorder
ADL	Activities of daily living
AED	Antiepileptic drugs
AFP	Alpha fetoprotein
AHI	Apnea–hypopnea index
AICA	Anterior inferior cerebellar artery
AIDP	Acute inflammatory demyelinating polyneuropathy
AJ	Ankle jerk
ALL	Anterior longitudinal ligament
ALS	Amyotrophic lateral sclerosis
ALT	Alanine aminotransferase
AMI	Autobiographical memory interview
AMPA	α-amino-3-hydroxy-5-methyl-4-isoxazolepropionic acid
ANA	Antinuclear antibody
anti-GAD	antibodies against glutamate decarboxylase
Anti-SRP	Anti-signal recognition particle
aPTT	Activated partial thrombin time
ASO Ab	Anti-streptolysin O antibody
AST	Aspartate aminotransferase
AV	Atrio-ventricular
AVM	Arteriovenous malformations
AZT	Azathioprine
B/L	Bilateral
BA	Brodmann area
Bid	Two times a day
BMP	Basic metabolic panel

BP	Blood pressure
BPH	Benign prostatic hyperplasia
BPNH	Bilateral periventricular nodular heterotopia
BSE	Bovine spongiform encephalopathy
BUN	Blood urea nitrogen
CA	Cancer antigen
CAD	Carotid artery dissection
CADASIL	Cerebral autosomal dominant arteriopathy with subcortical infarcts and leukoencephalopathy
CAG	Cytosine, Adenosine, Guanine
CAM	Cytokeratin
Caspr-2	Contactin-associated protein like 2
CBC	Complete blood count
CBD	Corticobasal degeneration
CBGD	Cortical basal ganglionic degeneration
CCA	Common carotid artery
CCM	Cerebral cavernous malformations
CCM-1	Cerebral cavernous malformation-1
CCM-2	Cerebral cavernous malformation-2
CCM-3	Cerebral cavernous malformation-3
CD3	Cluster of differentiation 3
CD4	Cluster of differentiation 4
CD 20	Cluster of differentiation 20
CDMS	Clinically definite multiple sclerosis
CEA	Carcinoembryonic antigen
CF	Complement-fixing
CGRP	Calcitonin gene-related peptide
CIDP	Chronic inflammatory demyelinating polyneuropathy
CIS	Clinically isolated syndrome
CJD	Creutzfeldt-Jakob disease
CK	Creatine kinase
CKMB	Creatine kinase (subunits: M=muscle; B=brain)
CM	Cavernous malformation
CMAP	Compound muscle action potential
CMT	Crisis Management Team
CMV	Cytomegalovirus
CNS	Central nervous system
CNs	Cranial nerves
COPD	Chronic obstructive pulmonary disease
CP	Cerebellopontine
CPAP	Continuous positive airway pressure
CPK	Creatine phosphokinase
CRDs	Complex repetitive discharges
CREST	Calcinosis, Raynaud phenomenon, esophageal dysmotility, sclerodactyly, and telangiectasia
CRP	C-reactive protein
CSD	Cortical spreading depression
CSF	Cerebrospinal fluid
CT	Computed tomography
CTA	Computed tomography angiography

CTG	Cytonsine,thymine, guanine
Cu/Zn	Copper/Zinc
CUGBP 1	CUG binding protein1
CVA	Cerebrovascular accident
CVS	Cardiovascular
CVT	Cerebral venous thrombosis
CXR	Chest X-ray
DBS	Deep brain stimulation
DHE	Dihydroergotamine
DHEA	Dehydroepiandrosterone
DIP	Drug-induced parkinsonism
DLB	Diffuse Lewy body
DM	Dermatomyositis
DMPK	Dystrophia myotonica-protein kinase
DNET	Dysembryoplastic neuroepithelial tumors
DREZ	Dorsal root entry zone
DSA	Digital subtraction angiography
DTI	Diffusion tensor imaging
DTR	Deep tendon reflexes
DVA	Developmental venous anomaly
DVT	Deep venous thrombosis
DWI	Diffusion-weighted imaging
EBV	Epstein-Barr virus
ECA	External carotid artery
ECHO	Echocardiogram
ECT	Electroconvulsive therapy
ED	Emergency department
EDS	Excessive daytime sleepiness
EEG	Electroencephalogram
EIA	Enzyme immunoassay
EITB	Enzyme-linked immunoelectrotransfer blot
EKG	Electrocardiogram
ELISA	Enzyme-linked immunosorbent assay
EMA	Epithelial membrane antigen
EMG	Electromyography
EMS	Emergency medical service
ENMC	European Neuromuscular Center
EOMI	Extraocular movements intact
EPC	Epilepsia partialis continua
ER	Emergency room
ESES	Electrical status epilepticus of sleep
ESI	Epidural steroid injections
ESR	Erythrocyte sedimentation rate
ESS	Epworth Sleepiness Scale
ETLE	Extratemporal lobe epilepsy
FACS	Fluorescence-assisted cell sorting
FALS	Familial ALS
FCD	Focal cortical dysplasia
fCJD	Familial Creutzfeldt-Jakob disease
FDA	Food and Drug Administration

FFI	Fatal familial insomnia
FHM	Familial hemiplegic migraine
FLAIR	Fluid–attenuated inversion-recovery
fMRI	Functional magnetic resonance imaging
FNF	Finger nose finger
FS	Febrile seizures
FSH	Follicle-stimulating hormone
FTD	Frontotemporal dementia
FVC	Forced vital capacity
GABA	Gamma-aminobutyric acid
GAD	Glutamic acid decarboxylase
GBM	Glioblastoma multiforme
GBS	Guilliain-Barré syndrome
GCS	Glasgow coma scale
GCSE	Generalized convulsive status epilepticus
Gd	Gadolinium
GDNF	Glial cell-derived neurotrophic factor
GERD	Gastroesophageal reflux disease
GH	Growth hormone
GI	Gastrointestinal
GKS	Gamma knife radiosurgery
GM 1	Monosialotetrahexosylganglioside
GMS	Gomori or Grocott methenamine silver
GPE	General physical examination
GRE	Gradient-echo MRI
GSS	Gertsmann Straussler Scheinker syndrome
GTP	Guanosine triphosphate
GTPases	Guanosine triphosphatases
H&E	Hematoxylin and eosin
HAART	Highly active antiretroviral therapy
HbA1c	Glycated hemoglobin
HBV	Hepatitis B virus
HcG	Human chorionic gonadotropin
HCV	Hepatitis C virus
HD	Huntington's disease
HDL	High density lipoprotein
HEENT	Head, eye, ear, nose, and throat examination
Hex A	Hexosaminidase A
Hg	Mercury
h-IBM	Hereditary inclusion body myositis
HIV	Human immunodeficiency virus
HKS	Heel-knee-shin
HLA	Human leukocyte antigen
HLD	Hyperlipidemia
HMB-45	Human melanoma black-45
HME	Hemimegalencephaly
HMG CoA	3-hydroxy-3-methylglutaryl-coenzyme A
HR	Heart rate
HRT	Hormonal replacement therapy
HS	Hippocampal sclerosis

HSV	Herpes simplex virus
HTLV	Human T-cell leukemia virus
HTN	Hypertension
Hz	Hertz
HZV	Herpes zoster virus
IBM	Inclusion body myositis
ICA	Internal carotid artery
ICAM	Intercellular adhesion molecule
ICAP-1	Integrin cytoplasmic domain-associated protein-1
ICM	Intracranial metastases
ICP	Intracranial pressure
ICU	Intensive care unit
IFN	Interferon
Ig	Immunoglobulin
IIH	Idiopathic intracranial hypertension
ILAE	International League Against Epilepsy
IM	Intramuscular
INO	Internuclear ophthalmoplegia
INR	International normalized ratio
IS	Infantile spasms
ISAT	International Subarachnoid Aneurysm Trial
IV	Intravenous
IVIg	Intravenous immunoglobulin
KJ	Knee jerk
KPS	Karnofsky performance status
KSS	Karolynska Sleepiness Scale
L 1–5	Lumbar vertebra (1–5)
LDH	Lactate dehydrogenase
LDL	Low-density lipoprotein
LE	Limbic encephalitis
LFTs	Liver function tests
LGI1	Leucine-rich glioma inactivated-1
LH	Luteinizing hormone
LLE	Left lower extremity
LMN	Lower motor neuron
LP	Lumbar puncture
LS	Lumbosacral
LT	Light touch
LUE	Left upper extremity
LVEF	Left ventricular ejection fraction
M1	First segment of the middle cerebral artery
mA	MilliAmperes
MAG	Myelin-associated glycoprotein
MAO-B	Monoamine oxidase B
MAP	Microtubule-associated protein
MBNL1	Muscle blind-like
MCA	Middle cerebral artery
MCD	Malformation of cortical development
MCTD	Mixed connective tissue disease
MCV	Mean corpuscular volume

MEG	Magnetoencepahlography
MEKK3	Mitogen-activated protein kinase kinase kinase 3
MELAS	Mitochondrial encephalomyopathy, lactic acidosis, and stroke-like episodes
MG	Myasthenia gravis
MGUS	Monoclonal gammopathies
MI	Myocardial infarction
MIBG	Metaiodobenzylguanidine
MLF	Medial longitudinal fasciculus
MM	Methionine
MMA	Maxillo-mandibular advancement surgery
MMN	Multifocal motor neuropathy
MMP	Matrix metalloproteinases
MMSE	Mini-Mental State Exam
MND	Motor neuron disease
MP-RAGE	Magnetization prepared rapid gradient echo
MPTP	1-Methyl-1,2,4,6 tetrahydropyridine
MRA	Magnetic resonance angiography
MRI	Magnetic resonance imaging
MRV	Magnetic resonance venography
MS	Multiple sclerosis
MSA	Multisystem atrophy
MSI	Magnetic source imaging
MSLT	Multiple Sleep Latency Test
MTMR1	Myotubularin related protein 1
mTOR	Mammalian target of rapamycin
MTS	Mesial temporal sclerosis
MUAPs	Motor unit action potentials
MV	Methionine-valine
MVD	Microvascular decompression
NAD	No apparent distress
NCC	Neurocysticercosis
NCHCT	Noncontrast helical computerized tomography
NCS	Nerve conduction study
NCSE	Nonconvulsive SE
NCV	Nerve conduction velocity
NF 1	Neurofibromatosis type 1
NF 2	Neurofibromatosis type 2
NIF	Negative inspiratory force
NIH	National Institutes of Health
NINDS	National Institute of Neurological Disorders and Stroke
NKDA	No known drug allergies
NMDA	N-methyl-D-aspartic acid
NMO	Neuromyelitis optica
NO	Nitric oxide
NPH	Normal pressure hydrocephalus
NREM	Non-rapid eye movement
NS	Normal saline
NSAID	Non-steroidal anti-inflammatory drugs
NSR	Normal sinus rhythm

nvCJD	New variant Creutzfeld-Jakob disease
O$_2$	Oxygen
OCB	Oligoclonal bands
OCD	Obsessive–compulsive disorder
OCP	Oral contraceptives
OD	Oculus dexter
ON	Optic neuritis
ONSF	Optic nerve sheath fenestration
OS	Oculus sinister, left eye
OSA	Obstructive sleep apnea
OSAHS	Obstructive sleep apnea–hypopnea syndrome
OU	Oculus uterque (both eyes)
P	Pulse
P1	First segment of the posterior cerebral artery
PAS	Periodic acid Schiff
PBP	Progressive bulbar palsy
PCA	Posterior cerebral artery
PCD	Paraneoplastic cerebellar degeneration
PCNSL	Primary central nervous system lymphoma
PCR	Polymerase chain reaction
PD	Parkinson's disease
PDGFR	Platelet-derived growth factor receptor
PDR	Posterior dominant rhythm
PE	Plasmapheresis
PEG	Percutaneous endoscopic gastrostomy
PEM	Paraneoplastic encephalomyelitis
PERRL	Pupils equal, round, react to light
PERRLA	Pupils equal, round, react to light and accomodation
PET	Positron emission tomography
PICA	Posterior inferior cerebellar artery
PIGD	Postural instability and gait difficulty
PK	Proteinase K
PLEX	Plasma exchange
PLL	Posterior longitudinal ligament
PLMI	Periodic leg movements of sleep (PLMS) index
PLS	Primary lateral sclerosis
PM	Polymyositis
PMA	Progressive muscular atrophy
PML	Progressive multifocal leukoencepahalopathy
pMRI	Perfusion MR imaging
PNH	Periventricular nodular heterotopia
PNS	Peripheral nervous system
PO	Per orally
POI	Perceptual Organizational Index
PP	Pin prick
PPD	Purified protein derivative
PPMS	Primary progressive multiple sclerosis
PPV	Positive pressure ventilation
PR	Progesterone receptor

PRL	Prolactin
PROMM	Proximal myotonic myopathy
PSG	Polysomnogram
PSI	Processing speed index
PSN	Paraneoplastic sensory neuronopathy
PSP	Progressive supranuclear palsy
PSVP	Positive spontaneous visual phenomena
PSW	Paroxysmal sharp waves
PT	Prothrombin time
PTH	Parathyroid hormone
PWS	Port-wine stain
qHS	Every night
QID	Four times daily
RA	Rheumatoid arthritis
RAM	Rapid alternating movements
RAP-1	Ras-proximate-1
RAS	Rat sarcoma
RBC	Red blood cells
RBD	REM sleep behavior disorder
RDI	Respiratory Disturbance Index
REM	Rapid eye movement
RERAs	Respiratory effort-related arousals
RF	Rheumatoid factor
RLE	Right lower extremity
RNA	Ribonucleic acid
RNS	Repetitive nerve stimulation
RPR	Rapid plasma reagin
RR	Respiratory rate
RRMS	Relapsing–remitting multiple sclerosis
RT	Radiation therapy
RUE	Right upper extremity
RYR1	Ryanodine receptor 1
S 1–3	Sacral segments (1–3)
S-100	Sangtec-100
SAH	Subarachnoid hemorrhage
SaO2	Saturation of oxygen expressed in %
SBH	Subcortical band heterotopia
SC	Subcutaneous
SCA	Spinocerebellar ataxia
SCG	Superior cervical ganglion
sCJD	Sporadic Creutzfeldt-Jakob disease
SCLC	Small cell lung cancer
SCM	Sternocleidomastoid
SE	Status epilepticus
SEGA	Subependymal giant cell astrocytoma
SEN	Subependymal nodules
SFEMG	Single-fiber electromyography
sIBM	Sporadic inclusion body myositis
SLE	Systemic lupus erythematosus
SMA	Sequential multiple analysis

SNAPs	Sensory nerve action potentials
SNRI	Serotonin-norepinephrine reuptake inhibitor
SOD	Superoxide dismutase
SOREMPs	Sleep Onset REM Periods
SOX-1	Sex determining region Y-box 1
SPECT	Single photon emission computed tomography
SPS3	Secondary prevention of small subcortical strokes
SS	Standard score
SSA	Sjogren syndrome A
SSB	Sjogren syndrome B
SSEP	Somatosensory evoked potentials
SSPE	Subacute sclerosing panencepahlitis
SSRI	Selective serotonin reuptake inhibitor
STIR	Short tau inversion recovery
SWI	Susceptibility-weighted imaging
SWS	Sturge-Weber syndrome
T1WI	T1-weighted image
T2WI	T2-weighted image
T3	Triiodothyronine
T4	Thyroxine
TBI	Traumatic brain injury
TCA	Tricyclic antidepressants
TCC	Trigeminocervical complex
TDP-43	TAR DNA-binding protein 43
TEE	Transesophageal echocardiogram
TFT	Thyroid function tests
TIA	Transient ischemic attack
tid	Three times daily
TLE	Temporal lobe epilepsy
TM	Transverse myelitis
TN	Trigeminal neuralgia
t-PA	Tissue plasminogen activator
TPO	Thyroperoxidase
TS	Tourette syndrome
TSC	Tuberous sclerosis complex
TSH	Thyroid-stimulating hormone
TTE	Transthoracic echocardiogram
UE	Upper extremities
UMN	Upper motor neuron
UPP	Uvulopalatopharyngeal
US	Ultrasound
V	Trigeminal (cranial nerve)
V1	Ophthalmic (cranial nerve)
V2	Maxillary
V3	Mandibular
VA	Vertebral artery
VAD	Vertebral artery dissection
VC	Vital capacity
VCI	Verbal comprehension index
vCJD	Variant CJD

VDRL	Venereal Disease Research Laboratory
VEEG	Video electroencephalogram
VEGF	Vascular endothelial growth factor
VEP	Visual evoked potentials
VGKC	Voltage-gated potassium channel
VMI	Visual motor integration
VMUAP	Voluntary motor unit action potentials
VNS	Vagal nerve stimulator
VPM	Ventral posterior medial (thalamic nucleus)
VS	Vital signs
WBC	White blood cells
WBR	Whole brain radiation
WFNS	World Federation of Neurological Surgeons
WHO	World Health Organization
WMI	Working memory index
ZNF9	Zinc finger protein 9

Poorly Controlled Headaches Since 8 Years of Age

Sara S. Shah and Sara C. Crystal

CHIEF COMPLAINT: **Severe headache despite using medications.**

HISTORY OF PRESENT ILLNESS

A 35-year-old, right-handed woman presented to the emergency room complaining of a persistent headache, similar in intensity and associated symptoms to her previous headaches.

At the onset of pain, she experienced nausea, and the pain increased from an intensity of 0 out of 10 to 10 out of 10 within a few minutes. The pain was constant and throbbing and was bifrontal or unilateral. It began behind her eyes and radiated posteriorly to the occipital nuchal areas. Associated symptoms included photophobia, phonophobia, nasal congestion, nausea, and vomiting. She denied any motor or sensory deficits. While the use of acute medications decreased her pain to 4 or 5 out of 10, it typically increased in severity again through the course of the day. The headaches lasted about 2 days, followed by several hours of fatigue and difficulty concentrating. Triggers included stress, changes in her sleep–wake cycle, cigarette smoke, chocolate, caramel, alcohol, and foods containing nitrates. Her menses did not seem to be a trigger.

The patient had her first headache at the age of 8. During her childhood, she experienced olfactory auras before the onset of her headaches, but these remitted by her teens. At the age of 30, she began experiencing visual auras, consisting of flashing wriggling lines across her visual field before her headaches. This was followed by a loss of vision in her right visual field and sometimes was accompanied by a metallic taste in her mouth and tingling of her tongue. Her last episode of visual and sensory aura was 2 years ago.

The patient's headaches were initially episodic but began increasing in severity and frequency in her 20s and again at the age of 32. She has had near-daily headache for the past 2 years. Past preventatives include gabapentin, topiramate, levetiracetam, and escitalopram, which were discontinued either for intolerable side effects or for inefficacy. Injections of local anesthetic to the greater occipital, supraorbital, and supratrochlear regions were helpful for acute exacerbations. She has had four previous admissions to the hospital within the past year for status migrainosus. In the past month, she has had 11 days of severe headache, with milder or residual headaches on the remaining days.

The patient denied any history of depression, but she endorsed anxiety due to her frequent headaches and guilt about not being able to spend time with her children because of frequent headaches.

PAST MEDICAL HISTORY

Past medical history included complex partial seizures, asthma, and anemia. Throughout her childhood, she had multiple episodes of staring and unresponsiveness, lasting approximately 2 minutes. At 22 years of age, when she was in her third trimester of pregnancy, she had a witnessed convulsive event, without a preceding aura. She was found to have uterine contractions, but no signs or symptoms of eclampsia, and she delivered a full-term healthy infant. For the past few years, she has had 1 to 2 episodes per year of staring and unresponsiveness, without convulsions, that last for 2 minutes.

PAST SURGICAL HISTORY

Tubal ligation.

MEDICATIONS

Clonazepam, 0.5 mg bid; divalproex sodium, 500 mg PO bid; nortriptyline, 75 mg PO daily; nadolol, 40 mg PO daily; oxcarbazepine, 150 mg PO bid; acetaminophen/butalbital/caffeine, 325/50/40 mg PRN (several times per week); butorphanol tartrate, 10 mg/mL nasal spray prn (approximately 1–2 times per week).

ALLERGIES

Aspirin, penicillins—rash; triptans, dihydroergotamine—arrhythmia; metoclopramide, prochlorperazine—dystonia; mushrooms—hives.

PERSONAL HISTORY

The patient is married with 2 children and works part time. She denied use of tobacco, alcohol, and illicit drugs.

FAMILY HISTORY

Family history was significant for migraines in her mother, sister, daughter, and maternal grandfather. Two aunts were diagnosed with epilepsy.

REVIEW OF SYSTEMS

Significant for Raynaud's phenomenon and back pain.

PHYSICAL EXAMINATION

Vital signs: Blood pressure, 103/77 mmHg; pulse, 100 bpm/regular; respiratory rate, 16/min; temperature, 97.2°F. The patient appeared anxious.

NEUROLOGICAL EXAMINATION

Neurological examination was normal, except that head and neck exam revealed tenderness over the bilateral greater occipital, supraorbital, supratrochlear, and auriculotemporal nerve regions.

DIAGNOSTIC TEST RESULTS

Complete blood count, chemistry, and hepatic panel were normal. Valproic acid level was <10 mcg/ml.
Magnetic resonance imaging of the brain with gadolinium was normal.

STOP AND THINK QUESTIONS

➢ Are there any red flags in this history that will warrant urgent imaging?

➢ What are the possible etiologies of chronic headache in this patient?

➢ What pharmacotherapy will you recommend to help her headaches?

POSSIBLE DIAGNOSIS: **Chronic intractable migraine with and without aura and intermittent episodes of status migrainosus, neuralgia, possible medication-overuse headache, and epilepsy**

DISCUSSION

Diagnostic criteria for migraine require five episodes all lasting 4 to 72 hours without adequate treatment and including two of the following characteristics: unilateral, pulsating, moderate to severe intensity, or worsened by or avoidance of routine physical activity (1). The patient must also have one of the following: nausea, vomiting, photophobia, or phonophobia (1). Migraines lasting longer than 72 hours are classified as status migrainosus and may require hospitalization.

Patients often respond to the pain by lying down in a dark, quiet room. Allodynia, defined as a painful response to non-noxious stimuli, and hyperalgesia, an increased pain response to noxious stimuli, may develop in some patients. Autonomic symptoms, such as lacrimation or ptosis, may be present in 45% of patients (3). The history is important in distinguishing migraines with autonomic symptoms from sinus headaches.

The patient's complaint of daily mild headaches punctuated by more severe headaches is consistent with the diagnosis of chronic migraine. Chronic migraine is defined as migraine that is present for ≥15 days in a month for at least 3 months without the overuse of medications (1). However, the patient's frequent use of combination analgesics suggests the possibility of medication-overuse headache. In this case, the offending medication must be tapered before improvement can be seen.

Migraines are preceded by an aura in 20% of patients. Typical auras consist of reversible visual, sensory, or speech disturbances that develop gradually, and may be characterized by positive and/or negative features. Common visual auras include flashing, wavy lines that move across the visual field, and scintillating scotomas, consisting of a dark semicircular region extending from the center of the visual field laterally. A typical sensory aura consists of numbness or tingling in one arm that progresses proximally to involve the same side of the face and sometimes the tongue (3). Symptoms last between 5 minutes and 1 hour with typical aura.

A prodrome, which should not be confused with aura, occurs in 80% of patients with migraine and may present up to 1 to 2 days before the onset of pain (3). Symptoms may include depression, restlessness, drowsiness, anxiety, irritability, trouble concentrating, anorexia, feeling cold, diarrhea or constipation, and thirst (3). A migraine may be followed by a residual period of confusion and fatigue.

Eighty-five percent of patients with migraine recognize certain triggers to their headaches (3). Possible triggers are changes in weather, the sleep–wake cycle, stress, foods such as chocolate, or alcohol, and hormonal changes. Half of women with migraines experience worsening of their headaches around their menses (3). Initiation of oral contraceptives might trigger migraines, while the frequency of migraines tends to decrease in pregnancy, especially in the second and third trimesters (3). Patients should be encouraged to keep a headache diary to help identify their triggers and menstrual periods, as well as use of acute medications.

The prevalence of migraine is highest in the United States and is calculated as 18% in women and 6% in men (2). Migraine is more common among Caucasians compared with black Americans. The peak age of onset of migraine with aura in females is between 12 and 14 years, and that of migraine without aura is between 14 and 17 years (2). The peak age of onset is earlier in males: 5 years with aura and 10 years without aura (2). Migraines are most prevalent between ages 25 and 55 (2). There is a distinct genetic component to migraines. Having a first-degree relative with migraine increases one's risk for migraine by 1.5 to 4 times (3). Migraine headaches have many comorbidities, including sleep disorders, epilepsy, vertigo, stroke, coronary artery disease, patent foramen ovale, Raynaud's disease, and asthma. The cost to society of migraine is estimated to be $13 billion a year (2).

Diagnosis of migraine requires a thorough history and physical and usually does not necessitate neuroimaging in the absence of atypical features. Secondary headaches must be ruled out when patients present with focal neurologic deficits or papilledema, or with a change in their previous headache pattern, such as an increase in intensity or frequency. Headaches that are worse in the morning may suggest increased intracranial pressure, and pseudotumor cerebri and intracranial masses should be ruled out. Exam may reveal papilledema and cranial nerve palsies. Subarachnoid hemorrhage is often described by the patient as "the worst headache of my life" and must be ruled out by imaging and lumbar puncture.

PATHOGENESIS OF MIGRAINES (6–8)

1. Cortical spreading depression

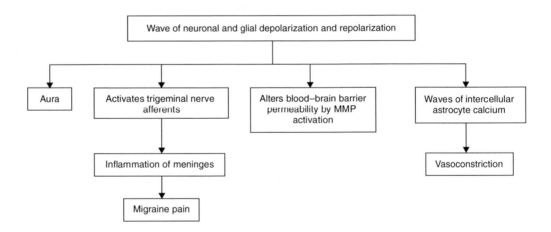

2. Neurogenic inflammation: unlikely to be the main mechanism of migraine pathogenesis

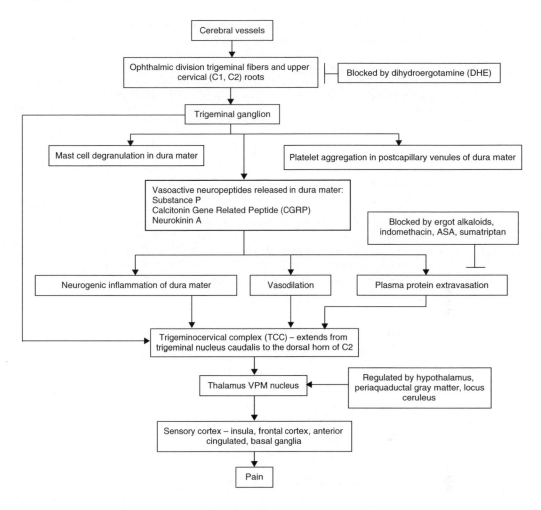

3. Central and peripheral sensitization

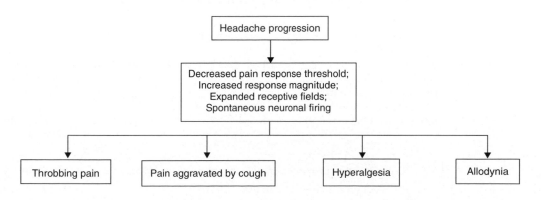

TREATMENT

Once the diagnosis of migraine is established, treatment should be initiated. Medications for migraine can be classified as acute, preventative, and transitional agents, the last of which refers to treatments for status migrainosus. First-line acute medications include the NSAIDs, combination analgesics, and triptans (Table 1.1). Triptans, which are migraine-

TABLE 1.1 *Abortive Treatment for Migraines*

Drug	Maintenance Dose	Maximum Dose	Side Effects
NSAIDs			Lightheadedness, fatigue, nausea, epigastric pain, indigestion, gastric erosions, interstitial nephritis, papillary necrosis; do not give to patients who have been diagnosed with gastritis, peptic ulcer disease, bleeding disorder, renal disease; avoid frequent use as this may lead to rebound headaches
Aspirin	325–650 mg PO q4–6h	4 g/d	
Indomethacin	25–50 mg/dose PO BID or TID	200 mg/d	
	Extended release tablet daily-BID	150 mg/d	
	Suppository 50 mg	—	
Ibuprofen	400 mg PO daily	400 mg/d	
Naproxen	500–750 mg PO initial dose; 250–500 mg PO q12h	1250 mg/d	
Piroxicam	10–20 mg PO daily	20 mg/d	
Flurbiprofen	100–300 mg PO daily or in divided doses	300 mg/d	
Sulindac	150–200 mg PO BID	400 mg/d	
Choline magnesium trisalicylate	500–1500 mg PO BID-TID or 3000 mg PO qhs	—	
Triptans			
Sumatriptan	Oral: 25, 50, or 100 mg/dose followed by second dose 2 h later if symptoms not adequately improved	200 mg/d	Angina, myocardial infarction, arrythmias, hypertensive episodes, paresthesias, flushing, diaphoresis; do not give to patients with known coronary artery disease, vascular disease, uncontrolled hypertension, pregnancy, basilar or hemiplegic migraine, or other uncommon forms of migraine
	Intranasal: 5, 10, or 20 mg followed by second dose 2 h later as needed	40 mg/d	
	Subcutaneous: 4–6 mg followed by second dose ≥1 h later as needed	12 mg/d	
Zolmitriptan	Oral: ≤2.5 mg followed by second dose 2 h later as needed	10 mg/d	
	Intranasal: 5 mg/dose		
Naratriptan	1–2.5 mg PO followed by second dose 4 h later as needed	5 mg/d	
Rizatriptan	5–10 mg PO followed by second dose 2 h later as needed	30 mg/d	
	If also on propranolol: 5 mg PO	15 mg/d	
Almotriptan	6.25–12.5 mg PO followed by second dose 2 h later as needed	2 doses/d or 25 mg/d	
Frovatriptan	2.5 mg PO followed by second dose 2 h later as needed	7.5 mg/d	
Ergot alkaloids			
Ergotamine	2 mg/tablet sublingual followed by subsequent tablets q30m as needed	6 mg/d, 10 mg/wk	Nausea, vomiting, coronary artery vasospasm, paresthesias, myalgias, uterine contraction; do not give to patients with vascular disease, uncontrolled hypertension, or pregnant women
Dihydroergotamine	Intranasal: 0.5 mg/puff 1 puff/nostril followed by second dose 15 min later as needed	3 mg/d, 4 mg/wk	
	Intramuscular /subcutaneous: 1 mg followed by subsequent doses q1h as needed	3 mg/d, 6 mg/wk	
	Intravenous: 1 mg repeat in 1 h as needed	2 mg/d, 6 mg/wk	
Others			
Acetaminophen	325–650 mg PO or rectal q4–6h, or 1000 mg q6–8h	4000 mg/d	Hepatotoxicity at high doses
Butorphanol	1 mg/puff nasal spray followed by additional puff 60–90 min later as needed, repeat this dosing sequence in 3–4 h as needed	—	Drowsiness, nausea, vomiting, nasal congestion

specific agents, are 5 HT agonists that cause cranial vasoconstriction and inhibition of neurons in the periphery and in the trigeminocervical complex (3). Triptans are contraindicated in patients with coronary artery disease or uncontrolled hypertension. Ergotamines are second-line agents given in sublingual, nasal, or injectable forms. Metoclopramide and prochlorperazine are antiemetics that are also effective at decreasing pain due to migraine. Patients should be warned about the possibility of rebound headaches with overuse of acute medications, especially those containing barbiturates. Nerve blocks may be used as abortive and transitional treatments for migraines. The procedure involves injections of a local anesthetic over the greater occipital, supraorbital/supratrochlear, and auriculotemporal nerve regions.

Prophylactic treatment should be initiated if the migraines significantly interfere with the patient's life, if patients are overusing acute medications, if the patient experiences 2 or more days of headache per week, or if complicated migraine types are present, such as ophthalmologic or basilar migraine. Beta blockers, antiepileptics, and tricyclic antidepressants are effective, as are some nonprescription supplements, including magnesium, riboflavin, and butterbur (petasides) (Table 1.2). Calcium channel blockers and gabapentin are also

TABLE 1.2 *Prophylactic Medications*

Drug	Maintenance Dose	Maximum Dose	Side Effects
Antihypertensives			
Propranolol	80 mg PO q6–8h initial dose; 160–240 mg/d q6–8h	240 mg/d divided	Bradycardia, atrioventricular block, hypotension, congestive heart failure, fatigue, depression, impotence, decreased libido, bronchospasm
Timolol	10 mg PO BID	30 mg/d	
Metoprolol	50–200 mg PO BID	400 mg/d	
Nadolol	40–120 mg/d PO	160–240 mg/d	
Atenolol	50–100 mg/d PO	100 mg/d	
Lisinopril	5–40 mg/d PO	40 mg/d	Hypotension, cough, angioedema, renal failure, hyperkalemia
Verapamil	80-120 mg PO BID	360 mg/d	Heart block, bradycardia, congestive heart failure, edema, constipation
Tricyclic antidepressants			
Amitriptyline	150 mg PO qhs	400 mg/d	Sedation, weight gain, blurry vision, dry mouth, constipation, urinary retention, tachycardia, sweating, orthostasis; use with caution in the elderly
Nortriptyline	75 mg PO qhs or 37.5 mg PO BID	150 mg/d	
Doxepin	25–150 mg PO qhs or divided BID or TID	300 mg/d	
Protriptyline	5–10 mg PO q6–8h initial dose; 15–60 mg PO q6–8h	60 mg/d; 30 mg/d in elderly	
Anticonvulsants			
Valproate	500 mg PO daily or 250 mg PO BID	1000 mg/d	Nasuea, vomiting, weight gain, hair loss, easy bruising, tremor, hepatotoxicity, teratogenicity
Gabapentin	300-900 mg PO TID	3600 mg/d	Somnolence, lightheadedness, ataxia
Topiramate	100 mg PO daily or in divided doses	200 mg/d	Lightheadedness, fatigue, ataxia, confusion
Vitamins/supplements			
Riboflavin	200 mg PO BID	—	Polyuria, turns urine bright yellow
Magnesium	400 mg PO daily	—	Diarrhea
Butterbur (Petasides)	75 mg PO BID	—	Burping

used but are somewhat less effective. Calcium channel blockers, however, may be especially useful in patients with prominent aura.

Equally important as medications are nonmedication approaches to migraine prevention and treatment, including biofeedback, acupuncture, and lifestyle modification, including changes to diet, maintenance of a regular sleep–wake cycle, and avoidance of triggers. Patients should be encouraged to keep a headache diary to help identify their triggers and menstrual periods, as well as use of acute medications.

Patients with unremitting migraine (status migrainosus) often require admission to the hospital. These patients might require a combination of prochlorperazine, metoclopramide, and dihydroergotamine. Subcutaneous sumatriptan may be of value, provided these patients were not treated with ergotamine in the previous 24 hours. The treatment of status migrainosus is outlined in Figure 1.1.

MIGRAINE IN CHILDREN AND ADOLESCENTS

As noted earlier, the peak age of onset of migraine is within the childhood and teenage years. The most common form of migraine in children is migraine without aura. This diagnosis of migraine is made by specific criteria that are similar to the ones applied to the adult population except with regards to the following: bilateral location for children aged 15 years or younger, and photophobia and phonophobia may be suggested by behavior, such as retreating into a dark and quiet room, rather than verbal affirmation (5). Medications approved for the acute treatment of migraine in children are triptans for adolescents and ibuprofen and acetaminophen for children younger than 12 years (5). Prophylactic treatment options include cyproheptadine (2–4 mg qhs, increased to BID or TID for children younger than 10 years), amitriptyline (1 mg/kg/d), and topiramate (50 mg BID

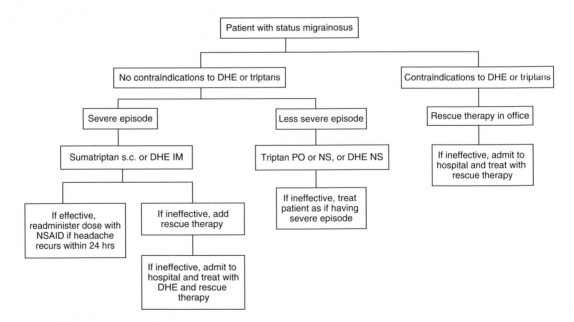

FIGURE 1.1 *Treatment of status migrainosus (4).*

Note: *Rescue therapy consists of analgesics (such as NSAIDs and acetaminophen), antiemetics (prochlorperazine 25 mg per rectum, 10 mg IM, or 10 mg IV), opioids (butorphanol NS, hydromorphine 2 mg PO or 3 mg per rectum, morphine 15–30 mg PO or 30 mg per rectum), and steroids (prednisone 80 mg taper).*

for teenagers) (5). In addition to pharmacotherapy, behavioral therapy is used. Specific measures include regulation of sleep, stress, and physical activity.

UNUSUAL MIGRAINE VARIANTS

Basilar migraine is an unusual form of migraine seen in both adults and children. It is preceded by an aura consisting of lightheadedness, vertigo, ataxia, visual phenomena, or diplopia. The pain following the aura is often occipital in location compared with the temporal or frontal pain of typical migraine. In order to be diagnosed with basilar migraine, one must meet the criteria for migraine with aura in addition to having at least two of the following: dysarthria, vertigo, tinnitus, hypacusia, and diplopia, visual phenomena in the temporal and nasal fields of eyes, ataxia, and decreased level of consciousness, double vision, decreased hearing, or simultaneous bilateral paresthesias (5).

Familial hemiplegic migraine (FHM) typically presents with an aura resembling a stroke and involving periodic hemiparesis and neurologic deficits. The symptoms begin between 30 minutes and 1 hour before the onset of the headache but may continue through the headache and remain even when the headache is over. These symptoms of aura occur contralateral to the side of the headache. Diagnosis of FHM requires patients meet the criteria for migraine with aura and have an aura involving motor weakness with at least one of the following: positive or negative visual phenomena, sensory symptoms, or dysphasia (5). These symptoms must entirely disappear upon termination of the aura. In addition, the patient must have a relative who has had an attack of FHM before, and other possible organic causes of the neurologic deficits must be ruled out (5).

REFERENCES

1. Olesen J. The international classification of headache disorders, 2nd ed. *Cephalalgia.* 2004;24(1):1–150.
2. Bigal ME, Lipton RB. The epidemiology, burden, and comorbidities of migraine. *Neurol Clin.* 2009;27(2):331–334.
3. Evans RW. Migraine: A question and answer review. *Med Clin North Am.* 2009;93(2):245–262.
4. Marcus DA. Treatment of status migrainosus. *Expert Opin Pharmacother.* 2001;2(4):549–555.
5. Lewis DW. Pediatric migraine. *Neurol Clin.* 2009;27(2):481–501.

Jasmin J. Gruber

CHIEF COMPLAINT: **Unable to walk.**

HISTORY OF PRESENT ILLNESS

A 64-year-old, right-handed female from Tobago presented with inability to walk when she woke up in the morning. She complained of gradually worsening back pain over the past 8 years with painful spasms in her legs and lower back. Over time, she had developed greater difficulty walking due to pain and weakness, and numbness in her legs. She started using a cane about 4 years ago. In the past 6 months, she had developed episodic urinary incontinence and rare bowel incontinence. She denied any history of trauma, fevers, or chills. She had no neck pain, radiating pains to arms, weakness or numbness of the hands. She denied losing weight or appetite, and denied having constipation and diarrhea. She did not notice changes in sensations in the perineal area.

PAST MEDICAL HISTORY AND PAST SURGICAL HISTORY

No other significant past medical or surgical history.

MEDICATIONS

None.

ALLERGIES

None.

PERSONAL HISTORY

She denied use of tobacco, alcohol, or drugs. She is heterosexual and was always in monogamous relationships. She moved to the United States 3 years ago.

FAMILY HISTORY

Her parents had history of hypertension and diabetes mellitus.

PHYSICAL EXAMINATION

Vitals: Blood pressure, 140/75 mmHg; heart rate, 75 beats per minute, regular; respiratory rate, 13/min; temperature, 98.5°F. General physical examination: Unremarkable.

NEUROLOGICAL EXAMINATION

Mental status: Normal.
CNs: I–XII: Normal.
Motor: Normal bulk in all four extremities without atrophy. Strength was 5/5 in both arms without pronator drift and 4/5 strength in bilateral hip flexors and quadriceps, 3/5 strength in bilateral anterior tibialis and gastrocnemius. Tone was increased in lower extremities. No fasciculations or abnormal movements were seen.
Sensory: Light touch, two-point discrimination, pain, and temperature sensation were diminished in both legs and the trunk to approximately 4 inches above the level of the umbilicus. Proprioception was diminished at ankles and knees bilaterally.

Reflexes: Biceps, brachioradialis, triceps 2+/4 bilaterally, and bilateral Hoffman's. Patellar and achillis 3/4, bilateral crossed adductors with spontaneous sustained clonus bilaterally. She had diminished rectal tone; perineal sensations were intact.

Coordination: Finger-to-nose intact bilaterally, rapid alternating movements normal in bilateral hands. She was unable to perform heel-to-shin maneuver or tap her heel repeatedly on a target.

Gait: The patient was able to stand briefly with a walker, which provoked painful spasms of the lower back and hips.

Straight leg raise test: Negative but range of motion was limited by increased tone.

STOP AND THINK QUESTIONS

➢ If the patient's reflexes were diminished with flexor plantar responses, where would you localize the lesion?

➢ What would be the differential if the patient's symptoms had developed over minutes, hours or days?

➢ What are the most likely diagnoses in this patient and which tests would help you properly diagnose, prognosticate, and treat the patient?

DIAGNOSTIC TEST RESULTS

CT of the total spine was normal without spondylosis, degenerative changes or compressive lesions. The cord appeared normal in caliber and position.

MRI of the total spine revealed diffuse spinal cord atrophy without abnormal signal changes or enhancement. MRI of the brain revealed mild nonspecific T2 hyperintensities in a microvascular distribution.

CSF revealed 10 white cells/mm^3 (90% lymphocytes), protein 56 mg/dl, glucose 46 mg/ml, and two oligoclonal bands in the CSF that were not present in the serum. Cultures of CSF were negative, including Mycoplasma; staining for ova and parasites was negative, as well as Mycobacterial (tuberculosis) cultures. PCR for viral (HSV, VZV) and Mycobacterial organisms was negative. HIV, syphilis, thyroid stimulating hormone, ACE, antithyroid, antinuclear, anti-Ro (SS-A), anti-La (SS-B), anti-cardiolipin antibody, and paraneoplastic antibody panel (including anti-amphiphysin) testing were all negative. Serum B12, copper, and vitamin E levels were normal. Schistosoma and Echinococcus antibodies were negative. Taenia solium IgG antibodies were positive but IgM antibodies were negative. HTLV-I antibody was positive with high titers in the serum and CSF.

DIAGNOSIS: HTLV-I–associated myelopathy.

HOSPITAL COURSE

She was referred for physical therapy and treated with baclofen up to 40 mg every 8 hours over the course of 6 weeks, which provided modest relief in painful spasms and allowed her to walk brief distances with a walker in her home. Oxybutynin 5 mg bid allowed greater bladder control and independence. Adequate fiber intake was encouraged to maintain a good bowel regimen. She was diagnosed with mild depression and received psychotherapy and sertraline.

DISCUSSION

The first priority in evaluation of myelopathy is to establish the acuteness of symptoms. Acute onset of symptoms over minutes to hours suggests an acute compressive, infectious, inflammatory or vascular myelopathy. Urgent CT scanning to evaluate for a compressive etiology is paramount as steroids and surgical decompression may prevent permanent deficits if a compressive etiology (fracture, extrinsic tumor, etc.) is found. If CT is negative, MRI and lumbar puncture should be considered to evaluate for the presence of inflammation to suggest an infectious (usually viral or autoimmune) etiology.

A very careful history and physical examination should lead to some clues to the potential diagnoses (Table 2.1). If symptoms have been gradually progressive, compressive etiologies are still the most common and most important to exclude, as urgent neurosurgical

TABLE 2.1 *Differential Diagnosis of Chronic Progressive Myelopathy*

Myelopathy	Red Flag	Diagnosis
Compressive	Trauma, focal back or neck pain, malignancy, dural AVMs	CT, MRI of spine
Intrinsic cord lesion		MRI spine-astrocytoma, ependymoma, hemangioblastoma, vascular malformation, rare spinal cavernoma (s)
Syrinx	Central cord syndrome	MRI of spine
B_{12} deficiency	History of gastric surgery, primarily posterior column involvement	Serum B_{12} <400 with elevated homocysteine or methylmalonic acid, positive intrinsic factor or parietal cell antibodies
Copper deficiency	Frequent use of dental adhesives (high in zinc)	Low serum copper
Folate deficiency	Gastric surgery, celiac disease, alcoholism	Serum folate
Nitric oxide toxicity	Onset after anesthesia, chronic NO exposure (health care, abuse)	Clinical
Heroin	Heroin abuse, posterior column involvement	Clinical
Lathyrism	Grass pea consumption	Clinical
Cassava	Cassava consumption	Serum thiocyanate
Superficial siderosis	Bleeding, co-existing cerebellar or eight nerve involvement	MRI evidence of iron deposition
Sarcoid	Erythema nodosum, hilar lymphadenopathy, arthralgia, + ACE	Noncaseating granulomas
Sjogren's	Dry mouth and/or eyes	SS-A (anti-Ro) or SS-B (anti-La) antibodies, positive lip biopsy
HIV	Risk factors	+ HIV, other causes excluded
Syphilis	Radicular pains, risk factors, primarily posterior cord symptoms, rapid plasma reagin positive	+ CSF VDRL
Tuberculosis	Exposure, abnormal CxR	+ PPD, culture
HTLV	Caribbean, Africa, South America, serum HTLV	+ CSF HTLV
Schistosomiasis	Sub-Saharan Africa, microscopic hematuria, eosinophilia	+ Serum IgM or evidence of parasite in urine, CSF
Primary progressive multiple sclerosis	No other cause found	>1 year of progressive symptoms and 2 of the following: nine brain lesions (or four plus abnormal visual evoked potentials), two or more spinal cord lesions, OCB or increased IgG index in CSF
Paraneoplastic	Malignancy	Anti-CRMP5, anti-amphiphysin, anti-GAD65 antibodies, anti-Ri
Inherited myelopathies	Family history of similar illness	Testing for SCA genes, Friedrich's ataxia, serum vitamin E, spinal muscular atrophy, hereditary spastic paraplegia, adrenomyeloneuropathy, Abetalipoproteinemia

intervention may prevent worsening of symptoms. CT followed by MRI should be undertaken to exclude both extrinsic and intrinsic cord lesions.

HTLV-I infection is endemic in Japan, the Caribbean, South America, and central Africa. Transmission can occur vertically from mother to child during birth or via breastfeeding or horizontally by sexual contact, blood transfusion, organ transplant or IV drug use. An estimated twenty million individuals are infected worldwide, 50,000 in the United States. HTLV-II is a closely related virus that can cause identical neurologic manifestations as HTLV-I, though it is believed that the vast majority of infected individuals remain asymptomatic. Approximately 2% of infected individuals will develop a gradually progressive myelopathy, predominantly affecting the thoracic cord, eventually resulting in paraplegia. Bowel, bladder, and sexual dysfunction are common and are also reported to occur in HTLV-infected individuals without other evidence of myelopathy. Symptoms usually begin in the third or fourth decade of life, and can occur in a stepwise fashion accompanied by multifocal lesions, mimicking relapsing-remitting or primary progressive multiple sclerosis. HTLV infection has also been associated with optic neuritis, peripheral neuropathy, polymyositis, an ALS-like illness, adult T cell leukemia, Sjogren's disease, and uveitis. Myelopathy is believed to be the result of chronic infection of the spinal cord with subsequent inflammation and degeneration. MRI can show multifocal enhancing lesions or be normal, but eventually shows diffuse atrophy. Treatable causes of chronic myelopathy should be ruled out; including neurosyphilis, schistosomiasis or neurocysticercosis; B12 and copper deficiency (see Table 2.1). Genetic causes of chronic myelopathy such as hereditary spastic paraparesis should also be considered. Chronic cyanide exposure (through raw consumption of cassava roots and leaves) can present as slowly insidiuous myelopathy. This condition is more common in African countries.

Another condition called lathyrism can be caused by eating certain legumes of the genus *Lathyrus sativa*, also known as grass pea or kesari dhal. HIV vacuolar myelopathy is clinically indistinguishable. The consumption of large quantities of *Lathyrus* grain causes toxic accumulations of high concentrations of the glutamate analogue, β-oxalyl-L-α, β-diaminopropionic acid (ODAP, also known as β-N-oxalyl-amino-L-alanine, BOAA). Ingestion of legumes containing this mitochondrial toxin results mostly from ignorance of their toxicity and usually occurs where the despair of poverty and malnutrition leaves few other food options. ODAP causes cell death because of mitochondrial injury; however, anterior motor neurons are especially vulnerable. A unique symptom of lathyrism is the emaciation of gluteal muscles. This disease is seen in Bangladesh, India, Nepal, and Ethiopia. It is unclear why this is more common is males than females.

HIV vacuolar myelopathy is associated with HIV infection. It occurs in about 10% of AIDS patients during late stages of HIV infection. It used to be more common before the introduction of highly active antiretroviral therapy. It is typically a painless myelopathy affecting the lower limbs but rarely asymmetric features and involvement of upper extremities have been described. Other associations such as AIDS dementia complex and peripheral neuropathies can be seen as well. Spinal cord atrophy is the most common abnormal finding involving the thoracic cord with or without cervical cord involvement. T2-weighted MRI often shows usually symmetric nonenhancing high-signal areas present on multiple contiguous slices, which may result from extensive vacuolation. This may be confined to the posterior columns or may be more diffuse. Histological findings are characterized by multifocal, extensive spongiform changes in the white matter and myelin pallor involving the dorsal and lateral tracts more than anterior and anterolateral tracts.

Primary progressive multiple sclerosis (PPMS) can also present with a slowly progressive myelopathy with or without superimposed episodic relapses and accounts for approximately 10% of cases of multiple sclerosis. The diagnosis is a clinical one and requires typical symptoms evolving over at least 1 year of observation and the absence of other identifiable causes. CSF oligoclonal bands are helpful, but not specific and can be seen in numerous other infectious and inflammatory myelopathies. Treatments effective in relapsing remitting multiple sclerosis have not shown benefit in the primary progressive form. Neuromyelitis optica usually presents with acute onset inflammatory myelopathy and longitudinally extensive (≥ 3 cord segments) lesions with cord swelling on MRI, with or without associated optic neuritis. Two-thirds of patients will have antibodies against aquaporin-4 in serum. Transverse myelitis may occur separately from neuromyelitis optica, but is also an acute inflammatory myelopathy, usually occurring after immune stimulation by infection or vaccination. ADEM is an acute, multifocal autoimmune disease of children affecting the brain and spinal cord, usually occurring after infection or vaccination and accompanied by fever and encephalopathic symptoms.

Paraneoplastic myelopathies (associated with antibodies against Ri, amphiphysin, and other cancer antigens) are extremely rare, but recognition of occult malignancy may accelerate diagnosis and improve oncologic outcome.

TREATMENT

Immunomodulatory and anti-viral treatments have not been proven effective in HTLV-associated myelopathy. Steroids have been reported to temporarily alleviate symptoms in patients with acute worsening and new or enhancing lesions on MRI. Fatigue, depression, pain, and bladder and sexual dysfunction are common symptoms that frequently impact quality of life. Fatigue and depression often respond to antidepressant therapy. Bladder and sexual dysfunction can be treated with anticholinergic agents and phosphodiesterase inhibitors. Painful spasticity should be treated, but the patient and physician should be aware that it may reduce functional strength. Regular physical activity is recommended to maintain function, and patients should be counseled on adaptation to permanent disability.

SUGGESTED READING

Araujo AQC, Silva MTT. The HTLV-1 neurological complex. *Lancet Neurol.* 2006;5:1068–1076.

Olivieira P, Matos de Castro N, Carvalho EM. Urinary and sexual manifestations of patients infected by HTLV-1. *Clinics.* 2007;62:191–196.

New Onset Focal Seizure, Headache, and Personality Changes

Samuel A. Goldlust

CHIEF COMPLAINT: **Seizure.**

HISTORY OF PRESENT ILLNESS

Patient is a 55-year-old, right-handed woman who was brought to the ER via ambulance 30 minutes after suffering a witnessed, generalized tonic-clonic seizure with focal onset in the left hand. She sustained a laceration on the back of the head, had urinary incontinence, and bit her tongue. She was confused for 10 minutes following the episode. When alert, she had obvious weakness on her left side. Upon arrival to the ER, she was given a 1000 mg dose of levetiracetam (Keppra) intravenously.

Her husband explained that he had noticed insidious changes in her personality. She "had not been herself" for the past few months. He noticed irritability and impulsivity. She was experiencing intermittent daily headaches for the past 2 months, described as dull and diffuse, and only partially responsive to over-the-counter medications. Headache also seemed to be worse in the morning. She denied nausea, vomiting, fever, weakness, or sensory change.

PAST MEDICAL HISTORY

Hypertension.

PAST SURGICAL HISTORY

Remote tonsillectomy.

MEDICATIONS

Prazosin.

ALLERGIES

Penicillin (hives).

PERSONAL HISTORY

Nonsmoker, rare alcohol use on social occasions, no recreational drugs.

FAMILY HISTORY

Significant for hypertension, diabetes, Alzheimer's disease. No family history of cancer.

PHYSICAL EXAMINATION

General physical examination: 2-cm scalp laceration on the left side, otherwise normal.

NEUROLOGICAL EXAMINATION

Higher mental functions: Awake, alert, and attentive. Oriented to place and person but could not provide the precise date. Good fund of knowledge for remote events, blunted affect. Speech fluent with intact comprehension, naming, repetition, reading, and writing.

Judgment and abstract thinking intact. 3/3 immediate but 2/3 delayed recall. Impaired serial 7's, slow processing, and slow registration.

CNs II–XII: PERRL, EOMI, marked papilledema bilaterally, face symmetric, V1-3 intact, tongue midline, symmetric shoulder shrug, and uvula moved symmetrically. Hearing and gag reflexes intact.

Motor: Subtle left hemiparesis, approximately 4/5. Left pronator drift, normal bulk, and tone.

Sensory: Left hemisensory deficit to all modalities.

Reflexes: 2+ symmetric throughout. No ankle clonus.

Plantars: Left-side extensor, right flexor.

Coordination: No dysmetria on finger-nose-finger or heel-knee-shin test.

Romberg: Negative.

Gait: Mild left hemiparetic.

STOP AND THINK QUESTIONS

➤ What is the differential diagnosis of new onset seizure in an adult?

➤ What classification of neurological disorder can cause the triad of seizure, headache, and mental status change?

DIAGNOSTIC TEST RESULTS

Routine labs: Normal.

MRI brain with gadolinium revealed a lesion in the deep gray structures and thalamus with mild dilatation of the lateral ventricles due to obstructive hydrocephalus. Postgadolinium

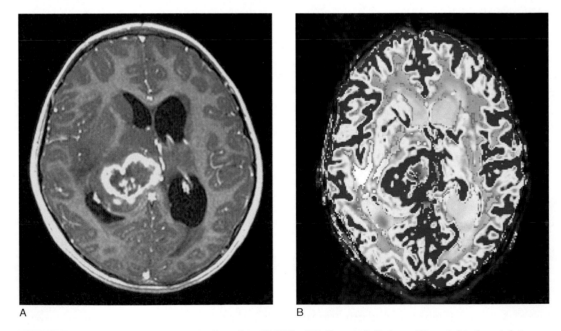

A   B

FIGURE 3.1 *Magnetic resonance imaging (MRI). (A) Postgadolinium T1-weighted axial image reveals a ring-enhancing deep right frontal lesion with associated mass effect, and midline shift. (B) Perfusion MR imaging reveals elevated relative cerebral blood flow at the tumor margin.*

T1 weighted axial image reveals a ring enhancing lesion with associated mass effect, and midline shift.

Perfusion MR imaging reveals elevated relative cerebral blood flow at the tumor margin.

DIAGNOSIS: **Astrocytoma WHO grade IV, GBM.**

DISCUSSION

In the above scenario, we encounter a middle-age woman without a history of epilepsy who presents with new onset seizure, personality change, and focal neurological deficits. Although possible with a variety of conditions including cerebrovascular disease, the triad of headache, mental status change, and seizure should raise suspicion for a mass lesion of the brain with associated increase in ICP.

The World Health Organization (WHO) has developed classification of glial brain tumors based upon the premise that each type of tumor results from the abnormal growth of a specific cell type. An outline of this classification is provided in Table 3.1. This classification provides a standard of communication amongst neurologists, neurooncologists, neurosurgeons, and radiation oncologists. The planning of therapeutic interventions and counseling to patients about their prognosis highly relies on this classification system.

Among primary brain tumors, 50% are gliomas, 50% of which are GBM, the most common and aggressive primary brain tumor with a mortality of nearly 100%. The peak age of onset is 45 to 65 years of age. The presenting symptoms are varied and depend upon the tumor size and location. The characteristic headache is often described as postural and dull, and may wake the patient at night or be exacerbated by cough or Valsalva. Seizure is the presenting symptom of nearly one third of high-grade glioma patients, and 10% to 20% of adults with new onset seizures will eventually be diagnosed with a malignancy of the CNS. Family members or patients may also describe alterations in concentration, memory, personality or initiative. Coupled with clinical suspicion, there are several characteristics on contrast enhanced MRI suggestive of GBM. A poorly defined, heterogeneously enhancing lesion GBM is frequently located in the frontal or temporal lobes, sparing the cortex and infiltrating deep structures. The heterogeneous signal intensity is due to cysts, hemorrhage, calcification, and necrosis, and is generally accompanied by perilesional vasogenic edema best demonstrated as hyperintensity on T2-weighted sequences. Characteristic spread across the corpus callosum may form a characteristic "butterfly lesion," though not requisite for diagnosis. Thick irregular rim of enhancement is typical, but enhancement can be solid, ring (Figure 3.1A), nodular, or patchy.

TABLE 3.1 *Histologic Classification of Glial Tumors*

Astrocytic Tumors	Oligodendroglial Tumors and Mixed Variants	Ependymal Tumors
Pilocytic (Grade I)	Oligodendroglioma, well differentiated (Grade II)	Myxopapillary ependymoma (Grade I)
Diffuse/Fibrillary (Grade II)	Anaplastic oligodendroglioma (Grade III)	Ependymoma (Grade II)
Anaplastic (Grade III)	Mixed oligodendroglioma/astrocytoma (Grade II)	Anaplastic (Grade III)
Glioblastoma Multiforme (Grade IV)	Mixed anaplastic oligodendroglioma/ astrocytoma (Grade II)	

Source: WHO, 2000.

pMRI (Figure 3.1B) and MRS are novel imaging techniques that are becoming increasingly common adjuncts to standard MRI. pMRI allows for a noninvasive assessment of cerebral blood flow, while MRS can detect specific biochemical compounds involved in metabolic processes in the CNS, such as lactate, creatinine, and choline.

Accordingly, radiologists have an increased ability to differentiate tumor from other diagnoses such as ischemia, necrosis, and abscess. pMRI study can help differentiate the radiation-induced changes (hypovascular) from recurrence of the tumor (hypervascular). pMRI and MRS are also helpful in selecting an appropriate target for stereotactic biopsy, as tissue of the highest histopathologic grade often also has the greatest vascularity and a unique biochemical composition.

The gross pathological examination shows a relatively circumscribed reddish gray rind of tumor surrounding the necrotic core, marked swelling of the brain with or without

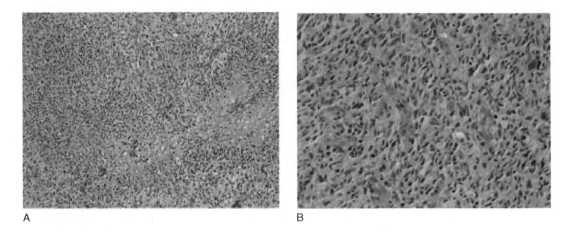

A   B

FIGURE 3.2 *Histopathology sections of glioblastoma from stereotactic-guided biopsy. (A) Pseudopalisading cells are seen organized around areas of necrosis adjacent to prominent vascular channels (H&E ×50). (B) Both vascular hyperplasia and abundant mitotic figures are recognized in a highly cellular and pleomorphic background (H&E ×200).*

TABLE 3.2 *Targets and Potential Novel Therapeutic Agents*

Endothelial growth factor receptor	Antibodies (including tagged to toxins/radioactive isotopes); tyrosine kinase inhibitors of EGFR (i.e., gefitinib, erlotinib)
Platelet-derived growth factor	Inhibitors of tyrosine kinase activity of PDGFR (imatinib)
Pl-3 kinase system	Small molecules targeting Pl-3 kinase and Akt[a]
mTOR inhibitors	Rapamycin
p53	Gene therapy
Ras pathway	Antisense oligonucleotides, farnesyl transferase inhibitors
Angiogenesis	Antibodies to VEGF, VEGF receptors, tyrosine kinase; inhibitors of VEGF

PI-3, phosphoinositol 3; VEGF, vascular endothelial growth factor; m-TOR, mammalian target of rapamycin; p53, tumor protein 53.
[a]This class of three genes in humans (Akt1, Akt2, and Akt3) codes for enzymes that are members of the nonspecific serine/threonine-protein kinase family.

gross hemorrhages. Microscopic examination shows high cellularity and mitoses, nuclear atypia and nuclear/cytoplasmic pleomorphism, coagulative necrosis, and vascular hyperplasia. The necrosis is described as "pseudopalisading" necrosis because areas of necrotic tissue are surrounded by anaplastic cells (Figure 3.2).

Prior to definitive therapy, corticosteroids are useful in stabilizing neurological deficits by reducing vasogenic edema. Dexamethasone is the drug of choice for its potency, long half-life, and lack of mineralocorticoid effects, but careful attention should be paid to common side effects of GI irritation, immunosuppression, and impaired glucose control. AED are reserved for patients with known seizure and should not be used for routine prophylaxis. Levetiracetam is the preferred agent because of a favorable pharmacokinetic profile and lack of drug-to-drug interactions.

Standard therapy for newly diagnosed GBM begins with maximal safe resection with the goal of gross total resection. Gross total resection may not be possible if the lesion is in eloquent cortex. Cytoreduction provides therapeutic benefit by alleviating increased ICP. With thorough preoperative planning and the utilization of intra-operative technologies, it is possible to minimize postoperative morbidity and increase the precision of tumor resection.

Within 4 weeks of resection, patients with GBM receive fractionated external beam radiation in conjunction with temozolomide, an oral alkylating chemotherapy drug. This is followed by temozolomide monotherapy for a minimum of 6 months, as long as the tumor is controlled.

Serial brain MRI is performed at regular intervals and for new or evolving neurological signs or symptoms, in addition to routine laboratory work. Unfortunately, the prognosis for GBM patients remains poor, and recurrence is nearly universal. Though there is no standard of care at the time of progression, re-resection should be considered. Following resection, therapeutic options include older cytotoxic chemotherapies (e.g., nitrosoureas, platinum compounds) or agents that target pathological angiogenesis, such as bevacizumab, which received an accelerated FDA approval in this setting. Angiogenesis, mediated by the VEGF, is thought to be an important factor in GBM tumorigenesis, and is an ongoing area of active research. Moreover, as scientists continue to unravel the molecular pathogenesis of malignant gliomas, the use of targeted molecular therapies has been increasing (Table 3.2).

SUGGESTED READING

Clark J, Butowski N, Chang S. Recent advances in therapy for glioblastoma. *Arch Neurol* 2010;67:279–83.
DeAngelis LM. Brain tumors. *N Engl J Med.* 2001;344:114–123.
Goldlust SA, Graber JJ, Bossert DF, Avila EK. Headache in patients with cancer. *Curr Pain Headache Rep.* 2010;14:455–464.

Sudden Speech Problems

Kristin M Waldron and Anuradha Singh

CHIEF COMPLAINT: **Acute onset of difficulty speaking.**

HISTORY OF PRESENT ILLNESS

An 18-year-old, right-handed man who was admitted to the hospital after a near-syncopal episode during a blood draw. He felt dizzy, warm, and flushed. These symptoms improved after a few minutes. An electrocardiogram was significant for a left bundle branch block, and a chest X-ray showed cardiomegaly. He was admitted to the hospital for further workup. He had similar episodes in the past, but denied ever losing consciousness. He reported that he had been seeing a cardiologist for the few months prior to admission, and had been started on Enalapril for presumed idiopathic cardiomyopathy. He denied any history of chest pain, shortness of breath, or palpitations.

On the morning of admission, while he was eating breakfast, he noticed that his face felt numb around his mouth on his right side and he was unable to speak but words were clearly formed in his head. He felt like his "tongue was swollen." He also noticed slight drooping of the face for few hours. He told the RN several hours later about his problem. He was able to communicate, understand others, and indicate that this had never happened before. He denied history of hypertension, diabetes, high cholesterol, or previous thrombotic events.

PAST MEDICAL HISTORY

Cardiomegaly.

PAST SURGICAL HISTORY

None.

MEDICATIONS

Enalapril (vasotec) 2.5 mg daily.

ALLERGIES

NKDA.

PERSONAL HISTORY

Occasional tobacco and alcohol use but denied any use of recreational drugs.

PHYSICAL EXAMINATION

Vital signs: 98.8°F; blood pressure, 100/60 mmHg; pulse, 105 min/regular; respiratory rate, 16/min.
General: No apparent distress, lying in bed.
CVS: Sinus tachycardia 102/min, no murmurs, S1 S2 normal.
Lungs: Clear to auscultation bilaterally, no wheezing, crackles, rales.
Abdomen: Soft, nontender, nondistended.
Extremities: No cyanosis, clubbing, or edema.
No carotid bruit.

NEUROLOGICAL EXAMINATION

Mental status: Alert, unable to produce speech. When he tried, he stuttered, and only got parts of words out. He could comprehend, as he followed all simple and complex commands; he could write well. He could not read out loud but could read in his mind. He could answer yes/no questions with head nods. He could name items, read and follow instructions, and could copy a figure. His memory was 3/3; he wrote the three objects correctly on a piece of paper.

CNs II–XII: OU 20/20, visual fields full, extra ocular movements intact, normal fundi, tongue midline, palate symmetrical, no facial asymmetry on smile, sternocleidomastoids strong bilaterally.

Motor: No pronator drift, fine finger movements fast and symmetrical, full strength to confrontation testing in all muscle groups. Able to stand on each leg independently and could do a full knee bend on each leg. Normal bulk and tone of the muscles.

Sensory: Intact to light touch, pin prick, vibration, and position.

Reflexes: 2+ throughout.

Plantars: Flexors bilaterally.

Cerebellar: Finger-to-nose and heel-knee-shin intact bilaterally.

Romberg: Negative.

Gait: Normal. He could walk on his toes and heel. His tandem walk was fine.

STOP AND THINK QUESTIONS

➤ What is the differential diagnosis of acute onset speech difficulties?

➤ Where will you localize his language deficits?

➤ What are the different types of aphasias? How will you distinguish them from one another?

➤ What are the common causes of stroke/TIA in a young person?

DIAGNOSTIC TEST RESULTS

CBC, SMA-20 and coagulation profile: Normal.

Noncontrast head CT: Normal.

MRI of brain: Small area of acute to subacute infarction, near the left superior temporal gyrus in the distribution of the left middle cerebral artery (see Figure 4.1).

Transthoracic echocardiogram: Mild left atrial dilatation, severe left ventricular dilatation, akinesis of inferior wall and interventricular septum; the remaining left ventricular wall segments were severely hypokinetic, LVEF <20%, right heart was normal in size and configuration; moderate-to-severe mitral insufficiency, no evidence of pulmonary hypertension.

Transoesophageal echocardiogram: No atherosclerosis in the aorta, no thrombus in the left heart, no atrial septal defect, no right to left shunt, akinesis of the inferior wall, LVEF exceedingly low (<20%).

Cardiac MRI: Significantly dilated left ventricle with severely decreased systolic function; LVEF <9% only. The study was consistent with nonischemic dilated cardiomyopathy.

Cerebrovascular duplex: 1% to 49% stenosis bilaterally.

He had negative hypercoagulable workup.

HIV test, negative; HbA1c, normal; lipid profile, normal.

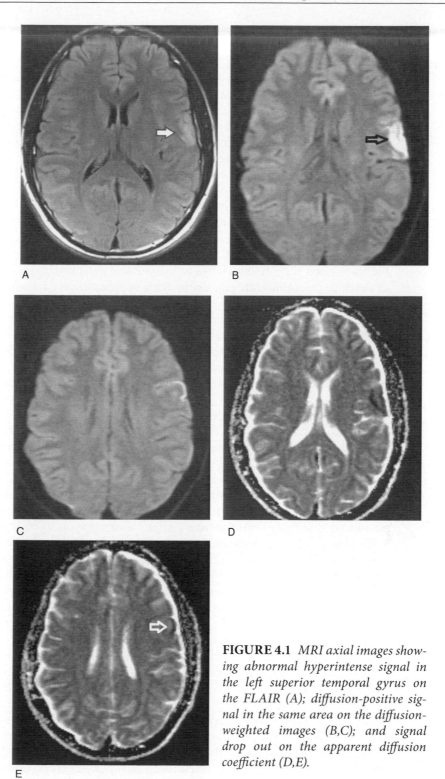

FIGURE 4.1 *MRI axial images showing abnormal hyperintense signal in the left superior temporal gyrus on the FLAIR (A); diffusion-positive signal in the same area on the diffusion-weighted images (B,C); and signal drop out on the apparent diffusion coefficient (D,E).*

DIAGNOSIS: Cardioembolic stroke leading to aphemia.

DISCUSSION

This case invites discussion about aphasias. It is beyond the scope of this book to discuss aphasias in detail. A brief introduction is provided below.

Speech is a mechanical function of one's ability to communicate that requires language production, phonation, and articulation. It consists of five parameters: hearing, speaking, repeating, reading, and writing. These five parameters allow us to symbolically express our thought processes. Speech output is based upon the syntax, the grammatical arrangement of words and sentences. Each spoken word is created out of the phonetic combination of a limited set of consonant and vowel speech sound units. Impairment of speech is a frequent complication of injury to the cerebrum. About 96% to 99% of humans have left hemispherical language dominance. The right hemisphere plays a role in language judging and expressing affective speech or what we call emotional content of speech (prosody). It helps us draw inferences, understand metaphors, and appreciate sarcasm and humor. Humans need their frontal lobes to initiate and maintain speech. Akinetic mutism or loss of drive to communicate can occur with supplementary motor area and anterior cingulated lesions.

The auditory comprehension of spoken speech takes place in the posterior end of the superior temporal gyrus. Karl Wernicke, the German neurologist, identified this area and called it receptive area of speech, BA 22. In 1865, Peirre Paul Broca, the French surgeon was able to demarcate the motor area for spoken speech (BA 44 and BA 45) in the posterior part of the left inferior frontal gyrus. How do these two vital areas of speech communicate with each other?

The arcuate fasciculus is a deep white matter tract that connects the motor and sensory areas of speech. There is an area in the brain just above Broca's area and slightly anterior to the primary motor control area. This area is important for writing and was first described as Seigmund Exner, BA 6. It is close to the area for hand movement. *Exner's writing area* is located within a small area along the lateral convexity of the left frontal lobe, close to the caudal area of the left middle frontal gyrus, somewhat, adjacent to Broca's expressive speech area, and the primary and secondary areas controlling the movement of the hand and fine finger movements. Exner's area appears to be the final common pathway where linguistic impulses receive a final motoric drive for the purpose of writing. Exner's area maintains extensive interconnections with Broca's area. Broca's area acts to organize impulses received from the posterior language zones and relays them to Exner's area for the purposes of written expression. The center for reading is posterior part of BA 17, an area of the brain just medial to the left occipital lobe and in the splenium of the corpus callosum. Lesions of the Broca's area or Wernicke's area, or their connections, may lead to a variety of speech disturbances classified as aphasias. A lesion to Broca's area will produce a motor, or expressive aphasia, in which patients can understand what is being said to them, but will have difficulty producing words. Their speech is hesitant and halting, they have trouble initiating speech, and writing is impaired. These patients express frustration at their deficit. A lesion in Wernicke's area produces a fluent aphasia. Their speech, while fluent, does not make sense. They make many paraphasic errors (word substitutions) and use neologisms (made up words). They cannot understand what other people are saying to them.

Conduction aphasias are due to lesions of the angular gyrus (which connects Wernicke's and Broca's areas). Speech is fluent with paraphasic errors, and comprehension is intact, but repetition is impaired. Transcortical sensory aphasia is due to a lesion of the linkage pathways around the auditory sensory areas (Heschl transverse gyrus). This area is thought to be responsible for assigning meaning to words. These patients will be able to repeat (via speech or writing), and speech will be fluent, but they will not be able to comprehend. In transcortical motor aphasia, there is a lesion in the anterior superior frontal lobe, near Broca's area. Their speech is nonfluent, but comprehension and repetition are intact. Writing is also impaired. Table 4.1 compiles different types of classical aphasia syndromes.

Table 4.1 *Different Types of Classical Aphasia Syndromes*

Type of Aphasia	Features	Lesion
Broca's aphasia	Speech: nonfluent, agrammatic Comprehension: intact Repetition: impaired Naming: poor Reading and writing: impaired Paraphasias: rare	Left inferior posterior frontal
Wernicke's aphasia	Speech: fluent Comprehension: impaired Repetition: impaired Naming: poor Reading and writing: impaired Paraphasias: common/mixed	Left posterior superior temporal
Conduction aphasia	Speech: fluent Comprehension: intact Repetition: impaired Naming: poor Reading and writing: good/impaired Paraphasias: common (literal)	Left supramarginal gyrus or left auditory cortex and insula (arcuate fasciculus)
Transcortical motor	Speech: nonfluent Comprehension: intact Repetition: intact Naming: poor Reading and writing: good/impaired Paraphasias: rare	Anterior or superior to Broca's area (extrasylvian)
Transcortical sensory aphasia	Speech: fluent Comprehension: impaired Repetition: intact Naming: poor Reading and writing: impaired Paraphasias: common (literal)	Left supramarginal gyrus or left auditory cortex and insula (arcuate fasciculus)
Anomic aphasia	Speech: fluent Comprehension: intact Repetition: intact Naming: impaired Reading and writing: maybe Paraphasias: rare	Left angular gyrus

(continued)

Table 4.1 *(continued)*

Type of Aphasia	Features	Lesion

Global aphasia	Speech: nonfluent
	Comprehension: impaired
	Repetition: impaired
	Naming: impaired
	Reading and writing: impaired
	Paraphasias: common
	  (literal and verbal)
		Large left perisylvian lesion, frontal,
		  temporoparietal lesion

Subcortical aphasia	Speech: fluent/nonfluent Comprehension: variable Repetition: intact Naming: poor Reading and writing: possible involvement Paraphasias: common	Head of caudate nucleus; anterior limb of internal capsule; thalamus

Aphemia	Disturbance of motor verbal
	  output alone
	Auditory comprehension: intact
	Written comprehension: intact
	Normal expression via written language
		Within Broca's area; subcortical,
		  disconnecting outflow

Our patient was a bit of a puzzle! He had nonfluent speech, he was able to name simple things (pen, watch), was able to write, and was able to repeat (although in a somewhat hesitant way). If he had a transcortical motor aphasia (intact comprehension and repetition with impaired speech production), he should have been unable to write. However, he was able to write very well. This brings us to a discussion of aphemia, also known as speech apraxia, which is a disorder of coordinated speech articulation that results in the severe impairment of verbal motor output. This is usually caused by small lesions of the motor system for articulation: pars opercularis, left precentral gyrus, inferior prerolandic gyrus, or white matter deep to those regions. This syndrome should be distinguished from Broca's aphasia, transcortical aphasia, and subcortical aphasia. Aphemia is not mild Broca's aphasia; it is severe dysarthria, at times in the setting of transient Broca's aphasia. Isolated aphemia may involve a disruption of the connections between Broca's area and the region of control of pharyngolaryngeal and tongue muscles, which is most likely the case with our patient. This area that controls articulation is adjacent to the facial motor cortex.

They have an isolated disorder of the planning of speech articulation. These patients are able to comprehend and can communicate via gestures and fluent writing. Sometimes, there is an associated right hemiparesis, limb apraxia, buccofacial apraxia, and a central right facial palsy (which our patient may have had transiently, early on in his presentation).

About 3% of the ischemic strokes in the United States occur between 15 and 45 years of age. African Americans (4×) and Hispanics (2×) have more strokes than whites. Intracranial hemorrhage, subarachnoid hemorrhage, and lacunar stroke are all more common in African Americans. Table 4.2 enlists some of the common predisposing factors for strokes.

TREATMENT

As documented above, a full workup of stroke in a young person was performed. MRI brain showed an acute infarct in the left MCA distribution. TEE was significant for severely impaired cardiac ejection fraction, and the diagnosis of dilated cardiomyopathy

TABLE 4.2 *Risk Factors for Strokes in Young Patients*

Cardioembolism	Rheumatic heart diseases
	Congenital cardiac defects
	Atrial fibrillation
	Patent foramen ovale
	Endocarditis
	Mitral valve prolapsed (low likelihood)
Fat embolism	Long bone fractures
Premature atherosclerosis	Family history
	Hypertension
	Hyperlipidemia
	Smoking
	Diabetes mellitus
	Hyperhomocysteinemia
	Homocystinuria
Prothrombotic	Factor V Leiden
	Antiphospholipids
	Protein C & S deficiency
	Antithrombin III deficiency
	Sickle cell disease
	Pregnancy
	Use of oral contraceptives
Genetic disorders	Fabry-Anderson disease
	Marfan syndrome (dissections more common)
	Homocystinuria
	Cerebral autosomal dominant arteriopathy with subcortical infarcts and leukoencephalopathy
	Mitochondrial encephalomyopathy, lactic acidosis, and stroke-like episodes
Arterial dissections	Traumatic and nontraumatic, aortic dissection with Marfan's syndrome
Noninflammatory vasculopathies	Moyamoya disease
	Fibromuscular dysplasia
Inflammatory vasculopathies	Meningitis
	Herpes Zoster Ophthalmicus
	Meningovascular syphilis
	Systemic lupus erythematosus, rheumatoid arthritis, Churg-Strauss vasculitis
	Cerebral autosomal dominant arteriopathy with subcortical infarcts and leukoencephalopathy

was confirmed. His hypercoagulable workup was negative for clotting abnormalities. The mainstay of treatment for stroke remains controling the underlying risk factors for stroke. The patient was started on carvedilol (coreg), digoxin, and lisinopril for his heart failure. Due to the fact that he had several infarcts, it was thought that he likely had a cardiac embolic source for his stroke (even though no clot in the atrium or on the valves was found). He was started on heparin and bridged to Coumadin. He was discharged from the hospital with a therapeutic INR, with plans to follow up in Coumadin clinic for management of his anticoagulation.

SUGGESTED READING

Ottomeyer C, Reuter B, Jäger T, Rossmanith C, Hennerici MG, Szabo K Aphemia: An isolated disorder of speech associated with an ischemic lesion of the left precentral gyrus. *J Neurol.* 2009;256(7):1166–8. Epub 2009 March 1.

Rheims S, Nighoghossian N, Hermier M. Aphemia related to a premotor cortex infarction. *Eur Neurol.* 2006;55(4):225–226.

Rowland L. *Merritt's Neurology.* 11th ed. Philadelphia, PA: Lippincott Williams & Wilkins; 2005.

Progressive Leg Weakness for the Past 6 Years

Rikki Racela

CHIEF COMPLAINT: **My legs are getting weaker and weaker.**

HISTORY OF PRESENT ILLNESS

A 65-year-old woman who comes into the neurologist's office complaining of weakness of both legs. She reported that her symptoms started about 6 years ago when she noticed some weakness lifting her legs at the hip. She would experience mild pain in the muscles at the end of the day. She could not tell if there was any worsening of the weakness at the end of the day. She found some relief with over-the-counter pain medication; however, the weakness persisted and slowly got worse. After 1 year, she began having difficulty rising from a chair and climbing stairs. She became less active and started gaining weight. She had been taking simvastatin, which was stopped. The patient's weakness continued to progress. By the time the patient came to our office, she was walking with a quad cane and was mostly sedentary. She did not have any complaints such as back pain, neck pain, or shooting pains down to her arms or legs. She had no other common neurological symptoms such as drooping of the eyelids, double vision, slurred or nasal speech, or difficulty chewing or swallowing. She denied any sensory symptoms or bladder or bowel problems. She had not noticed "fluttering" of muscles. She had no history of thyroid disease or parasitic infections. She denied any rash, arthralgias, weight loss, or difficulty swallowing.

PAST MEDICAL HISTORY

Right eye cataract, hypertension, hypercholesterolemia, coronary artery disease.

PAST SURGICAL HISTORY

Coronary stent, Lap cholecystectomy.

MEDICATIONS

Lisinopril/hydrochlorothiazide (Prinzide), metoprolol, aspirin.

ALLERGIES

No known drug allergies.

PERSONAL HISTORY

No smoking, social alcohol, no drug use.

FAMILY HISTORY

No history of neurological disorders.

REVIEW OF SYSTEMS

No shortness of breath, fever, neck stiffness, weight loss, difficulty swallowing, bowel or bladder disturbances, muscle pains, joint pains or swelling, rash, exotic travel, or weird dietary habits.

PHYSICAL EXAMINATION

Vitals: Blood pressure, 140/82 mmHg; pulse, 80; respiratory rate of 15.

General: Obese, sitting up comfortably in chair in no apparent distress.

Head, eye, ear, nose, and throat examination: No rashes on face, ear canals, and tympanic membranes normal, no lymphadenopathy.

Cardiovascular: Regular rate and rhythm.

Pulmonary: Clear to auscultation bilaterally.

Abdomen: Soft, nontender, nondistended.

Musculoskeletal: Patient with diffuse, slight joint, and muscle tenderness.

Skin: No rashes.

NEUROLOGICAL EXAMINATION

Mental status: Awake, alert, and oriented × 3. Good knowledge of current events, normal affect, and normal language comprehension and expression. Normal immediate and recent memory.

CNs: II–XII intact.

Motor: 4/5 finger abduction and wrist flexion B/L, 5/5 wrist extension, shoulder flexion/abduction, 3/5 hip flexion, 4+/5 knee ext B/L, no pronator drift, normal muscle bulk and tone.

Sensory: Normal to light touch, pain, temperature, vibration, proprioception.

Reflexes: Areflexic throughout, negative jaw jerk, toes down, no clonus.

Coordination: Normal finger-to-nose test, heel-to-shin, negative Romberg.

Gait: Required help to rise from chair, short waddling gait using quad cane.

STOP AND THINK QUESTIONS

➢ What are the signs of proximal muscle weakness? What are some potential causes?

➢ Does it make a difference that there is both proximal and distal weakness in this case?

➢ What was the significance in stopping the statin in this case?

DIAGNOSTIC TEST RESULTS

NCS/EMG of all four extremities (another facility): Bilateral ulnar neuropathy and L4/5 radiculopathy as per patient.

MRI of the entire spine was normal.

CK 826, ESR 36, ANA positive. Routine laboratory tests were normal.

NCS of upper and lower extremities: The sensory and motor NCSs of both upper and lower extremities showed normal latencies, normal amplitudes of SNAPs, and CMAP with normal conduction velocities. F-waves latencies of both upper and lower extremities were normal.

EMG interpretation: The insertional activity was normal in all muscle groups. There were abundant positive sharp waves and fibrillation potentials bilaterally in both upper and lower extremities, as well as abundant CRDs in different muscle groups (right vastus lateralis, right iliopsoas, right gastrocnemius, and right tibialis anterior, bilateral first dorsal interossei, bilateral abductor pollicis brevis, and left extensor digiti communis). There were signs of fibrillations and positive waves in both L2–L5 and S1 paraspinal muscles and C5–C7 and T1 paraspinal muscles.

The VMUAP were of short duration and amplitude, with early recruitment indicating a myopathic pattern. The findings were consistent with a myopathy of both proximal and distal muscles with predominant involvement of distal muscles.

DIAGNOSIS: **Inclusion body myositis (IBM).**

DISCUSSION

Once it is determined that the patient has predominant muscle weakness, a neurologist should try to tease out the differential diagnoses of myopathy. Table 5.1 lists some common causes of myopathy.

TABLE 5.1 *Causes of Myopathy*

Inflammatory	Polymyositis
	Dermatomyositis (juvenile and adult forms)
	IBM
	Overlap syndromes or mixed connective tissue disorders (rheumatoid arthritis, systemic lupus erythematosus, Sjogren, Scleroderma)
	Vasculitis
Endocrine disorders	Hypothyroidism
	Cushing's syndrome
	Iatrogenic (exogenous steroids use)
Electrolyte disorders	Hypokalemia
	Hypophosphatemia
	Hypocalcemia
	Hyponatremia or hypernatremia
Drugs	Alcohol
	Corticosteroids
	Illicit drugs: cocaine, heroin
	Penicillamine
	Colchicine
	Antimalarial drugs
	3-Hydroxy-3-methylglutaryl-coenzyme A reductase inhibitors (Statins)
	Zidovudine
Infections	Viral: any virus
	Bacterial: Lyme, pyomyositis
	Fungal
	Parasitic: trichinosis, toxoplasmosis
Metabolic	Disorders of carbohydrate, lipid, and purine metabolism
Rhabdomyolysis	Seizures, crush injuries, delirium tremens with alcohol abuse, malignant hyperthermia, exertion, vascular surgery

This patient has IBM. IBM is a slowly progressive myopathy that affects both proximal and distal musculature and is frequently asymmetric. It is more common in males. There are both s-IBM and h-IBM forms with the sporadic form being the most common acquired myopathy in patients over 50 years old. h-IBM patients would have a positive family history. There is a slow rate of decline of weakness in IBM patients. Our patient had 3 to 6 months period of stabilization. Patients with later age of onset have a worse prognosis.

Early on, finger and wrist flexors, knee extensors, and ankle dorsiflexors are typically involved. Forearm flexor compartment may look "scooped out" in IBM patients. The pattern of weakness, age of onset, presence or absence of cutaneous manifestations, and neuropathological features on muscle biopsy help differentiate the three common inflammatory myopathies (see Table 5.2). The dysphagia can be seen in ~60% of patients with IBM. There is an increased association with various autoimmune and connective tissue disorders such as SLE, Sjögren's syndrome, scleoderma, interstitial pneumonitis, psoriasis, and sarcoid. Isolated erector spinae weakness resulting in "droopy neck" has been reported.

The pathophysiology of the disease is unknown. CK is usually elevated in this diagnosis but rarely above 12× of normal. EMG will show a diffuse myopathic process. The gold standard of diagnosis is muscle biopsy, where pathology would reveal intracytoplasmic vacuoles and non-necrotic myofibers with mononuclear inflammatory infiltrates predominantly in the endomysium. The inflammatory infiltrates consist mainly of T cells and macrophages. The presence of rimmed vacuoles is a characteristic feature of s-IBM (see Figure 5.1). However, rimmed vacuoles can be seen in other conditions such as distal myopathies, oculopharyngeal muscular dystrophy, and chronic upper motor neuron disease.

TABLE 5.2 *Differential Diagnosis of Common Inflammatory Myopathies*

Types	Clinical Features	Laboratory Data	Neuropathology
Polymyositis	Insidious over 3–6 months	Elevated serum creatine phosphokinase	Lymphocytic inflammation: mononuclear cells
	Female: male=2:1		
	Bimodal distribution: 10–15 years; 45 60 years	Aspartate aminotransferase, alanine aminotransferase, and lactate dehydrogenase are elevated in most cases	CD8 T cells
	Shoulder and pelvic girdle muscles involvement		
	Neck flexors (~50%)	Myopathic changes on EMG	Endomysial infiltrate
	Ocular, facial, and distal muscles are spared		
	Dysphagia and dysphonia +/−		Myonecrosis
	Cardiac +/−		
	Respiratory +/−		Patchy and focal
	Systemic symptoms +		
Dermatomyositis	Features of PM+ cutaneous manifestations: Gottron's sign; heliotrope rash; shawl sign; dysphagia; increased risk of malignancy	Myositis-specific autoantibodies: anti-Jo1; anti-signal recognition particle; anti-Mi-2	B cells, macrophages
			CD4 T cells
			Decreased capillaries
			Perifascicular atrophy
			Perivascular infiltrate
IBM	Older individuals	Increased creatine phosphokinase (not > 12× normal)	Same as PM; also rimmed vacuoles and eosinophillic cytoplasmic inclusions
	Insidious onset		
	Slow progression or plateau		
	Weakness is focal, distal, and often asymmetric		
	Finger and wrist flexors weakness		
	Ankle dorsiflexors and knee extensors weakness		
	Dysphagia (~60%)		

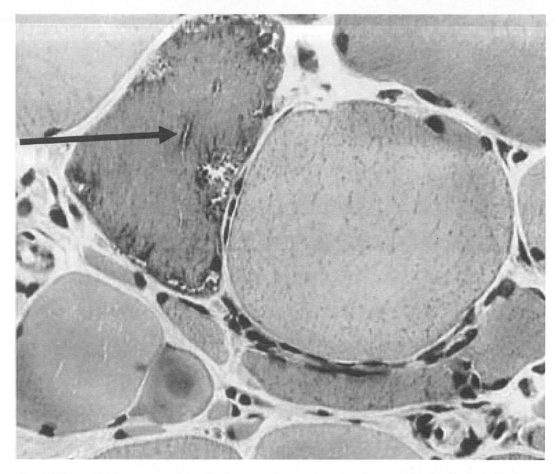

FIGURE 5.1 *IBM—section of muscle from another patient shows rimmed vacuoles (arrow). Notice atrophic fibers amid hypertrophic fibers as well. (Reprinted with permission from the textbook,* Motor Disorders, *edited by David S. Younger, Lippincott Williams and Wilkins, Philadelphia, 1999.)*

Electron microscopy shows intranuclear and intracytoplasmic 15- to 21-nm tubulo-filaments. TDP-43, a nucleic acid binding protein is found in IBM muscle sarcoplasm. Patients with h-IBM would have similar features on the muscle biopsy except lack of inflammation.

MRI of the thighs with STIR and T1 sequences can help differentiate the PM from sIBM. PM shows inflammation and atrophy in a symmetrical and fascial distribution favoring the posterior muscle group. IBM is more likely being asymmetrical and involves the anterior thigh and more distal musculature with fatty replacement. MRI may not be very useful unless there are large areas of inflammation.

TREATMENT

Patient had been given two prednisone trials each lasting 1 month at starting doses of 24 mg and 32 mg daily with no improvement. Unfortunately, there is no treatment for IBM. Supportive treatment such as referral to physical therapist and physiatrist should be made to improve patient's abilities. Our patient did not have dysphagia but patients with dysphagia require referral to a speech therapist to assess aspiration risks. Botox injections and cricopharyngeal myotomy may be indicated.

SUGGESTED READING

Askanas V, Engel W. *Inclusion-Body Myositis and Myopathies: Different Etiologies, Possibly Similar Pathogenic Mechanisms. Curr Opin Neurol* 2002;15(5):525–53.

Dalakas MC. Inflammatory, immune, and viral aspects of inclusion-body myositis. *Neurology.* 2006;66 (2 Suppl 1):S33–S38.

Dion E, Cherin P, Payan C, et al. MR imaging criteria for distinguishing between inclusion body myositis and polymyositis. *J Rheumatol.* 2002;29:1897–1906.

Karpati G, O'Ferrall EK. Sporadic inclusion body myositis: Pathogenic considerations. *Ann Neurol.* 2009;65(1):7–11.

Oldfors A, Fyhr I-M. *Inclusion Body Myositis: Genetic Factors, Aberrant Protein Expression, and Autoimmunity. Curr Opin Rheumatol* 2001;13(6):469–475.

Peng A, Koffman BM, Malley JD, Dalakas MC. Disease progression in sporadic inclusion body myositis: observations in 78 patients. *Neurology.* 2000;55(2):296–298.

Tawil R, Griggs RC. *Inclusion Body Myositis. Curr Opin Rheumatol* 2002;14:653–657.

Brijesh Mallami, Ninghan Zhang, and Sara G. Crystal

CHIEF COMPLAINT: **Neck pain on the right side of the neck and left leg weakness.**

HISTORY OF PRESENT ILLNESS

A 57-year-old, right-handed, African American male from California with progressively worsening right-sided head and neck pain accompanied by left leg weakness for the past several months. Patient was in his usual state of health until 6 months prior to admission when he started experiencing right shoulder pain and weakness. The pain progressively involved the right side of his neck that would come in spasms and occur several times a day. This would radiate to the back of his neck and get exacerbated by chewing and yawning. He did not suffer from any trauma to the neck. Over the past 2 months, his pain got progressively worse. He noticed left leg weakness and difficulty ambulating. Pain was recalcitrant to pain medications like morphine and oxycodone. He denied difficulty with bowel or bladder function. There was no associated fever, night sweats, weight loss, cough, or shortness of breath. He denied hypophonia, dysarthria, dysphagia, visual disturbances, and back pain.

PAST MEDICAL HISTORY

Asthma.

PAST SURGICAL HISTORY

None.

MEDICATIONS

Morphine sulfate 20 mg per orally q8h.

ALLERGIES

NKDA.

PERSONAL HISTORY

Active smoker with history of one pack per day for over 40 years; no history of alcohol or recreational drug abuse.

FAMILY HISTORY

Father had prostate cancer.

PHYSICAL EXAMINATION

Acutely ill-appearing male, appeared in distress because of frequent neck spasms.
Vital signs: Pulse, 73; respiratory rate, 12/min; blood pressure, 98/70 mmHg; temperature, 98°F; O_2 saturation, 98%.
Neck: Supple, no jugular venous distension, tenderness on the right side of the neck.
Lymph: No lymphadenopathy.
Heart: Regular rate, normal S1, S2, no murmurs, or rubs.

Lungs: Clear to auscultation bilaterally.

Abdomen: Nondistended, bowel sounds present, nontender.

Musculoskeletal: Midline and paraspinal tenderness to palpation of cervical spine, R>L.

Skin: No ulcers or excoriations.

NEUROLOGICAL EXAMINATION

Mental status: Normal.

CNs II–XII: Normal.

Motor: No pronator drift. RUE 5/5 RLE 5/5 LUE 5/5 LLE 5/5.

Sensory: Intact to pin prick, light touch, position, and vibration.

Reflexes: 1+ biceps b/l, 2+ triceps b/l, 2+ patellar on the right, 3+ on the left patellar, Achilles trace b/l, no Hoffman's, bilateral down-going toes, no clonus.

Coordination: Negative Romberg's sign; finger-nose-finger intact.

Gait: Antalgic, unable to tandem.

STOP AND THINK QUESTIONS

➢ What is the differential diagnosis for neck pain?

➢ Which diagnostic tests would you consider for this patient?

➢ How does the patient's smoking history change your differential diagnosis?

DIAGNOSTIC TEST RESULTS

WBC 5.9/Hgb 13.9/Hct 41.1%/MCV 95.1/Platelet 249/Neut 65.4%/Lymp 23.5%/Mono 6.9%/Eos 3.0%/Baso 1.2%; Normal basic metabolic and coagulation profile.

Protein electrophoresis of urine with reflex immunofixation: No protein observed.

Cancer antigen 19.9: 7.82 (ref ≤ 31); CEA: 1.1 (ref ≤ 5); Free Immunoglobulin Light Chain: Kappa 21.8 (ref: 3.3–19.4), Lambda 19.1 (ref: 5.7–26.3), Kappa/Lambda ratio: 1.14 (ref: 0.26–1.65); AFP: 3.8 (ref: 0–10).

Cryoglobulin qual w/ reflex to total protein: Negative; HIV-1/HIV-2 EIA: Nonreactive.

Chest X-ray and CT of the head without contrast: Normal.

His previous work-up included MRI of the cervical spine that reportedly showed abnormal T2 signal at C1, C2, and he was found to have a lesion in the pelvis on CT, but no biopsy was performed.

CT of the neck: Asymmetric increased haziness of the fat adjacent to the right subclavian vessels with several asymmetrically prominent right supraclavicular lymph nodes, measuring up to 0.8 cm in the short axis, likely inflammatory or infectious in nature but no evidence of epidural abscess.

MRI of the cervical spine with gadolinium: Abnormal T1 and T2 marrow signal intensity at the right arch and lateral mass of C1 and base of C2 that extends to the lamina with enhancement. There is no significant epidural extension of disease. There is associated abnormal enhancement of the surrounding soft tissues, but there is no evidence for a fluid collection or abscess. There is no other level of osseous involvement identified in the cervical spine. There is mild discogenic degenerative disease without disc herniation, central canal stenosis, or foraminal stenosis. The spinal cord demonstrated normal signal intensity and morphology without abnormal enhancement. There is no abnormal leptomeningeal enhancement.

Flexion/extension cervical spine X-ray: There is a lucency in between the posterior aspect of the C2 vertebral body and posterior elements potentially related to a pathologic destruction of the bone, which was better seen on the MR study. There is no evidence for instability in flexion or extension at this level.

Bone scan: Abnormal radiotracer uptake in the right upper cervical spine, which likely corresponds to lesions seen in the right arch and lateral mass of C1 and base of C2 of the MRI. Metastatic bone disease cannot be excluded.

Follow-up MRI of the cervical spine with and without gadolinium (Figure 6.1).

Abnormal process centered at the right C1–2 facet joints involving the right lateral C1 and right lateral C2 vertebral bodies. There is low signal intensity throughout the right lateral C1 and C2 vertebrae. There is subtle abnormal enhancement within the right lateral C1 and C2 vertebrae. There is abnormal enhancement within the C1–2 facets synovial space, which is somewhat expanded with abnormal increased T2 signal intensity. Irregular bony contour is present at the facet margins although the remainder of the atlas and axis cortical margins is grossly intact. There is increased T2 signal intensity and prominent enhancing soft tissue within the right peril-vertebral space consistent with inflammatory change. Findings are most consistent with an infectious process at the right C1 and C2 facet joint with secondary osteomyelitis and perivertebral inflammatory changes. It is similar or somewhat progressed compared with the previous studies consistent with an indolent infection. It is not consistent with metastatic prostate carcinoma. Remainder of the cervical spine and spinal cord is normal. No epidural extension.

CT chest/abdomen/pelvis with contrast showed mediastinal lymphadenopathy in the superior mediastinal right paratracheal region measuring 2.2 cm, lower left paratracheal lymph node measureing 1.3 cm in short axis, and mildly enlarged subcarinal, perivascular lymph nodes. Also, the hila demonstrated mild adenopathy with an 11 mm node in the left hilum. There is bilateral diffuse bronchial wall thickening and centrilobular emphysema. Central airways appear grossly patent. A nodular density in the left upper lobe measures 0.7 cm, which is nonspecific. Metastatic disease cannot be excluded. There are other small nonspecific lung nodules, measuring less than 4 mm.

Transbronchial aspiration biopsy of the left lower paratracheal lymph node shows abundant necrotic debris and scattered lymphocytes, rare aggregates of epithelioid histiocytes,

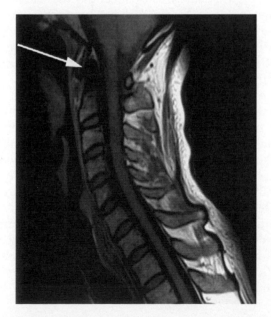

FIGURE 6.1 *Sagittal MRI cervical spine FLAIR sequence showing T2 marrow signal intensity at the right arch and lateral mass of C1 and base of C2 that extends to the lamina.*

and a few multinucleated giant cells. These findings are suggestive of necrotizing granulomatous inflammation. In addition, scattered large round structures of unknown source or nature are noted. Cell block sections show few clusters of benign bronchial epithelial cells, and red blood cells and a few of those round structures similar to the ones seen on the smears. No acid fast bacilli detected.

Most of the round structures noted in the smears and cell block show single or double rims without internal contents. There are two to three such structures that do show some denser internal contents probably degenerated; therefore a clear visualization of the details becomes impossible. The traditional GMS stain and PAS stains highlight the outer rim. Given the clinical presentation, these cytologic findings are highly suggestive of infection of Coccidioides. Recommend correlation with serum test.

Coccidioides Total Antibody with Reflex Testing: 6.35 (Reference rage < 0.90).

DIAGNOSIS: Coccidioidomycosis.

TREATMENT

Fluconazole 400 mg daily for minimum of 6 months. Morphine and percocept 30 tabs prescription provided. Patient was asked to repeat MRI C-Spine in 2 months to re-evaluate the lesion and assess response to treatment.

DISCUSSION

Most fungi are inhaled by humans and begin as a primary pulmonary infection that is often self-limited. On occasion, hematogenous dissemination of the organism can lead to extrapulmonary disseminated infection that may involve the CNS. In recent years, there has been an increase in diagnosis of fungal infections of the CNS that may be attributable to the widespread use of antibacterial agents and the rapid growth of the immunocompromised population. However, pathological fungi, such as coccidioidomycosis, can also infect immunocompetent individuals. In the CNS, fungal infections can produce three main types of infection: meningitis, meningoencephalitis, and localized brain infection such as a brain abscess or granuloma. Table 6.1 lists the common fungal infections.

Hyphae or molds, such as aspergilli, usually cause focal disease with vascular thrombosis that can cause hemorrhagic necrosis. Yeasts, such as Cryptococcus, generally cause a more diffuse process with the base of the brain being primarily affected. Unlike a primary infection, disseminated disease is often fatal if not treated with systemic antifungal therapy. Fungal infections of the CNS can result in neurological complications such as obstructive hydrocephalus, infarcts, seizures, and dementias.

Coccidioides immitis is a dimorphic fungus that is endemic to certain semiarid parts of the southwestern United States and northwestern Mexico. Humans inhale the windborne arthrospores from dry soil. Seasonal outbreaks have been observed after dust storms, droughts, and earthquakes, which result in extremely dry, hot, dusty conditions. Approximately 60% of infected people remain asymptomatic, whereas others may develop a mild flu-like illness or a severe pneumonia that resolves spontaneously over a period of weeks to months. Only about 0.5% to 1.0% of infected individuals develop extrapulmonary dissemination of the disease affecting the meninges, bone, joints, soft tissues, or skin.

Disseminated disease generally occurs during the first year of primary infection. Systemic risk factors include corticosteroid use and HIV infection. Patients of African and Asian (South Pacific) descent are at a higher risk of developing disseminated disease as compared to Caucasian patients. The mechanism of this increased risk remains unknown, but is suspected to be due to differences in cell-mediated immunity. Dissemination

TABLE 6.1 Fungal Infections of the CNS

Fungus	Common Types of Infection (Davis 1999)	Diagnostic Tests (Davis 1999)	Treatment (see references)
Candida Albicans[a]	Meningitis	Laboratory Tests: Cerebrospinal fluid examination	Amphotericin B combined with Flucytosine
Mucor, Rhizopus, Absidia, and Cunninghamella[a]	Rhino-orbital-cerebral infection	Hemogram and urinalysis Liver and renal function tests	Surgical debridement and Amphotericin B
Aspergillus[a]	Brain abscess or granuloma	Fungal Cultures: Cerebrospinal fluid	Voriconazole
Cryptococcus neoformans[a]	Meningitis; meningoencephalitis	Suptum or tracheal aspirate Urine Bone marrow aspirate Skin biopsy Joint aspirate	Induction: Amphotericin B and Flucytocine Consolidation/maintenance: Fluconazole
Coccidioides immitis[b] (Southwestern United States)	Meningitis; meningoencephalitis; brain abscess or granuloma	Sinus Meningeal biopsy Serologic Tests: Antibody tests of cerebrospinal	Fluconazole or Itraconazole (skeletal involvement)
Blastomyces dermatitidis[b] (Midwestern United States, St. Lawrence waterway)	Meningitis; brain abscess or granuloma	fluid and serum Radiologic Tests: Chest radiograph MRI, CT of head Joint radiographs Bone scan	Amphotericin B or Voriconazole
Histoplasma capsulatum[b] (Mississippi Valley)	Meningitis		Amphotericin B or Itraconazole

[a]Saprophytic fungi—infect only immunocompromised hosts. Distribution is ubiquitous.
[b]Pathogenic fungi—can infect any host. Distribution is endemic (Perdiagao 2004).

after primary coccidioidomycosis is infrequent but is associated with significant morbidity and mortality and can have a wide spectrum of clinical presentations. Meningitis is the most lethal complication of coccidioidomycosis. Disseminated lesions are also frequently seen in the head and neck. Its involvement can be cutaneous, laryngeal, mucosal, and otological and may consist of suppurative, necrotic, or granulomatous tissue. In a recent retrospective analysis of 150 cases with extrapulmonary nonmeningeal disease, skeletal involvement was documented in nearly half of the patients, with increased risk in African Americans and males. Disease in the axial skeleton has a predilection to vertebral infection and osteomyelitis of the skull. A primary concern in vertebral dissemination is the compromise of spinal integrity or vertebral stability, with surgical debridement and stabilization necessary in some cases. This group lacked mortality but had extremely high morbidity, often requiring multiple surgical debridements.

Diagnosis of disseminated coccidioidomycosis is usually made by cultures and serological testing. Recovery of the organism confirms the diagnosis. Cultures of cerebrospinal fluid or other tissue specimens typically show the double-walled spherule containing numerous endospores surrounded by a granulomatous reaction (see Figure 6.2). Serological testing detects CFIgG antibodies. However, there is a high rate of false-negative serologic tests in immunocompromised (37%) and immunocompetent patients (13%) in disseminated disease. For vertebral involvement, MR imaging with gadolinium

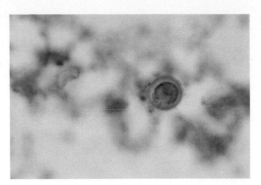

FIGURE 6.2 *Diff Quik Stain showing Coccidioides in the bronchial aspirate.*

has been found to be useful for determining the extent of the lesion. The involvement of the intervertebral disc, vertebral body marrow, and adjacent epidural and soft tissue can be seen clearly. Where there is no immediate threat of cord impingement, patients can be managed medically with antifungal agents and repeated MRI imaging to track disease regression.

Both itraconazole and fluconazole have been used in treatment, but patients with skeletal infections have been noted to respond twice as frequently to itraconazole as to fluconazole, with respective responses of 52% and 26% at 12 months. However, there is significant potential for relapse once the antifungal treatment is discontinued. Comparing fluconazole and itraconazole treatment, relapse rates after 12 months of therapy were 28% and 18%, respectively. Discontinuing therapy at least once would seem reasonable, since over two-thirds of patients do not relapse. This practice is supported by the observation that most relapses occur at the site of a previous lesion. However, in cases of vertebral infection, the site of the initial lesion is particularly critical, and treatment durations are often extended beyond 12 months.

SUGGESTED READING

Adam RD, Elliott SP, Talijanovic MS. The spectrum of presentation of disseminated coccidioidomycosis. *Am J Med.* 2009;122:770–777.

Arnold MG, Arnold JC, Bloom DC, Brewster DF, Thiringer JK. Head and neck manifestations of disseminated coccidioidomycosis. *Laryngoscope.* 2004;114(4):747–752.

Bakleh M. Successful treatment of cerebral blastomycosis w/voriconazole. *Clin Infect Dis.* 2005;40(9): P69–P71.

Davis, LE. Fungal infections of the central nervous system. *Neurol Clin.* 1999;17(4):P761–P781.

Galgiani JN, Catanzaro A, Cloud GA, et al. Comparison of oral fluconazole and itraconazole for progressive, non-meningeal coccidioidomycosis. A randomized, double-blind trial. Mycoses Study Group. *Ann Intern Med.* 2000;133:676.

Groll AH, Giri N, Petraitis V, et al. Comparative efficacy and distribution of lipid formulations of amphotericin B in experimental Candida albicans infection of the central nervous system. *J Infect Dis.* 2000;182:274.

Herron LD, Kissel P, Smilovitz D. Treatment of coccidioidal spinal infection: Experience in 16 Cases. *J Spinal Discord.* 1997;10(3):215–222.

Murthy JMK. Fungal infections of the central nervous system: The clinical syndromes. *Neurol India.* 2007;55(3): P221–P224.

Pappas PG. Clinical practice guidelines for the management of candidiasis. Update by the Infectious Diseases Society of America. *Clin Infect Dis.* 2009;48(5): 503–535.

Perdigao J, Rojas R, Verzelli LF, Castillo M. Fungal infections of the central nervous system. *Sem Roentgenol.* 2004 Oct;39(4):505–518.

Perfect JR, Dismukes WE, Dromer F, et al. Clinical practice guidelines for the management of cryptococcal disease: 2010 Update by the Infectious Diseases Society of America. *Clin Infect Dis.* 2010;50:291.

Spellberg B. Recent advances in the management of mucormycosis: From bench to bedside. *Clin Infect Dis.* 2009;48(12):1743–1751.

Walsh, TJ. Treatment of aspergillosis: Clinical practice guidelines of the Infectious Diseases Society of America. *Clin Infect Dis.* 2008;46:327.

Wheat LJ, Freifeld AG, Kleiman MB, et al. Clinical practice guidelines for the management of patients with histoplasmosis: 2007 update by the Infectious Diseases Society of America. Clin Infect Dis. 2007;45:807.

Shuhsaul Raza and Amrmulha Singh

CHIEF COMPLAINT: **Right-sided headaches, blurring of vision, and nausea.**

HISTORY OF PRESENT ILLNESS

A 65-year-old woman presented to the ER with complaints of recently worsening right-sided headaches. She had a history of "dull" right-sided headaches for the past 5 years. Her headaches became more intense over the last couple of months. She got partial relief of pain with ibuprofen. Initially, the headaches used to occur two to three times a week, but since last month, she had been suffering from headaches at least three to five times a week. She has had periods of blurring of vision in the right eye, with or without headaches. She presented to the ER with worsening headaches and persistent nausea for 5 days prior to admission. She denied any other common neurological complaints such as double vision, difficulty with her balance, weakness or numbness, bladder or bowel symptoms, or swallowing and speech difficulties. She had no other constitutional symptoms such as fever, neck pain, vomiting, arthralgias, and changes in her appetite, night sweats, or chronic cough.

PAST MEDICAL HISTORY

Hypothyroidism for 10 years.

PAST SURGICAL HISTORY

Brain tumor surgery in 1998.

MEDICATIONS

Synthroid 75 mcg once daily; ibuprofen 400 mg prn for headaches.

ALLERGIES

Codeine, Parlodel.

PERSONAL HISTORY

Nonsmoker, alcohol use socially, no drugs. Postmenopausal, not on hormone replacement therapy.

FAMILY HISTORY

No family history of cancer.

PHYSICAL EXAMINATION

Caucasian female who was well nourished and was in no apparent distress. General physical exam was unremarkable.

Vital signs: pulse, 66/min; temperature, 97°F; blood pressure, 110/70 mm Hg; respiratory rate, 14/min.

No postural hypotension; Kernig's and Brudzinski's signs were negative; skin: no rash.

NEUROLOGICAL EXAMINATION

Higher mental functions: Alert, awake, oriented to time, place, and person. Her knowledge of current events, judgment, abstract thinking, calculation, and praxis were fine. Recall 3/3 after 5 minutes. She had normal linguistic skills.

CNs II–XII: OD 20/25, OS 20/20, no nystagmus, pupils 4 mm both eyes, possible visual field cut in the left inferolateral quadrant; other cranial nerves exam was unremarkable.

Motor: No sign of atrophy, normal tone, strength 5/5, no pronator drift.

Sensory: Intact to all modalities of sensation.

Reflexes: Biceps (2+), brachioradialis (2+), triceps (2+), patellar (2+), Achilles (2+), Hoffman's negative, no clonus.

Plantars: Flexors.

Coordination and gait: Normal.

Romberg's: Negative.

STOP AND THINK QUESTIONS

➢ Is it migraine with auras? She has headaches, visual symptoms, and nausea and a previous history of headaches. Do migraines start around this age?

➢ Would you worry about space-occupying lesion with recurrence?

➢ What is Parlodel? What is it used for? Does that make you think about certain kinds of brain tumors?

DIAGNOSTIC TEST RESULTS

Routine labs: nl, EKG = NSR; TSH, T3, and T4: nl.

Serum PRL = >400 μg/dL (↑↑); urinalysis = normal; serum ACTH: nl.

MRI brain with gadolinium: A homogenously enhancing pituitary mass that extended into the suprasellar cistern, slightly more on the right (Figure 7.1A and B). There had been interval enlargement of the suprasellar component, which measured 1.5 × 1.2 × 1.0 cm at present (previously 1.3 × 1.0 × 0.7 cm in mediolateral, anteroposterior, and craniocaudal dimensions, respectively). The mass seemed to compress the optic chiasm, which was not well delineated. There was another 0.8 × 0.6 nodular enhancing lesion noted within the fourth ventricle, attached to the posterior aspect of the superior medulla (Figure 7.2A and B).

Pathology: Immunostains revealed positivity for PRL and chromogranin. Immunostains for LH, FSH, ACTH, GH, TSH, and alpha subunit were noncontributory. The labeling index (proliferation index) MIB-1 was approximately 10%. Immunostains for cytokeratins (CK7, CK20, and CAM 5.2) were not contributory. Stains for EMA, progesterone receptors, S100 protein, and HMB-45 were negative. Blood vessels were highlighted with vimentin immunostain (refer Figure 7.3 for histopathology of prolactinoma).

DIAGNOSIS: Prolactinoma.

DISCUSSION

The pituitary, called the "master gland," is located at the base of the skull. It lies in the sella turcica. In females, it is usually larger and its superior border tends to be convex. In males, it is smaller and its superior border tends to be concave. It is composed of an

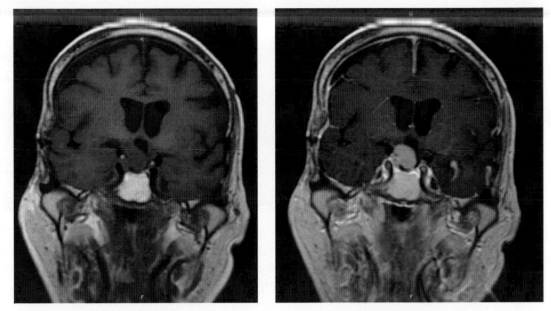

A: PRE-CONTRAST   T1   B: POST-CONTRAST   T1

FIGURE 7.1 *(A) Coronal T1WI showing a pituitary adenoma (showing the lesion); (B) coronal T1WI postgadolinium image showing a homogenously enhancing pituitary mass that extends into the suprasellar cistern, slightly more on the right.*

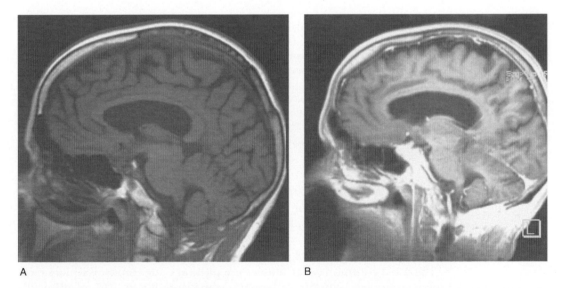

A   B

FIGURE 7.2 *(A) Sagittal T1WI MRI brain showing another 0.8 × 0.6 nodular lesion within the fourth ventricle, attached to the posterior aspect of the superior medulla in the same patient; (B) MRI brain, sagittal T1WI postgadolinium image showing homogeneous enhancement of the same lesion.*

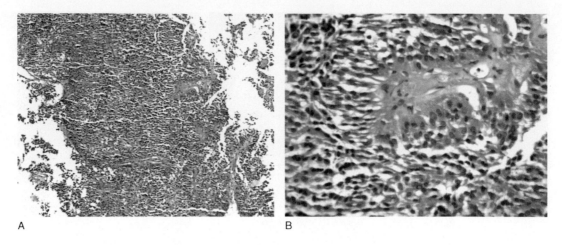

FIGURE 7.3 *Histopathology of prolactinoma; sections (A) low power and (B) high power show sheets of monotonous cells with round nuclei, prominent nuclei, and moderate blue-gray cytoplasm, displacing the normal pituitary architecture.*

TABLE 7.1 *Differential Diagnosis of a Sellar Mass*

Pituitary adenoma
Rathke's cleft cyst
Craniopharyngioma
Meningioma
Germinoma
Chordoma
Carcinoma
Epidermoid, dermoid cysts, teratomas
Pituitary sarcoid
Aneurysm
Abscess
Hypothalamic hamartoma, glioma, and gangliocytoma
Metastases
Histiocytosis X
Infiltrative lesions (hereditary hemochromatosis)
Lymphocytic hypophysitis

anterior and a posterior part. Posterior pituitary is an extension of the hypothalamus and forms the pituitary stalk or infundibulum. Anterior pituitary secretes various trophic hormones (GH, PRL, ACTH, LH, FSH, and TSH) and responds to releasing factors secreted by hypothalamus.

Differential diagnosis of mass lesions in the sellar region is quite wide (see Table 7.1).

The most common sellar masses are pituitary adenomas, Rathke's cleft cysts, and craniopharyngiomas. Pituitary adenomas constitute about 10% of clinically detected brain tumors. These tend to present in the fourth to sixth decades. Based on its size, a pituitary adenoma can be classified as a microadenoma (<10 mm in diameter) or a macroadenoma (>10 mm in diameter). About 30% of adenomas can invade adjacent bone or dura. Table 7.2 enlists different kinds of pituitary adenomas that typically grow in the sella turcica.

TABLE 7.2. *Different Types of Pituitary Adenomas*

Type	Frequency (%)	Symptoms
Prolactinomas	20–30	Amenorrhea, infertility, galactorrhea, bitemporal hemianopsia, osteopenia
GH cell adenomas	5	Gigantism (prepuberty), acromegaly (after epiphyseal closure), abnormal glucose tolerance, muscle weakness, HTN, CHF, arthritis, CTS
Mixed GH-PRL adenomas	5	Combined symptoms of prolactinomas and GH cell adenomas
ACTH cell adenoma	10–15	Hypercortisolism (Cushing' syndrome), hyperpigmentation (ACTH precursor molecule stimulates melanocytes)
Gonadotroph cell adenomas	10–15	Visual impairment, hypogonadism
Null cell adenomas	20	Hypopituitarism
TSH cell adenomas	1	Symptoms of hyperthyroidism
Others	15	

Bitemporal hemianopsia, hormonal effects, symptoms of increased intracranial tension (headache, nausea, vomiting) due to space-occupying effects, and pituitary apoplexy (acute hemorrhage) can be the presenting symptoms of pituitary adenomas. Prolactinomas are the most common hormone-secreting pituitary tumors. The exact frequency with which prolactinomas occur in the general population is not clearly established. In nonselected surgical series, this tumor accounts for approximately 25% to 30% of all pituitary adenomas. Although research continues to unravel the mysteries of disordered cell growth, the cause of pituitary tumors remains unknown. Most pituitary tumors are sporadic—they are not genetically passed from parents to offspring. They tend to be soft solid lesions, often with areas of necrosis or hemorrhage as they get bigger. As they grow, they first expand the sella turcica and then grow upward. They usually indent at the diaphragm sellae, giving them a "snowman" configuration. The enlargement of the sella turcica generally occurs with pituitary macroadenomas that originate in the sella. As they grow in size, they can extend into the sphenoid or cavernous sinus.

Prolactinomas can cause symptoms secondary to the hormonal effects of excess PRL and/or the space-occupying effects of the tumor itself. Women in the reproductive-age group can present with amenorrhea, loss of libido, and/or infertility. Galactorrhea is observed in 30% to 80% of these women. Features of hypoestrogenism such as vaginal dryness, dyspareunia, and a decline in bone mineral density (i.e., osteopenia or osteoporosis) can be seen.

Postmenopausal women and elderly men can have subtle symptoms, thereby delaying the diagnosis. However, this group tends to present more with symptoms of space-occupying effects of the tumor. Major symptoms include headache secondary to stretching of the pain-sensitive structures around the pituitary gland and visual disturbances. Assessment of the visual fields by confrontation method and formal visual field testing, visual acuity, and fundi examination can help determine if the tumor has caused any compression of the visual pathways, especially the chiasma. Modest increases in the serum PRL levels on one or more occasions should make you think of a prolactinoma. TSH and free thyroxine should also be checked. In a patient with a history suggestive of adrenal insufficiency, basal and cosyntropin-stimulated cortisol levels are checked.

After performing biochemical testing, MRI scan of the pituitary hypothalamic area (with gadolinium) or a CT scan of the region (with contrast) can help exclude a mass lesion.

TABLE 7.3 *Causes of Hyperprolactinemia*

Physiological Reasons	Drugs	Pathological Conditions
Breast feeding	Antihistamines	Hypothyroidism
Breast stimulation	Antihypertensives: α-methyldopa, reserpine, verapamil	Pituitary adenomas
Pregnancy	Monoamine oxidase inhibitors	Polycystic ovarian disease
Sexual intercourse	Oral contraceptives, estrogen supplements	Seizures
	Opiates	Stress from trauma, surgery, illness
	Phenothiazines: trifluoperazine, halperidol	Chest wall burns

Good correlation exists between the size of the prolactinoma and the degree of elevation of the serum PRL. A serum PRL level of 200 ng/ml or greater in the presence of a macroadenoma is virtually diagnostic of prolactinoma. There are several other causes of high PRL levels ranging from physiological reasons to iatrogenic causes (Table 7.3).

TREATMENT

Treatment is indicated if mass effects from the tumor and/or significant effects from hyperprolactinemia are present. Bromocriptine mesylate or Parlodel, a dopamine agonist, used in the treatment of Parkinson's disease is considered the drug of choice to shrink prolactinomas. As a dopamine receptor agonist, it decreases the synthesis and secretion of PRL. Our patient developed cardiac arrhythmia after 3 months of drug administration, and the medication had to be discontinued. If a decision is made to withdraw medical treatment, especially in microprolactinoma patients, PRL levels and radiological imaging with MRI or CT scanning should be periodically performed to monitor recurrence and growth of prolactinoma.

Transsphenoidal hypophysectomy is indicated if medical therapy fails; patient should be made aware of possible complications of surgery (summarized in Table 7.4). Additional treatments for prolactinoma include radiation therapy, which is indicated in recurrent prolactinoma. Our patient had a second recurrence of the pituitary adenoma that required RT in addition to surgery. The major complication of RT is hypopituitarism. It occurs in 33% to 70% of patients; the incidence increases with the length of follow-up.

Open (transcranial or craniofacial) approach is more invasive, expensive, and associated with higher surgical risks but provides maximal exposure of many structures. Small pituitary tumors can be effectively targeted by focused beam of RT referred to as "stereotactic radiosugery." It is a reasonable option for very invasive, highly vascularized, and nonfunctioning macrodenomas. There should be at least 5-mm separation between the tumor and chiasma/optic nerve before considering radiosurgery as an option.

TABLE 7.4 *Risks of Transsphenoidal Surgery*

Postoperative infarction or hemorrhage
Diabetes insipidus
Fluid and electrolyte disturbances
Cerebrospinal fluid rhinorrhea
Meningitis
III, IV, VI cranial nerve palsies

Complications of radiosurgery and radiotherapy include

- delayed panhypopituitarism
- cognitive impairment
- optic nerve and temporal lobe radionecrosis
- possible radiation-induced tumors

Despite all treatments, recurrence rate of macroprolactinoma is still about 15% to 20%. Patients with microprolactinoma generally have an excellent prognosis. In up to 95% of patients, these tumors do not enlarge over a 4- to 6-year follow-up. Macroprolactinomas have a tendency to grow with time and require aggressive treatment to prevent complications. The growth rate varies with the individual and cannot be reliably predicted. Careful monitoring of clinical signs and symptoms, coupled with pituitary imaging and with serial measurements of serum PRL levels (i.e., to detect any major change in tumor behavior), remain the cornerstones of follow-up for these patients.

SUGGESTED READING

Kreutzer J, Buslei R, Wallaschofski H, et al. Operative treatment of prolactinomas: indications and results in a current consecutive series of 212 patients. *Eur J Endocrinol.* 2008;158(1):11–18.

Serri O. Progress in the management of hyperprolactinemia. *N Engl J Med.* 1994;331(14):942–944.

CHIEF COMPLAINT: **My legs have been getting weak.**

HISTORY OF PRESENT ILLNESS

A 53-year-old, right-handed male carpenter presented to the clinic with complaints of progressive leg weakness for the past 5 months. It came to his notice that he had difficulty climbing up stairs and standing for a long time. Two months earlier, he noticed that his left leg was getting weaker. There was slow progression of weakness that affected his right leg and then both shoulders. He encountered difficulty carrying his grocery bags; his hands became weak. He had difficulty writing and gripping tools. He complained of mild pain in his muscles. On direct questioning, patient admitted to difficulties with swallowing food, and a concurrent 30-pound weight loss over the past 6 months. He denied any new skin lesions or rash, any problems with his speech, or difficulty breathing. He did not have any fever or chills, or problems with his vision. The weakness had no diurnal variations. He denied suffering from any recent infections or history of travel.

PAST MEDICAL HISTORY

Hypertension.

PAST SURGICAL HISTORY

None.

MEDICATIONS

Baby aspirin 81 mg; denied use of statins in the past.

ALLERGIES

NKDA.

PERSONAL HISTORY

Fifteen-year history of smoking one pack of cigarettes per day but quit a few years ago. No alcohol, no other illicit drugs.

FAMILY HISTORY

Mother was diagnosed with breast carcinoma.

REVIEW OF SYSTEMS

No skin problems, no joint pains, no chest pain, no shortness of breath, no dyspnea, no arthralgias, dry eyes or dry mouth, no thryroid disease.

PHYSICAL EXAMINATION

Vital signs: Blood pressure, 150/97 mmHg; heart rate, 116/min; respiratory rate, 18/min; temperature, 99.5°F; pain scale, 8/10.

No apparent skin lesions.

Lungs clear, heart sounds within normal limits, abdomen is soft, nontender.

Proximal more than distal muscle atrophy in limbs. Normal joints.

NEUROLOGICAL EXAMINATION

Mental status: Alert and oriented, normal language functions, memory 3/3, good consolidation with normal affect, attention and concentration and good judgment.

CNs I–XII: Grossly intact, including gag reflex, no dysarthria; no ptosis.

Motor: Deltoids L 4-/5, R 4/5.

Triceps and biceps 4+/5 bilaterally.

Wrist extensors and flexors 4+/5.

Interossei and finger flexors 4+/5 bilaterally.

Hip flexors 3+/5 bilaterally.

Hip abductors R 3-/5, L 2+/5.

Quadriceps L 3+/5, R 4/5.

Hamstrings 4/5 bilaterally.

Dorsiflexion L 4-/5 R 4+/5.

Plantar flexion 5/5 bilaterally. Notably, patient could not get out of chair without using arms and could not climb up stair, with either leg, to get up onto the examination table. Neck flexors and extensors showed normal strength.

Sensory: Mild loss of pin prick over L anterolateral thigh. Light touch, vibration, and proprioception were all intact throughout distribution.

Reflexes: 1+ in upper extremities symmetrical, absent in lower extremities.

Plantars: Down (flexors).

Coordination: FNF and RAM intact. No resting, postural, or intention tremor.

Gait: Scissors on walking, short stride. Did not pick up legs and feet completely off floor, especially on the left side.

STOP AND THINK QUESTIONS

➤ What are the possible etiologies of the patient's complaints?

➤ What is the significance of weight loss, swallowing problems, and this pattern of muscle weakness?

➤ How will you work up the case?

DIAGNOSTIC TEST RESULTS

Labs: CPK = 5500, aldolase = 64, B12 = 858, AST 169, ALT 162, ESR = 3. Normal ACE, ANA, HIV, and Hep B and Hep C negative. T3, T4, and TSH values normal. Anti-Jo negative. Stool cultures negative for trichinosis. PPD negative.

EMG: Fibrillation potentials, positive sharp waves, short duration, and small amplitude motor unit action potentials.

CXR/CT chest: Nonspecific ground glass opacities in both lungs may reflect areas of inflammation or atypical adenomatous hyperplasia, no lymphadenopathy.

Skeletal survey: no evidence of lytic/blastic lesions. Pelvis, hip joint, femoral head all intact on both sides.

Muscle biopsy left quadriceps: Moderate perimysial and endomysial fibrosis. CD 8+ T cells were seen to invade the muscle fascicles and surround the healthy fibers resulting in phagocytosis and many necrotic fibers with macrophages in them (Figure 8.1). Atrophic fibers were found in groups. Some vacuoles suggestive of rimmed vacuoles in fibers were seen, however, these did not stain with congophilic stains for amyloid deposits. Electron microscopy did not show any tubulo-reticular structures.

DIAGNOSIS: **Polymyositis (PM).**

DISCUSSION

This case demonstrates an asymmetric proximal muscle weakness with early involvement of distal muscles. Pain was not the prominent complaint, but left anterolateral thigh sharp pain and numbness were present. This presentation was in the setting of dysphagia to solid foods and significant weight loss progressing over months.

Based on the findings, the differential should include the acquired myopathies, chronic demyelinating polyneuropathy, and myasthenia gravis. The presence of a high CPK confirmed a myopathy. There are three important idiopathic inflammatory myopathies, namely:

- PM
- DM
- IBM

PM and DM both exhibit proximal more than distal muscle involvement, usually symmetrical. Patients have normal sensations. Ocular muscles are spared, and tendon reflexes are usually preserved (2).

DM usually presents with hallmark skin lesions as follows:

- Heliotrope rash (purplish discoloration on the upper eyelids with edema), Gottron's papules (raised scaly violaceous rash over proximal interphalangeal and metacarpophalangeal joints)
- Erythematous rash on knees, elbows, neck and anterior chest (V sign), back, and shoulders (shawl sign)

sIBM is the most common of the myopathies presenting after age 50. It is usually more insidious in its progression than PM, developing over months to years. sIBM is distinguished clinically from PM based on early involvement of wrist and finger flexors and other distal muscles such as the anterior tibialis (1). Hence, patients may complain of falls due to foot drop or difficulties with grasping objects. As demonstrated in this case, the clinical line between sIBM and PM is not always clear and so a biopsy is of prime importance. As opposed to earlier beliefs that rimmed vacuoles can be seen in both diseases. However, only sIBM biopsies demonstrate degenerative protein aggregates such as amyloid inclusions and p-tau helical filaments in affected muscle fibers (2). Therefore, ruling out such histological findings can help secure a diagnosis of PM. Finally, one must rule out other infective forms of myopathies such as those caused by trichinosis, viral disease, and other idiopathic generalized myopathies such as eosinophilic myositis.

PM is a rare disorder with an incidence of 5 to 10 cases per 100,000 individuals. It can occur at any time after the second decade of life and is associated with other connective tissue diseases (RA, scleroderma) and in rare cases with an underlying occult cancer. When associated with connective tissue disease, the female-to-male ration can be 9:1 (1). PM progresses subacutely, usually over weeks, and is usually proximal and symmetrical, involving distal muscles only late in the disease. Therefore, patient's complaints pertain to difficulties with brushing hair, getting out of chairs, and climbing stairs. The association

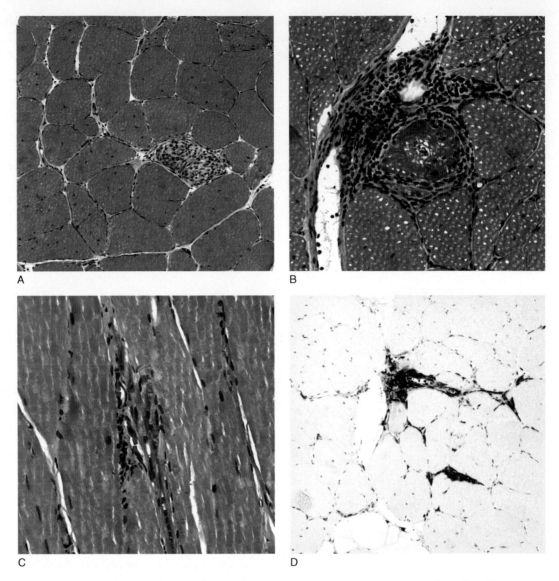

FIGURE 8.1 *Photomicrographs of cryostat sections, H&E stain showing muscle with inflammation characterized by myofiber atrophy and necrosis (A); H&E stain showing internal nuclei, angulated necrotic muscle fibers with inflammation (B); Paraffin section stained with H&E, also showing muscle with inflammation, along with some regenerating basophilic muscle fibers (C) and; Special anti-CD3 immunostains, showing T cell invasion into myofibers (D). (Images courtesy of Douglas C. Miller, MD, PhD, Clinical Professor of Pathology & Anatomical Sciences, University of Missouri School of Medicine.)*

with other autoimmune disease may explain findings such as nonspecific interstitial lung disease in many patients; however, one should always rule out an underlying malignancy, especially when there is concurrent weight loss. Surprisingly, ESR is normal in 80% of patients, while a CPK > 12× normal is highly supportive of the diagnosis. Aldolase is also frequently elevated in PM. EMG is helpful to support the diagnosis of a myopathy, but is nonspecific (1).

The biopsy is of great help and should be done early in the disease before the initiation of steroids. This is crucial as failing to do so may make the biopsy noninterpretable. Our patient's biopsy findings include perimysial fibrosis (acid phosphatase stain) and invasion of mononuclear cells into non-necrotic fibers (see Figure 8.1).

DIFFERENTIAL DIAGNOSIS OF INFLAMMATORY MYOPATHIES INCLUDES THE FOLLOWING

- Spinal muscular atrophy, ALS (EMG can be an important diagnostic tool)
- Muscular dystrophies (develop over longer time)
- GBS, polio, West Nile virus (acute onset)
- Drugs (AZT, amphotericin B, amiodarone, colchicines, steroids, statins, cyclosporine, gemfibrozil, heroin, cocaine, phencyclidine)
- Polymyalgia rheumatica, fibromyalgia
- Connective tissue diseases (SLE, RA, scleroderma, Sjogren's, overlap syndromes)
- Hypothyroidism

PM patients respond very well to steroid treatment as opposed to sIBM patients who fail to respond or even worsen. This case demonstrates that one cannot rely on the clinical presentation to distinguish between PM and sIBM, and therefore a pretreatment biopsy is essential (2).

TREATMENT

Treatment is initiated at 50–75 mg of prednisone daily or alternate day for 4–8 weeks while following serial CPKs. At 2 months, the dose should be decreased at a rate of 5 mg/week to reach a dose of 25–35 mg/d. Muscle power improvement lags behind CPK reductions; however, this should not discourage continuation of tapering of steroids. On the other hand, too fast of a tapering could lead to relapse of disease. Maintenance should be for at least 12 months of complete suppression of disease. Once the decision is made to take the patient off steroids, tapering is at a rate of 1 mg/d per month (i.e., over a period of 2 years) with careful monitoring of CPK and strength. Alternative treatments are with steroid sparing medications such as methotrexate or azathioprine, and some advocate IVIG for cases that fail to respond to these treatments. The overall 5-year and 10-year survival rate is close to 95% and 84%, respectively (3). The prognosis does not correlate well with the CPK levels, the degree of muscle weakness at presentation, and the degree of disability.

REFERENCES

1. Greenberg SA. Inflammatory myopathies: Evaluation and management. *Semin Neurol.* 2008;28(2): 241–249.
2. Chahin N, Engel AG. Correlation of muscle biopsy, clinical course and outcome in PM and sporadic s-IBM. *Neurology.* 2008;70:418–424.
3. Mastaglia FL, Phillips BA, Zilko P. Treatment of inflammatory myopathies. *Muscle Nerve.* 1997;20:651–664.

History of Headaches and Seizures

Geneviève Legault and Anuradha Singh

CHIEF COMPLAINT: **Routine visit for follow-up headaches and seizures.**

HISTORY OF PRESENT ILLNESS

This is a 45-year-old, right-handed female with a history of seizures and migraines. Patient reported that she has been suffering from migraines since her teenage years. Her headaches tend to occur three to four times a month and last for a few hours. These are very debilitating, and she often has to miss her work. She gets throbbing headaches on her temples. Her headaches used to be associated with nausea and vomiting during high school years. She had dealt with headaches all her life, which would be triggered by menstrual periods and sleep deprivation. She denied visual complaints, balance problems, weakness, or numbness in any of the four extremities. She tried a few prophylactic medications such as verapamil and topamax (topiramate) for her headaches without any relief. She is currently using nasal spray Imitrex (sumatriptan) for acute attacks with good relief.

She also gave history of seizures since 19 years of age. Her last seizure was in September 2009. She has had at least 10 to 12 complex partial seizures with secondary generalization with or without aura. Her typical aura was described as a "strange feeling" followed by speech arrest, deviation of eyes to the right, loss of consciousness, and convulsive movements. Convulsions would last only 2 to 3 minutes. Patient often would have no recollection of events. The frequency of seizures could be very variable, from one to three times a year. She had previous CT scan of the brain that revealed cavernous angiomas and several normal EEGs.

She denied any history of head trauma with loss of consciousness prior to onset of headaches or seizures. She did not have meningitis or encephalitis in the past. She was told that her CT scan of the brain was abnormal.

PAST MEDICAL HISTORY

Migraines, partial seizures with secondary generalization.

PAST SURGICAL HISTORY

Breast biopsy (right side; pathology consistent with fibrocystic disease), pilonidal cyst excision.

CURRENT MEDICATIONS

Vimpat (Lacosamide) 150 mg two times a day and Keppra (levetiracetam) 1500 mg two times a day.

PAST MEDICATIONS

Carbamazepine, Topamax (topiramate) (developed renal stones), Cymbalta (duloxetine), Inderal (propranolol), Calan (verapamil).

ALLERGIES

None.

PERSONAL HISTORY

Denied any smoking, drugs, and alcohol.

FAMILY HISTORY

Her mother who is deceased now had history of seizures and was diagnosed with cavernous angiomas and brain tumor in the eloquent cortex that could not be resected and was treated with radiation therapy alone.

GENERAL PHYSICAL EXAMINATION

Unremarkable.

NEUROLOGICAL EXAMINATION

Higher mental functions: Alert and oriented to time, place, and person; affect, attention, and concentration, judgment were normal; her immediate recall was 3/3 and recall of three objects after 5 minutes was 3/3. Comprehension, expression (fluency), repetition, reading, and writing were normal.

CNs II–XII: OU 20/20, pupils equal and reactive, fundi normal, visual fields full by confrontation method, muscles of mastication and facial muscles symmetric; face symmetric, hearing normal by whispering, uvula moved symmetrically, tongue midline, no tongue atrophy, no tongue fasciculations, sternocleidomastoids, and trapezii muscles showed normal strength.

Motor: Normal tone, strength proximally and distally in both upper and lower extremities was normal and is 5/5.

Sensory: Intact to light touch, pin prick, temperature, vibration, and position sense. Cortical sensations were intact.

Reflexes: Biceps, triceps, brachioradialis, patellar, and ankle jerks were 2+ and symmetrical; there was no ankle clonus or Hoffman's.

Plantars: Flexors bilaterally.

Romberg: Negative.

Cerebellar: Finger-nose-finger in upper extremities and knee-shin-heel did not show any dysmetria.

Gait: Normal.

STOP AND THINK QUESTIONS

➢ Does this patient have focal or generalized seizures? What do auras signify?

➢ Do patients with epilepsy commonly suffer from migraines?

➢ What are the risk factors for seizures?

DIAGNOSTIC TEST RESULTS

CBC and differential, SMA-20, ESR, CRP, and RF: unremarkable.

MRI brain: Multiple cerebral and cerebellar cavernomas, more prominent in the left uncus, left posterior temporal and left insula, and right temporal and parietal lobes (the largest cavernoma in the left temporal lobe); the thalami, basal ganglia, and cerebellum showed multiple cavernomas (see Figure 9.1).

Ambulatory EEG for 72 hours: Normal.

DIAGNOSIS: Cerebral cavernous malformation (CCM).

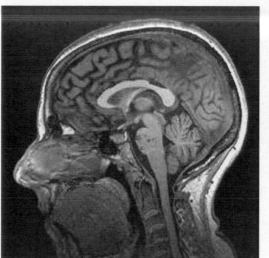

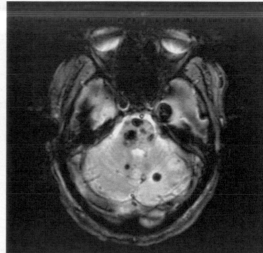

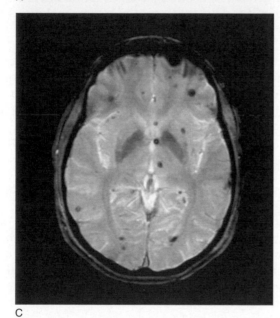

FIGURE 9.1 *Magnetization-prepared rapid gradient echo (MP-RAGE) sagittal section of brain showing multiple cavernomas in the pons (A); Hemoflash T2 axial MRI images (B,C) showing multiple cavernomas in the pons, cerebellum, and left temporal—typical "India ink" blotch appearance (B) and bilateral multiple cavernomas in the supratentorial regions (C).*

DISCUSSION

Cavernoma is a member of the cerebral vascular malformations family. Initially introduced by McCormick in 1966 and a few years later by Russell and Rubenstein in 1977, vascular anomalies are subdivided into AVM, defined by the presence of arteriovenous shunting without intervening capillary bed, venous malformations, consisting of anomalous veins separated by normal brain parenchyma, capillary telangiectasias, determined by a cluster of capillaries interspersed with normal brain tissue, and finally CCM. This classification still holds today.

Cavernomas are themselves classically defined as a cluster of tightly packed capillary-like vessels (or channels, or caverns) containing a single layer of endothelium without intervening brain parenchyma or mature vessel wall components. They have been given several names, including cavernous angiomas, cavernous hemangiomas, cavernomas, and cavernous malformations. Their size can vary from a few millimeters to several centimeters, with a mean of 8 mm (range described of 1 to 90 mm).

The channels of a given cavernoma have been shown to increase both in size and number with time, refuting their initial attribute of congenital lesions and affirming their dynamic nature. The vast majority of CCM (70%–90%) can be found anywhere in the supratentorial location, but are most commonly subcortically located. They also exhibit a predilection for the rolandic and temporal areas. An infratentorial lesion is not infrequently diagnosed (15%–25% of all CCMs), with the majority of them being located in the pons or cerebellar hemispheres. Spinal cord cavernomas are rare and constitute 5% of all cases. Cavernous malformations have also been described in other organs, including the thyroid gland, liver, retina, and skin.

The gross pathology evaluation of CCMs discloses a mulberry appearance with engorged purplish clusters. On microscopy, dilated thin walled capillary-like tunnels with a simple endothelial lining and a thin fibrous adventitia are found, with no elastic fiber or smooth muscle into the vessel walls. The classical definition advises for no intervening brain tissue, although some reports mention it may be present. Microscopy analysis of the immediate surrounding brain unveils the presence of gliosis and hemosiderin-laden tissue. In addition, dilated capillaries may be seen, which some have suspected as being part of a spectrum with capillary telangiectasias. Other findings such as inflammation, calcification and rarely ossification may be present in various proportions, although thought to be more frequent in larger lesions. DVA may be present in up to 25% of specimen, with a higher frequency reported in posterior fossa lesions in comparison to supratentorial CCMs.

Different etiologies lead to the development of cavernomas. The vast majority of patients presenting with cavernomas are sporadic cases. Up to 25% of them can remain asymptomatic throughout their life, while the majority will present with seizures (40%–70%), focal neurological deficits (9%–50%), nonspecific headaches (4%–30%), or cerebral hemorrhages (32%). Most patients exhibit a single lesion, but multiple cavernomas can be demonstrated in up to 12% to 20% of patients.

Some cavernomas are iatrogenic and encountered following cranial or craniospinal radiation therapy. The latency period before cavernoma emerged ranges from 1 to 41 years postradiation, with a mean of 19.5 years. A distinction can, however, be made according to the age at which the patient was treated. Lesions appear sooner for patients treated at a younger age: for patients irradiated during their first decade of life, the mean number of years postradiation before lesions are seen is 4.75 to 16 years, while it is 24.5 years if patients received their radiotherapy in their second decade of life. From a retrospective review of 189 patients with cavernomas including five postradiation cases, 23% of the CCM diagnosed before 15 years of age (3 out of 13 patients) were postradiation, whereas only 1.1% of the patients older than 15 years of age at diagnosis had received prior radiation treatment(1). Radiation-induced cavernomas possibly result from microvascular changes generated by radiation. More specifically, it has been recognized that radiation can induce microvascular narrowing and fibrosis, leading to ischemia and microinfarcts. This promotes reactive neoangiogenesis, which leads to the release of VEGF. The exact mechanism of formation of these radiation-induced lesions has yet to be fully elucidated.

Familial cavernous malformations represent another setting where cavernomas, and especially multiple ones in 50% to 75% of the time, can be found. Typically, five or more lesions are enumerated in affected individuals, but the count can climb to many dozen distinct lesions. Together, these cases are rare but can constitute 6% to 20% of encountered patients with cavernomas. Three genetic loci have been discovered so far and a mutation in one of the known causative genes can be identified in 70% to 80%. All cases are following an autosomal dominant inheritance with incomplete penetrance numbered to approximately 60%. A first locus, CCM1, has been located to 7q11.2-q21. This mutation is identifiable in 30% to 40% of patients, although it represents 70% of the mutated genes in families of Hispanic heritage due to a founder effect. The mutated gene encodes KRIT1 (krev interaction trapped 1), which has been shown to bind to ICAP1alpha (integrin cytoplasmic domain associated protein alpha), a beta1 integrin associated protein, and to RAP-1A (Krev-1), a member of the RAS family of GTPases(2). CCM1 has been associated with an impairment of interendothelial junction stabilization. A function in the inhibition of endothelial proliferation, apoptosis, migration, lumen formation, and sprouting angiogenesis has also been proposed. A second locus has been discovered on 7p15-13, MGC4607, and its gene encodes the malcavernin protein. A CCM2 mutation is present in 20% to 40% of affected families. Its exact function remains unclear but it has been found to form a complex with CCM1 protein and ICAP1alpha, suggesting a final common pathway. A possible role as a scaffolding protein for MAP kinases including MEKK3 and MKK3 for downstream p38 MAPK signaling has been observed, possibly in response to hyperosmotic stress, while other studies have witnessed binding to Rac and actin. Patients exhibiting a mutation at this locus often have less lesions than with other loci, and lesions seem to progress at a slower pace. A third causative gene, CCM3, has been situated to 3q25.2-q27 and is identified in 10% to 20% of familial CCM. The PDCD10 (programmed cell death 10) gene has been suggested to be involved in vasculogenesis, apoptosis, and tumor signaling. CCM3 seems to participate in a protein complex also containing CCM1 and CCM2 although its precise role remains unclear. Mice studies have proposed an essential role for early embryonic vascular development through stabilization of VEGF receptor 2 (VEGFR2) signaling. Patients are more likely to present before 15 years of age and with hemorrhage than carriers of another mutated locus. No mutation can be detected in 20% to 40% of families with cavernous malformations. There is a strong suspicion for more not yet identified genes, and a potential locus has been proposed at 3q26.3-27.2 for CCM4. Rare reports of patients with familial cavernomas have revealed a coexisting benign CNS tumor (meningioma or astrocytoma).

Cavernous malformations can present in infants and children, but more commonly between the second and fifth decades, with a mean age of 30 to 40 years at diagnosis. Familial cases tend to present at a younger age than sporadic cases. There is no sex predisposition, but females have been associated with an increased frequency of hemorrhage and neurological deficits. The incidence in the general population is 0.5%. CCM represents 5% to 15% of all vascular malformations, being second only to DVA. CCM is the culprit in 5% of intractable temporal lobe epilepsy patients. Other types of vascular malformations including capillary telangiectasias, AVM, and DVA may be found in association in 8% to 44% of CCMs.

CCMs appear with a wide spectrum of clinical manifestations, ranging from asymptomatic cases (incidental or autopsy finding) to patients presenting with a fatal hemorrhage, and any combination of headaches, seizures, focal neurological deficits that depend on the involved site, and hemorrhagic strokes. Periods of remission and exacerbation in association with progressive insidious deteriorations lead to an extremely diverse combination of acute and/or chronic deficits, especially when multiple lesions are present.

Cavernous malformations appear on CT scan as nonspecific, irregular, and hyperdense masses with variable amounts of calcifications. Faint and nonspecific contrast enhancement may be identified in postcontrast injection studies. This specific type of vascular malformation is typically angiographically occult, due to its low flow and small vessel composition, yielding a normal study in the majority of cases. A capillary blush or early draining vein can be seen in 10% of the cases. Alternatively, another type of vascular malformation that may coexist with a CCM can be disclosed. MRI is the most revealing radiological tool. The occurrence of evolving blood products of diverse age leads to signals of varying intensities and the so-called characteristic "popcorn" appearance. A dark hemosiderin rim on T2-weighted sequences, GRE or SWI denotes hemosiderin from prior hemorrhages and is typical of cavernoma lesions. Different patterns of T1 and T2 characteristics have lead to the classification of MRI lesions into four groups(3). The type 1 lesion has a core that is hyperintense on T1 and hyper or hypointense on T2. It correlates with subacute hemorrhage histopathologically and clinically with a high frequency of bleeding relapses. The second type of lesion exhibits a core with mixed-signal intensities on T1 and T2, in combination with a hypointense rim, representing lesions with hemorrhages and thromboses of varying ages. Chronic hemorrhage with hemosiderin within and around the lesion constitutes the third type of lesion and is visually identified by an iso- or hypointense T1 appearance with hypointense core and rim on T2-weighted images. Finally, a lesion not visualized on T1 and T2 sequences, but only readily identified by a punctuate hypointensity on GRE signifies a tiny CCM or telangiectasias and possibly represent a true new lesion. Contrast-MRI can reveal the presence of a coexisting DVA and may show a variable and inconsequential contrast enhancement.

The annual bleeding rate for any supratentorial lesion is 0.25% to 1.1% while it reaches 2% to 3% in infratentorial lesions. Lesions with previous hemorrhage have an increased risk of subsequent bleed, and recurrent hemorrhages happen in 17% to 21% of patients. Familial CCM share a similar symptomatic annual bleeding rate of 1.1% per lesion-year, but the existence of multiple lesions makes the rate of symptomatic hemorrhage per patient-year rise to 6.5%. The asymptomatic hemorrhage rates climb to 2% and 13% per lesion-year and patient-year respectively.

Handling these lesions should include a combination of conservative and more invasive approaches. Patients presenting with acute neurological complaints, seizures, or hemorrhage to the emergency department should be managed in a timely manner, potentially requiring emergent surgical evacuation of the lesion and hematoma, and treatment of a prolonged seizure, the specifics of which are beyond the scope of this text.

Asymptomatic lesions are observed, regardless of their location. For symptomatic cavernomas, whether they are giving rise to progressive neurological deficits, intractable epilepsy, and/or recurrent hemorrhages, a surgical approach is usually entertained for accessible lesions. Surgical studies report a poor outcome of 1.5% with an overall mortality of 1.5%. A series of 168 patients with symptomatic epilepsy observed 65% of patients being seizure-free at 3 years post-treatment(4). Good outcome predictors included a mesiotemporal location, a size smaller than 1.5 cm, and the absence of secondarily generalized seizures, while another series reported long pre-operative seizure history and poor pre-operative seizure control as unfavorable prognostic factors(5). Brain stem cavernomas are certainly one of the many neurosurgical challenges, and recent advancements in microsurgical techniques have redefined a more aggressive approach. A retrospective review of 300 patients with a mean follow-up of 51 months found 56% of new or worsening neurological deficits, which were permanent in 35%, 28% of perioperative complications, and 6.9% of rehemorrhage(6). The overall risk of postoperative hemorrhage was 2.0% per year.

Patients with symptomatic lesions entirely surrounded by eloquent tissue such as the motor cortex, thalamus, basal ganglia, or inaccessible brain stem cavernomas are usually observed despite the poor natural history associated with untreated brain stem and thalamic lesions. Stereotactic radiosurgery constitutes a potential alternative to conservative therapy in symptomatic patients with surgically inaccessible lesions. This approach offers a reduced risk of hemorrhage 2 years after treatment, but the bleeding risk during the latency period may be as high as 10%. Initial studies observed a high complication rate and a potential for radiation-induced injury with 3% mortality and 16% of permanent neurological deficits, leading to mixed enthusiasm regarding this approach. More recent reports have been associated with more optimistic figures including a reduction in the risk of permanent neurological deficit to 11%. Therefore, controversy remains as it carries a non-negligible risk of neurological sequelae in these eloquent surgically inaccessible sites without offering the expected reduction in hemorrhage. This method is being used to treat selected patients with CCM. Unraveling the pathophysiology of CCMs may lead to specific molecular therapies and thus ultimately improve patient outcome. Much research is still needed.

In conclusion, CCMs are angiographically occult vascular malformations that vary from remaining asymptomatic throughout life to being associated with fatal hemorrhages or significant neurological impairments. Usually single, lesions can be multiple, especially in familial cases, and are best identified on MRI, GRE, or SWI. Three mutated loci have been identified with familial cases, CCM1, CCM2, and CCM3. CCMs carry a risk of hemorrhage of 1.1% (2%–3% in the posterior fossa) per lesion-year. Asymptomatic lesions are observed. Symptomatic lesions are surgically resected if accessible. Stereotactic radiosurgery may be considered for symptomatic surgically inaccessible lesions.

REFERENCES

1. Heckl S, Aschoff A, Kunze S. Radiation-induced cavernous hemangiomas of the brain: A late effect predominantly in children. *Cancer.* 2002;94(12):3285–3291.
2. Yadla S, Jabbour PM, Shenkar R, Shi C, Campbell PG, Awad IA. Cerebral cavernous malformations as a disease of vascular permeability: From bench to bedside with caution. *Neurosurg Focus.* 2010;29(3):E4.
3. Zabramski JM, Wascher TM, Spetzler RF, et al. The natural history of familial cavernous malformations: Results of an ongoing study. *J Neurosurg.* 1994;80(3):422–432.
4. Baumann CR, Acciarri N, Bertalanffy H, et al. Seizure outcome after resection of supratentorial cavernous malformations: A study of 168 patients. *Epilepsia.* 2007;48(3):559–563.
5. Cohen DS, Zubay GP, Goodman RR. Seizure outcome after lesionectomy for cavernous malformations. *J Neurosurg.* 1995;83(2):237–242.
6. Abla AA, Lekovic GP, Turner JD, de Oliveira JG, Porter R, Spetzler RF. Advances in the treatment and outcome of brain stem cavernous malformation surgery: A case series of 300 surgically treated patients. *Neurosurgery* 2011;68(2):403–14.

Aditi D... ... and Amarendra Singh

CHIEF COMPLAINT: **Slurring of speech.**

HISTORY OF PRESENT ILLNESS

Patient is an 85-year-old, left-handed female in her usual state of health until the day she presented to the ER. At home, she woke up in the morning around 6 a.m. and felt a little "out of balance." She was holding on to walls, but she did not feel weakness on one side or the other. She reported no falls. She had her breakfast and then made a call to her friend around 8:30 a.m. who noticed that her speech was not clear. She could think clearly and knew what she had to say but her "words are not clear to others." She immediately called 911 and was brought to the hospital around 10 a.m. She could give a detailed history but her words were hard to comprehend because of continued slurring of speech. She denied other common neurological symptoms. She denied having nausea, vomiting, double vision, vertigo, headaches, or any swallowing difficulties. The staff in the ER noticed slight drooping on the right side of her face. She could not tell if she was weak on one side or the other. She denied any sensory symptoms. She had never experienced any previous TIAs or strokes.

PAST MEDICAL HISTORY

Hypercholesterolemia, GERD.

PAST SURGICAL HISTORY

Tonsillectomy.

MEDICATIONS

Aciphex, aspirin.

ALLERGIES

None.

PERSONAL HISTORY

She denied use of tobacco, alcohol, or drugs.

FAMILY HISTORY

Heart diseases run in her family, one of her brothers was diagnosed with lung carcinoma; other brothers were diagnosed with heart problems.

PHYSICAL EXAMINATION

Blood pressure, 144/88 mm Hg; pulse, 72/min, regular; respiratory rate, 16/min; afebrile; no carotid bruits.
Cardiovascular: S1 and S2 normal, no cardiac murmurs.
Lungs: Clear, no rales or ronchi.
Abdomen: Soft, nontender, and no visceromegaly.

NEUROLOGICAL EXAMINATION

Higher mental functions: Alert and oriented ×3, normal affect; attention, concentration, judgment were normal, she had significant dysarthria but normal comprehension, no phonemic or semantic paraphasias, she could read well, she could name and repeat; she was not able to write legibly because of mild right hand dexterity problems, but she could write a sentence without making any grammatical mistakes. She had no visuospatial apraxia; memory 3/3 on immediate recall.

CNs II–XII: Right upper motor neuron facial, rest unremarkable.

Motor: Right subtle pronator drift, no motor weakness in all four extremities.

Sensory: Intact to all modalities of sensation.

Reflexes: UE 2+ and symmetrical, LE: right KJ 3+, left KJ 2+, trace AJ bilaterally.

Plantars: Rt. extensor, left flexor.

Cerebellar: Unremarkable.

Gait: Normal for age.

Romberg: Negative.

STOP AND THINK QUESTIONS

➤ Is she a t-PA candidate?
➤ What is the difference between aphasia and dysarthria?
➤ Does she seem to suffer from a stroke from a large vessel or small vessel disease?

DIAGNOSTIC TEST RESULTS

Labs: CBC and metabolic profile: normal; ESR 27.

TSH 5.97 (increased); HbA1C 6.5.

ALT 78; RPR, nonreactive.

Coags profile: Normal.

EKG: sinus rhythm with short PR (88 ms).

CT stroke series: Precontrast head CT and postcontrast CT perfusion demonstrate mild microvascular disease. No evidence of infarction or intracranial hemorrhage. CT angiogram demonstrates atherosclerotic changes with no evidence of intraluminal clot or dissection. A moderately severe focal stenosis at the origin of the left vertebral artery is noted.

MRI brain (see Figure 10.1A and B): Acute left paramedial pontine infarct and mild moderate microvascular ischemic changes, volume loss, and mild focal stenosis of the proximal right PCA.

Carotid Doppler: The duplex scan shows stenosis in the right internal carotid artery at the high end of 16% to 49%, and in the left internal. Carotid artery at the low end of 16% to 49%. The vertebral arteries shows antegrade flow. The subclavian arteries are patent.

Abdominal US: Bilateral renal cysts as described above with mildly complex cyst in the right kidney.

Video esophagogram/swallowing study: Abnormal oropharyngeal swallow with mild risk of aspiration.

Doppler lower extremities: No evidence of deep vein thrombosis.

DIAGNOSIS: **Lacunar stroke, left paramedian pons.**

HOSPITAL COURSE

She was not a t-PA candidate, as the onset of symptoms was not very clear. She was switched to Plavix because of GERD. She was also started on Lipitor 40 mg once daily.

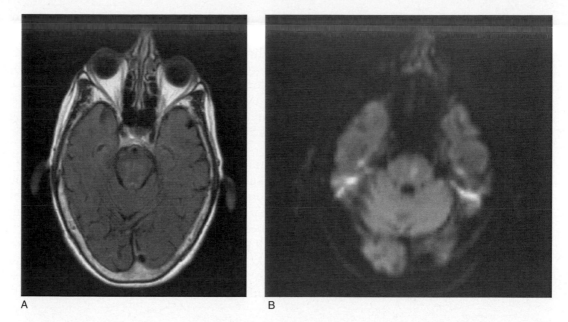

A   B

FIGURE 10.1 *(A) MRI Brain FLAIR sequence showing chronic microvascular disease in the pons; (B) MRI DWI showing wedge-shaped focus of abnormally increased diffusion restriction at the para-median left pons. Lipid profile: Serum cholesterol 222; LDL 141. 2-D ECHO: Essentially normal.*

DISCUSSION

Lacunar strokes describe a set of clinical stroke syndromes with typical signs and symptoms caused by small subcortical or brain stem lesions. This subset of strokes account for approximately 25% of ischemic strokes, though the prevalence varies depending on the definition used for diagnosis and the population under study. Lacunar strokes as a stroke subtype were first recognized by French neurologists and neuropathologists in the nineteenth century. The term "lacunae" was used at that time to describe small holes in the brain appreciated at autopsy. In the modern era, C. Miller Fisher rediscovered lacunar infarcts.

There are different types of lacunar strokes: TIA, asymptomatic lacunar infarcts, and symptomatic lacunar syndromes. The lesions are classically located in the following regions: lenticular nucleus, thalamus, frontal lobe white matter, pons, basal ganglia, internal capsule, and caudate nucleus. The arteries giving rise to lacunar infarcts are deep or penetrating arteries ranging from 100 to 400 μm in diameter originating from large cerebral arteries. They do not have collateral branches or terminal anastamoses and provide blood supply to the deepest and nearest territories to the middle cerebral hemispheres and brain stem. Branches of the anterior and middle cerebral arteries, including lenticular branches and the long deep perforator medullary branches, are affected, as are branches of the posterior cerebral artery including the thalamoperforator and thalamogeniculate branches. The paramedian branches of the basilar artery may also be affected.

Small infarcts that do not cause acute stroke symptoms are much more common than symptomatic syndromes. These silent infarcts were approximately five times more common than infarcts presenting with stroke. In TIAs, focal neurologic deficits last less than 1 hour. By the classical definition, TIAs are the result of a cerebral dysfunction of an ischemic nature lasting no longer than 24 hours. Lacunar infarctions may account for 29% to 34% of all TIAs.

Lacunar infarcts cause clinically evident strokes when they occur at strategic sites; locations at which descending and ascending long tracts are concentrated, subcortically, or in the brain stem. The time course for the lacunar infarcts is short, occurring over minutes to hours. However, symptoms may evolve over the course of several days especially in larger artery thrombosis. Lacunar infarcts can thus be associated with worsening motor deficits after hospital admission. Lacunar strokes tend to occur most frequently at night between midnight and 6 a.m.

The following features are characteristically absent in lacunar strokes: aphasia, apraxia, agnosia, negligence, amnesic disturbances, vomiting, and vegetative symptoms, visuospatial disturbances including oculomotor deficits, disturbances of brain stem function such as pupil abnormalities, decrease in consciousness, seizures. While 20 lacunar syndromes have been described, five have been validated as highly predictive of lacunar strokes. A lacunar syndrome has an overall positive predictive value of 87% for detecting the lacunar infarct on MRI. See Table 10.1 for descriptions of the five most common lacunar syndromes, the locations of the lacunar infarct, and the positive predictive value of clinical findings associated with each clinical syndrome.

Pure Motor Hemiparesis

Pure motor hemiparesis is the most common of the lacunar syndromes accounting for approximately 50% to 66% of all lacunar syndromes. The most common topographies include the posterior limb of the internal capsule, corona radiate, and pons. Infarcts in the mesencephalus or meduallary pyramids are less common. Clinical features of hemiplegia involve the face and arm (brachiofacial) or the arm and leg (braciocrural) in the absence of any sensory deficits. Focal deficits, such as paralysis of a hand, are more likely to be of cortical origin.

TABLE 10.1 *Lacunar Syndromes*

Lacunar Syndrome	Location	Clinical Findings
Pure motor hemiparesis	Posterior limb of internal capsule, corona radiate, basal puns, medial medulla	Unilateral paralysis of face, arm and leg, dysarthria and dysphagia may be present
Pure sensory syndrome	Thalamic ventroposterolateral nucleus, pontine tegmentum, corona radiata	Unilateral sensory deficit or irritative sensory disturbance of face, arm, and leg without motor deficits
Ataxic hemiparesis	Corticopontocerebellar, dentatorubrothalamocortical or somesthetic propiopoceptive pathways of posterior limb of internal capsule, or pons, corona radiata, thalamus	Unilateral weakness and limb ataxia
Sensorimotor syndrome	Thalamocapsular, maybe basal pons or lateral medulla	Hemiparesis or hemiplegia of face, arm, and leg with ipsilateral sensory impairment
Dysarthria-clumsy hand syndrome	Anterior limb and genu of internal capsule, pons, cerebellar peduncles, corona radiata	Unilateral facial weakness, dysarthria, and dysphagia with mild hand weakness and clumsiness

Pure Sensory Syndrome

Pure sensory syndrome presents with sensory deficits (hypoesthesia) and/or irritative sensory disturbances of superficial and deep sensations. Complete hemisensory syndromes tend to occur involving the face, arm, and leg. This syndrome is most commonly caused by infarction of the thalamic ventroposterolateral nucleus. In addition, the brain stem or thalamocortical projection areas may also be involved. Pure sensory syndromes without evidence of lacunar infarction occur in fewer than 7% of cases and can be caused by nonlacunar infarcts, cerebral hemorrhages, multiple sclerosis, and arteriovenous malformations.

Ataxic Hemiparesis

Ataxic hemiparesis is characterized by the simultaneous presence of a pyramidal syndrome with a homolateral ataxic syndrome. A transient sensory deficit may also be observed in some cases. This syndrome is predominantly caused by infarcts to the corticopontocerebellar, dentarubrothalamocortical, or somesthetic proprioceptive pathways of the posterior limb of the internal capsule or pons. In fewer than 7% of cases, the syndrome is caused by nonlacunar infarcts, cerebral hemorrhages, tumors, or infections.

Sensorimotor Syndrome

Sensorimotor syndrome presents as a complete or incomplete pyramidal syndrome with complete or partial sensory deficit of the ipsilateral side of the body involving the face, arm, and leg. It is most commonly caused by nonlacunar infarctions.

Dysarthria-Clumsy Hand Syndrome

This syndrome presents with moderate to severe dysarthria with central facial weakness, homolateral hyperreflexia with Babinski's sign, and weakness of the hand with impairment of tasks requiring manual ability without an associated motor deficit. Infarcts are typically present in the anterior limb and/or genu of the internal capsule and the pons. This lacunar syndrome has the most favorable outcome, with no neurologic disability reported in 46% of patients. Our patient seems to have this syndrome.

PATHOPHYSIOLOGY

Lacunar strokes are produced by an alteration of blood flow in the distribution of a penetrating arteriole. The lacunar hypothesis suggests that particular syndromes are caused by small infarcts of the brain owing to single perforating artery occlusion. Much of the clincopathological evidence detailing the vascular basis of lacunar infarcts is drawn from the work of C. Miller Fisher. Most symptomatic lacunar infarcts investigated in Fisher's study were the result of occlusion of perforating arteries by atheromatous plaques and thrombus formation.

Several pathophysiological mechanisms for the development of lacunar infarcts have been suggested. While many mechanisms may be responsible, most lacunar infarctions are due to disease of the cerebral small vessels. Atherosclerosis, cardioembolism, and cryptogenic stroke account for only 25% of cases. Two pathologic types of small artery disease are responsible for most lacunes: microatheroma and lipohyalonisis.

Microatheroma describes the pathologic changes that precipitate the development of larger subcortical infarcts. In microatheromas, the proximal segment of perforating arterioles, of larger size in diameter, undergo atheromatous alterations leading to arterial stenosis. These penetrating arteries tend to originate from the middle cerebral artery, the Circle of Willis, distal basilar, or vertebral artery. The subsequent occlusion of these arteries causes lacunar infarcts. Histologically, this mechanism of lacunar infarction is similar to atherosclerosis of larger arteries, in which a plaque occludes the lumen of the artery.

Lipohyalinosis refers to a process that produces smaller subcortical infarcts. In lipohyalinosis, resulting from long-standing hypertension, smaller perforating arteries, those less than 200 μm in diameter, are affected. The arteries undergo arteriolar wall disorganization with vessel wall thickening and subsequent luminal narrowing. Fibrinoid necrosis is an additional type of thrombotic arteriopathy that may be responsible for lacunar infarction. In fibrinoid necrosis, arterioles and capillaries of the brain are predominantly affected by sudden increases in blood pressure that occurs in hypertensive encephalopathy or eclampsia. This is thought to be due to disordered cerebrovascular autoregulation in response to sudden high blood pressure levels. Arterial walls are unable to constrict and subsequently overdistend in a segmental fashion with resultant necrosis. Leukoaraiosis, a term describing diffuse white matter abnormalities on CT and MRI brain scans, is common findings in patients with lacunes. Lacunar infarctions, more so than other subtypes of ischemic strokes, are most strongly predicted by leukoaraiosis. The association of lacunar infarcts and white matter changes further supports the concept of small vessel disease as the underlying mechanism of both leukoaraiosis and lacunar infarcts.

Though embolic mechanisms of lacunar infarction are less common, they are also a potential source of arterial occlusion. Embolic occlusion of perforating arteries may result from one of two mechanisms: embolization of cardiac origin either from atrial fibrillation, rheumatic valve disease, and nonbacterial thrombotic endocarditis. The embolism may also be of arterial origin from carotid or aortic atheromatosis. Microemboli may dislodge from the larger atheromatous plaques leading to lacunar infarcts. Both embolic mechanisms are exceptional causes of lacunar infarcts.

Other rarer mechanisms include hemodynamic disorders, arterial dissection, and hematologic disorders and infections. Hemodynamic disorders may cause aberrant flow and low distal perfusion characterized by previous TIAs or progressive or graded stroke symptomatology. Arterial dissection resulting from chronic hypertension may precipitate the development of Charcot-Bouchard aneurysms (these are microaneurysms of brain vasculature that occur in small blood vessels of less than 300 micrometer diameter), intracerebral hemorrhage, or thrombosis leading to lacunar infarcts. Finally, hematological disorders and infections, including conditions that increase red cell volume as in polycythemia vera or infections altering small arteries as in chronic vasculitides such as neurosyphilis, may result in lacunar infarcts.

Wardlaw et al. proposed an additional hypothesis, arguing that lacunar infarcts are a focal manifestation of a diffuse and progressive vascular disease of small-sized cerebral arterioles. This disease process may ultimately lead to cognitive impairment and dementia. This process may result from compromise of the blood brain barrier, from hypertension, diabetes, or other processes altering the arteriolar endothelium. Toxic blood components including plasmin and other proteases may cross the increasingly permeable blood brain barrier leading to neuronal and glial damage and altering interstitial fluid which may disrupt axonal signal transmission. This gradual and asymptomatic process may account for the formation of silent lacunar infarcts, leukaraiosis (periventricular white matter disease), cognitive impairment, and dementia.

Vascular risk factors for lacunar stroke are similar to those for atherothrombotic stroke, including aging, hypertension, and diabetes. Hyperlipidemia, however, is not associated with small subcortical strokes. Precise diagnosis of lacunar infarcts can be difficult given the nature of the vascular lesion. Ischemic strokes resulting from occlusion of an artery as small as 0.2 to 0.8 mm in diameter cannot reliably be diagnosed in vivo and can only truly be determined by neuropathological examination. Therefore, lacunar infarcts are practically diagnosed by extrapolating from different sources of information both clinical and radiologic. Probability assumptions are made based on clinical features and neuroimaging of brain parenchyma.

Ancillary investigations such as ultrasonography both cardiac and carotid are used to rule out other potential causes of ischemia. As two of the most effective treatments in stroke depend on an accurate diagnosis, carotid surgery for severe symptomatic carotid stenosis, and warfarin for atrial fibrillation, patients should be screened with ultrasonography, EKG, and holter monitoring.

Lacunar strokes acutely are typically <15 mm in diameter; however, they can extend up to 20 mm in some cases. The infarcts will then shrink up to 50% when progressing from the acute to chronic stages with most lacunar infarcts ultimately less than 5 mm in diameter.

In terms of sizing criteria, the following four specific criteria demonstrated on MRI are being utilized in the SPS3 study to define lacunar strokes radiographically.

- On DWI, the lesion must be ≤2 cm in size at the largest dimension with a positive apparent diffusion coefficient image
- On FLAIR or T2, the lesion must be a well-delineated focal hyperintensity ≤2 cm in size at the largest dimension. If the DWI is negative and the study was carried out within 30 days of the index event, this criteria alone is insufficient to qualify as a lacunar infarct
- On FLAIR or T1, multiple (at least 2) hypointense lesions 0.3 to 1.5 cm in size at the largest dimension in the cerebral hemispheres qualify if the patient's event is clinically hemispheric
- On FLAIR or T1, the lesion must be well-delineated and hypointense, ≤1.5 cm in size and correspond to the clinical syndrome with the MRI carried out within 1 month of the event

DWI has a higher sensitivity for acute lesions than T2-weighted MRI or FLAIR. With DWI, a hyper intense signal is apparent whenever there is an area of restricted water diffusion, this occurs in acute ischemic regions. In a study examining the efficacy of DWI in helping to differentiate lacunar from nonlacunar stroke in patients with lacunar syndrome, 40.5% with lacunar syndrome had nonlacunar infarcts on DWI. This study suggests that clinical examination is insufficient and at times inaccurate; therefore, clinical and radiologic evidence should be employed simultaneously to arrive at a diagnosis. In this study, CT on admission provided little extra information.

Noncontrast head CT has a low sensitivity for detecting lacunar strokes. Approximately 30% to 44% for lacunar strokes are detected by noncontrast head CT; this detection rate may be worse in the hyperacute phase (<6 h). Noncontrast CT is limited in its utility and is predominately useful in identifying posterior fossa infarcts and defining the degree of cortical extension in subcortical infarcts.

TREATMENT

Current stroke guidelines do not differentiate between lacunar and nonlacunar strokes with regard to treatment or risk modification. In addition, many of the major secondary stroke prevention trials have not distinguished between different stroke subtypes. Different antiplatelet drugs may have distinct influences on stroke prevention and treatment depending on the stroke subtype. Table 10.2 includes some of the medications used for secondary stroke prevention.

TABLE 10.2 *Medications Used in Secondary Stroke Prevention*

Medications	Mechanism of Action	Dose	Side Effects
Aspirin	Inhibits cyclooxygenase, reducing production of thromboxane A2; therefore, interfering with the formation of thrombi	50 to 325 mg/d for secondary stroke prevention	Gastrointestinal hemorrhage or milder gastrointestinal symptoms; intracranial bleeding
Clopidogrel (Plavix)	Thienopyridine that inhibits adenosine diphosphate (ADP)–dependent platelet aggregation	75 mg once daily	Rash and diarrhea, decreased frequency of gastric upset and gastrointestinal bleeding compared with aspirin
Ticlopidine (Ticlid)	Thienopyridine, ADP receptor inhibitor	250 mg two times daily	Severe neutropenia in 1% of patients, rash, diarrhea
Dipyridamole	Impairs platelet function by inhibiting activity of adenosine deaminase and phosphodiesterase	75 mg three times daily	Headache (incidence of headache declines over 7 days after initiation of therapy)
Aggrenox (aspirin 25 mg + extended release dipyridamole 200 mg)	Same as aspirin and dipyrdamole	One tab two times daily	Headaches, mild gastrointestinal irritability

The use of the medications listed above in secondary stroke prevention has not been exclusively studied in patients with lacunar strokes. Table 10.3, taken from Benavente et al.'s article "Small Vessel Strokes," details the outcomes of secondary stroke prevention trials for subgroups of participants with small subcortical strokes.

The management of hypertension also plays an important role in primary and secondary stroke prevention. Hypertension is a well-known risk factor for lacunar strokes, and it has been shown that even a modest reduction in blood pressure has significant benefit in reducing stroke incidence and recurrence.

The SPS3 phase III trial enrolling 2,500 patients with symptomatic small subcortical strokes confirmed by MRI is the first study of secondary stroke prevention focusing specifically on patients with small vessel disease. This study is examining whether combination antiplatelet therapy of aspirin plus clopidogrel is superior to aspirin alone as well as whether intensive blood pressure management for reducing stroke recurrence, cognitive decline, and major vascular events. The results of this study will help to inform the management of many patients with cerebral small vessel disease.

PROGNOSIS

Overall, the long-term survival of patients with lacunar strokes is more favorable than those with other stroke subtypes (Table 10.3). The early mortality associated with lacunar strokes is approximately 0% to 2% of case fatalities 30 days following a lacunar stroke. The long-term risk of death is only slightly higher at 3% per year. While the mortality associated with stroke is generally low, the risk of recurrence is 4% to 11% per year among patients with a lacunar stroke exposed to different therapeutic interventions. Approximately, 60% of recurrent strokes were additional small subcortical strokes. Whereas mild disability may result from one subcortical stroke, multiple lacunar infarcts may precipitate the development of vascular dementia among other disabling pathologies. Lacunar infarcts, more so than other stroke subtypes, most commonly predispose patients to the development of vascular dementia.

TABLE 10.3 *Stroke Prevention Studies That Identified Lacunar Strokes as Index Events*

Study	Patients, n	Patients with Lacunar Stroke Enrolled, n (%)	Interventions	Relative Risk Reduction in Patients with Lacunar Stroke as Index Event, %
AICLA	604	98 (16)	Aspirin vs. aspirin +dipyridamole vs. placebo	69
CATS	1072	275 (26)	Ticlopidine vs. placebo	50
CAST	20,655	6102 (30)	Aspirin vs. placebo	10
Cilostazol Stroke Prevention Study	1095	810 (74)	Cilostazol vs. placebo	43
WARSS	2206	1237 (56)	Aspirin vs. warfarin	NS
AAASPS	1809	1221 (68)	Ticlopidine vs. aspirin	NA
MATCH	7599	3148 (52)	Clopidogrel vs. clopidogrel +aspirin	NA

Note: AAASPS, African American Antiplatelet Stroke Prevention Study; AICLA, Accidents, Ischemiques Cerebraux Lies a l'Atherosclerose; CAST, Chinese Acute Stroke Trial; CATS, Canadian American Ticlopidine Study in thromboembolic stroke; MATCH, Management of Atherothrombosis with Clopidogrel in High-Risk Patients; NA, results not reported separately for lacunar stroke patients; NS, results not significant; WARSS, Warfarin-Aspirin Recurrent Stroke Study.

Source: Adapted from Benavente, O., et al., Small vessel strokes. *Curr Cardiol Rep*, 2005; 7(1): 23–28.

SUGGESTED READING

Arboix A, Marti-Vilalta JL. Lacunar stroke. *Expert Rev Neurother.* 2009;9(2):179–196.

Benavente O, White CL, Roldan AM. Small vessel strokes. *Curr Cardiol Rep.* 2005;7(1):23–28.

Benavente OR, White CL, Pearce L, et al. The secondary prevention of small subcortical strokes (SPS3) study. *Int J Stroke* 2011;6(2):164–175.

Fisher CM. Lacunar infarcts: A review. *Cerebrovas Dis.* 1991;1:311–320.

Gan R, Sacco RL, Kargman DE, Roberts JK, Boden-Albala B, Gu Q. Testing the validity of the lacunar hypothesis: The Northern Manhattan. Stroke Study experience. *Neurology.* 1997;48:1204–1211.

Norrving B. Lacunar infarcts: No black holes in the brain are benign. *Pract Neurol.* 2008;8(4):222–228.

Rajapaske A, Rajapaskse S, Sharma JC. Is investigating for carotid artery disease warranted in non-cortical lacunar infarction? *Stroke.* 2011;42(1):217–220.

Wardlaw JM. What causes lacunar stroke? *J Neurol Neurosurg Psychiatry.* 2005;76:617–619.

Left-Sided Neck Pain and Ptosis

CASE 11

Ritvij Bowry, Anuradha Singh, and Daniel Sahlein

CHIEF COMPLAINT: **Neck pain for two weeks.**

HISTORY OF PRESENT ILLNESS

A 33-year-old, right-handed man was referred to the ER for evaluation of sharp left-sided neck and head pain for 11 days after playing tennis the day prior to the onset of symptoms. He noticed a strange feeling of "fullness" and drooping of the left eye a few days ago that pushed him to go to the ER. He did not notice any worsening of the drooping of the left eye in the evening hours. Patient denied ever having similar symptoms before. There is no history of previous thrombotic events. He denied any history of trauma, speech problems, or swallowing difficulties. There was no associated nausea, weakness, numbness, spinning sensation, visual disturbances, headaches, or tearing from his eyes. He did not notice any incoordination, imbalance, hearing loss, tinnitus, or trouble walking. He denied any systemic symptoms such as cough, fevers, chills, night sweats, fatigue, weight loss, shortness of breath, or any bowel or bladder problems. He stated that until now he had been in perfect health.

PAST MEDICAL HISTORY AND PAST SURGICAL HISTORY

None.

MEDICATIONS

None.

ALLERGIES

None.

PERSONAL HISTORY

No history of smoking or illicit drug use; one Etoh drink per week on the weekends.

FAMILY HISTORY

Noncontributory.

PHYSICAL EXAMINATION

Vital signs: Blood pressure, 148/103 mm Hg; pulse, 86/min; respiratory rate, 18/min; O_2 saturation, 99%; temperature, 99.0°F.
Average statured young man in no acute distress, droopy eyelid on the left, no rash, normal musculoskeletal examination.

NEUROLOGICAL EXAMINATION

Mental status: Alert, following commands, oriented to time, place and person, fluent speech, intact language, no dysarthria, recalls 3/3 objects, intact attention and concentration.
CNs II–XII: Conjugate eye movements intact, no nystagmus, full visual fields, visual acuity 20/20 bilaterally, +left ptosis, +anisocoria (prominent in the dark): left pupil 1 mm, right

pupil 3 mm, bilaterally reactive, reactive to accommodation and convergence, symmetric facial strength and sensation, equal hearing bilaterally, palate symmetric, uvula and tongue midline, equal shoulder shrug bilaterally.

Motor: 5/5 bilaterally both upper and lower extremities, no drift, normal bulk and tone.

Sensory: Symmetric light touch, pin prick, temperature, position and vibration sense in all four extremities.

Reflexes: 2+ symmetrical upper and lower extremities, no clonus or Hoffman's sign.

Plantars: Flexors bilaterally.

Coordination: Normal FNF bilaterally, normal RAM, normal fine finger movements, normal HKS bilaterally.

Gait: Steady, normal stride, and arm swing; he was able to tandem walk and walk on heels and toes.

STOP AND THINK QUESTIONS

➢ What do abnormal eye findings indicate in this case?

➢ Where will you localize the lesion after review of the history and examination?

➢ How will you work up this young patient to reach the diagnosis?

DIAGNOSTIC TEST RESULTS

CBC, SMA-20, RPR, Lyme, ESR, ACE: Normal.

Chest X-ray showed no evidence of cardiopulmonary disease.

MRI of the brain without contrast gadolinium: Normal evaluation of the brain. No evidence of diffusion abnormality or intracranial hemorrhage. However, MP-RAGE T1-weighted axial images at the skull base demonstrate marked abnormality of the right vertebral artery and left internal carotid artery, in both cases demonstrating luminal narrowing and a crescentic T1 hyperintense collection surrounding the vessel (hematoma in the form of methemoglobin within the vessel wall/pseudolumen) (Figure 11.1A). There is a focal 1.5 cm outpouching of the cervical segment of the left internal carotid artery at a level just below the skull base representing a pseudoaneurysm (Figure 11.1B).

MRA of the neck and brain without contrast: 3D Time-of-Flight angiography of the neck shows luminal narrowing and irregularity as well as a discrete intimal flap within the right vertebral artery extending from C6 (the inferior margin of the study) to C2 (Figure 11.2A and B). The left cervical internal carotid artery demonstrates 50% to 60% narrowing associated with intimal flap, luminal wall irregularity, and a focal 1.5 cm outpouching at the level of the skull base. The remainder of the study is unremarkable.

Four-vessel cerebral angiogram: On day 2, the patient underwent a cerebral angiogram to further assess the right vertebral and left internal carotid artery dissections and to better understand the flow dynamics. Contrast injection of the right subclavian artery demonstrated a severe focal stenosis (90%) 1 cm distal to the origin of the right vertebral artery with an associated 5 mm post-stenotic dilatation or outpouching (Figure 11.3A). Distal to this outpouching, the cervical vertebral artery demonstrated luminal irregularity with varying degrees of mild to moderate stenosis to the level of the C2 foramen transversarium, most significant at the C2 level where there was approximately 60% stenosis (Figure 11.3B). The left internal carotid artery demonstrated luminal irregularity with associated varying degrees of stenosis of up to 60% within a 3.5 cm section of the cervical segment (Figure 11.3C). The 1.5 cm pseudoaneurysm seen on MRI at the level of the skull base was not seen angiographically, though a 0.5 mm "beak" or psuedoaneurysm neck

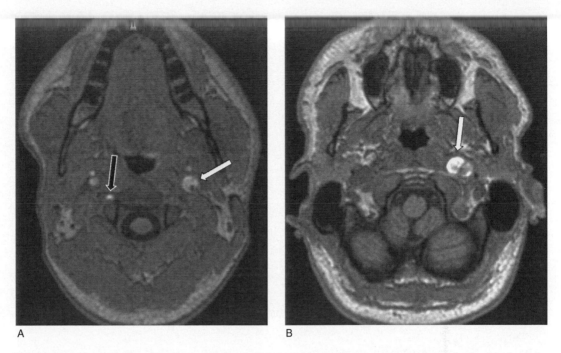

FIGURE 11.1 *(A) Transaxial T1-weighted MP-RAGE noncontrast image through the level of the inferior aspect of C2. Note the crescentic T1 hyperintense collection surrounding the right vertebral artery (solid black arrow) and, to a greater extent, the left internal carotid artery (white arrow). (B) Transaxial T1-weighted MP-RAGE noncontrast image through the level of the skull base. The left internal carotid artery demonstrates an irregular 1.5 cm outpouching (white arrow) that is predominantly T1 hyperintense though heterogeneous in signal intensity.*

remnant was seen, suggesting that the pseudoaneurysm had thrombosed off and therefore could not be opacified with contrast (Figure 11.3D).

The left ICA stenosis was hemodynamically significant, though well compensated. The external carotid artery supplied collateral support to the supraclinoid left internal carotid artery via the anterior deep temporal artery (Figure 11.3E). The posterior distribution supplied collateral support via a large posterior communicating artery (Figure 11.3F). The right ICA supplied collateral support via the anterior communicating artery (Figure 11.3G). No endovascular intervention was performed because the study showed adequate collateral circulation.

DIAGNOSIS: Cervical artery dissections.

HOSPITAL COURSE

Based on the above findings of right vertebral artery and left internal carotid artery dissections, the patient received aspirin 325 mg and was started on a Heparin drip. He did remarkably well. His left Horner's syndrome and headache improved without any neurological sequelae, while being maintained on a Heparin drip. Patient was placed on dual antiplatelet therapies with Plavix and aspirin. A repeat MRA in 3 months was planned to assess for vessel patency and resolution of the dissections. The patient was discharged home in stable condition and advised to refrain from engaging in heavy lifting, neck

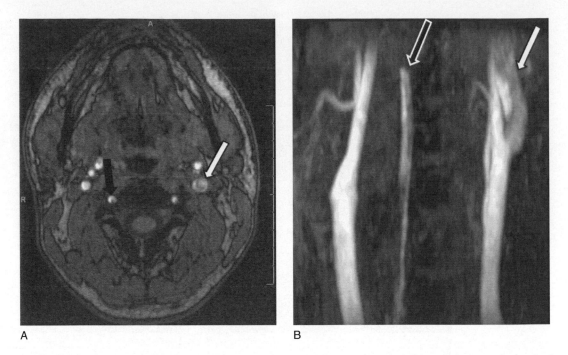

A   B

FIGURE 11.2 *(A) Noncontrast transaxial MRA utilizing 3D Time-of-Flight technique at the level of the inferior aspect of C2. Note the discrete intimal flaps seen in both the right vertebral artery (black arrow) and left internal carotid artery (white arrow). The signal within the lateral compartment of the right vertebral artery is brighter, suggesting that this is the "true lumen" with rapidly flowing blood, and the medial compartment is the "pseudolumen," containing thrombus, which is also somewhat bright on these images. (B) Reformatted maximum intensity projection in the left anterior oblique position from noncontrast MRA utilizing 3D Time of Flight technique. Note the stenosis and luminal wall irregularity throughout the visualized right vertebral artery (extending from C2-C6) (black arrow). An intimal flap (discreet longitudinal black line) can be seen throughout much of the course of the right vertebral artery. The proximal left internal carotid artery is also abnormal (white arrow) with a an intimal flap (faint longitudinal black line). Increased hyperintensity seen along the antero-medial aspect of the vessel (part of the vessel farthest from the white arrow) likely represents true lumen and darker, more heterogeneous signal intensity along the posterolateral aspect of the vessel (closest to the white arrow) likely represents pseudolumen.*

manipulations, and strenuous activities that could cause neck hyperextension or flexion, and educated about common symptoms of a stroke.

DISCUSSION

Before getting into the clinical discussion, it is important to brief our readers about the basic anatomy of two vessels—the vertebral and the internal carotid arteries. Both arteries have four main divisions that are summarized in Table 11.1. Dissection of the intracranial part of the internal carotid artery is rare at any age because the intracranial carotid artery is less mobile and the skull absorbs most of the force of trauma. Spontaneous dissection of the vertebral artery usually occurs in the tortuous distal extracranial atlantoaxial segment, V3, but may extend into the intracranial portion, V4.

This patient presented with a sudden onset of head and neck pain and developed a left-sided partial Horner's syndrome, one day after playing tennis. Horner's syndrome has mainly four components that can be remembered by the mnemonic SPAM (sunken eyeballs/

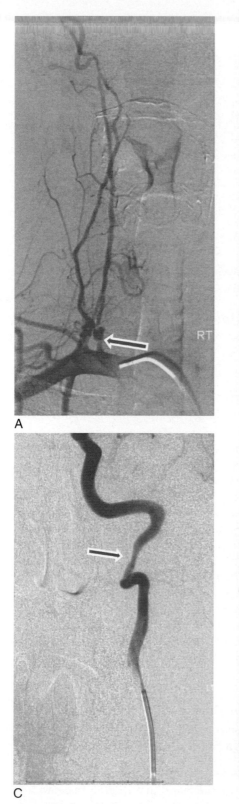

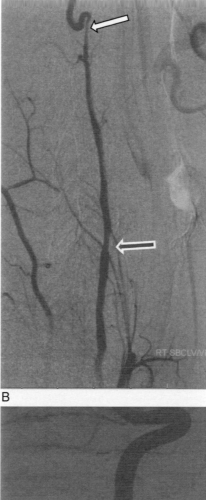

A

B

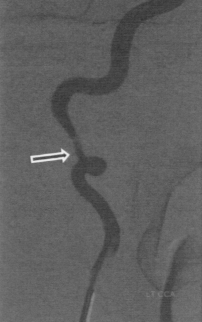

C

D

FIGURE 11.3 *(A) Conventional digital subtraction angiography, frontal view. Right subclavian injection. Note the severe stenosis and focal 5.0 mm outpouching (black arrow) within the proximal right vertebral artery. The luminal irregularity extending through the right vertebral artery to the level of C2 (seen better on 11.3B). (B) Conventional digital subtraction angiography, lateral view. Right subclavian injection. Note the luminal wall irregularity throughout the cervical vertebral artery with areas of mild to moderate narrowing (black arrow) with more severe narrowing (white arrow) at the level of the C2 foramen transversarium. (C) Conventional digital subtraction angiography, frontal view. Left internal carotid artery injection. Note the segmental stenosis and luminal wall irregularity (black arrow) with the cervical segment of the left internal carotid artery. (D) Conventional digital subtraction angiography, lateral view. Left internal carotid artery injection. Note the small "beak" (black arrow) extending from the posterior aspect of the cervical internal carotid artery at the level of the skull base. This represents a 0.5 mm neck remnant from the pseudoaneurysm seen on the MRA. Absence of contrast filling of the pseudoaneurysm suggests that it is thrombosed.*

(continued)

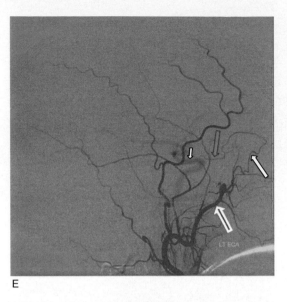

E

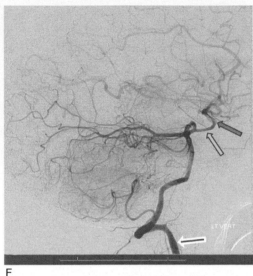

F

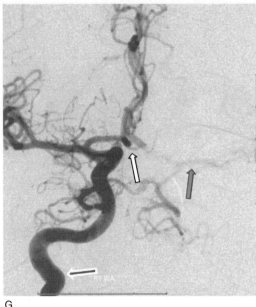

G

FIGURE 11.3 (*continued*) *(E) Conventional digital subtraction angiography, lateral view. Left external carotid artery injection. ICA collateral support from the ECA. There is filling of the normal left internal maxillary artery (black arrow) and a branch of the left internal maxillary artery, the anterior deep temporal artery (large white arrow). The anterior deep temporal artery fills the ophthalmic artery in retrograde fashion (gray arrow), which then fills the left internal carotid artery (faint opacification, small white arrow). (F) Conventional digital subtraction angiography, lateral view. Left vertebral artery injection. Normal contrast opacification of the left vertebral artery (black arrow). There is a large posterior communicating artery on the left side (white arrow), which fills the supraclinoid segment of the left internal carotid artery (gray arrow). Filling of numerous ICA and MCA branches is then seen (faint opacification). (G) Conventional digital subtraction angiography, frontal view. Right internal carotid artery injection. There is normal opacification of the right internal carotid artery (black arrow). There is a prominent anterior communicating artery (white arrow), which supplies the left anterior cerebral artery and, to a lesser extent, the left middle cerebral artery (gray arrow).*

sympathetic plexus affected, *p*tosis, *a*nhydrosis, and *m*iosis). The interruption of the cervical sympathetic plexus to pupillomotor pathways causes a constellation of symptoms as below:

- **Ptosis:** Weakness of Muller's smooth muscle (elevates the upper eyelid)
- **Miosis:** Loss of sympathetic innervations to the papillary dilator muscles and unopposed action of the iris constrictor, that is greatest in dim illumination. There

TABLE 11.1 *Four Divisions of the Vertebral and Internal Carotid Artery*

VA	ICA
Proximal V1: From subclavian origin (ostium) to the C6 transverse foramen	Cervical/C1: from the bifurcation of CCA (opposite the superior border of the thyroid) until it enters the carotid canal Branches: None
Intraforaminal V2: The vertical course from C6 to C2 within the transverse foramina	Petrous/C2: Extends from base of skull to the apex of the petrous bone; enters the cranial vault at the foramen lacerum; entry point of the artery is the carotid canal in the petrous portion of the temporal bone Branches: caroticotympanic, cavernous and hypoglossal
Atlantoaxial V3: C2 to C1 to the foramen magnum	Cavernous: passes through the cavernous sinus with the Abducens nerve Branches: supply posterior pituitary
Intracranial V4: from the foramen magnum to the lower pons where it joins the other vertebral artery to form the basilar artery	Supraclinoid/C4: begins after penetrating the dura and continues until the bifurcation into the middle cerebral artery and anterior cerebral artery Branches: ophthalmic, posterior communicating and choroidal

could be slight elevation of the lower lid due to denervation of the lower lid muscle analogous to the Muller muscle in the upper eyelid causing sunken eyeballs (upside-down ptosis).

- **Anhydrosis +/−:** Loss of sweating on half of the side of the ipsilateral body (central) or face (preganglionic).

- **Loss of the Cilospinal Reflex:** Pinching the skin of the neck should cause dilatation of the ipsilateral pupil under normal conditions. This reflex is lost in Horner's syndrome.

Please note that *iris heterochromia* is another finding that can be seen in congenital Horner's or Horner's occurring before 2 years of age or with long standing Horner's syndrome.

Horner's syndrome can be of three kinds:

1. **Central Sympathetic Fibers (First-order neurons):** Arise in the hypothalamus, descend through the lateral brain stem and cervical spinal cord alongside the spinothalamic tracts till they terminate in the intermediolateral cell columns of the spinal cord at the level of C8-T2 (see Figure 11.4). This is called the Ciliospinal Center of Budge.

2. **Preganglionic Pupillomotor Fibers (Second-order neurons):** These exit the interomediolateral cell column at the ventral aspect of the T1-T2 level, enter the cervical sympathetic chain, where they are in close proximity to the apex of the lung and the subclavian artery and synapse in the superior cervical ganglion (SCG).

3. **Postganglionic Pupillomotor Fibers (Third-order neurons):** The fibers then exit the SCG but soon after their exit, vasomotor and sudomotor branches are given off, which travel with the ECA to supply the blood vessels and sweat glands of the face. The pupillomotor fibers continue to ascend up with the ICA through the carotid plexus to go to cavernous sinus. These leave the carotid plexus briefly and run with the abducens (cranial nerve VI) in the cavernous sinus and then enter the orbit through the superior orbital fissure along with the ophthalmic branch of the trigeminal nerve (V1).

Thus, a Horner's syndrome can present as a pathology of the lateral hypothalamus, brain stem, spinal cord, first or second thoracic roots, sympathetic chain, carotid

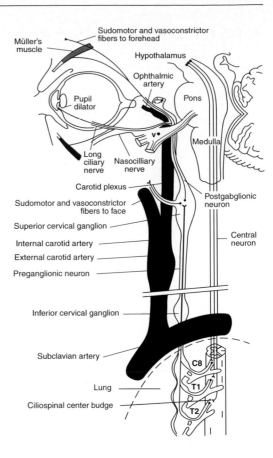

FIGURE 11.4 *Sympathetic pathway for pupillary innervation. (Reproduced with permission from TJ Martin, JJ Corbett. The Pupil. In* Neuro-ophthalmology: the requisites in ophthalmology, *JH Krachmer [Ed], Mosby, St. Louis 2000. Copyright © 2000 Elsevier.)*

plexus, cavernous sinus or orbit. Table 11.2 lists some of the causes of Horner's syndrome.

Based on the patient's presenting signs and symptoms, and given the patient's history of sudden onset of left-sided head and neck pain with left-sided Horner's syndrome after playing tennis (which can involve repeated hyperextension and flexion of the neck), the most likely diagnosis would be a VA and/or ICA dissection. The frequency of spontaneous VA dissections is one third that of spontaneous ICA dissections.

Cervical artery dissections can occur either spontaneously, or with major or minor head or neck trauma causing hyperextension or hyperflexion of the neck (such as chiropractic neck manipulation, coughing, or sneezing) that causes a small tear to form in the intimal surface of the carotid or vertebral arteries and allowing for blood to seep into the vessel wall. A flap then protrudes into the lumen of the vessel, which predisposes it to thrombus formation and distal embolization causing cerebral ischemia. Subintimal dissection tends to cause stenosis, whereas subadventitial dissections can result in aneurysmal formation. Arterial dissections occur when there is a breakdown in the vessel wall of the artery causing blood to flow into the tissue layers. Dissection in the arterial wall causes clot to form with possible embolic events. Predisposing factors for arterial dissections can range from various non-trivial neck traumas, to sports-related injuries, or a genetic predisposition to connective tissue disorders, and hypertension. Some of the common predisposing factors are listed in Table 11.3.

The annual incidence of spontaneous carotid artery dissections is approximately 2.5 to 3 per 100,000 people. However, the overall incidence of vertebral artery dissections is unclear. The incidence of vertebral artery dissections or occlusion attributable to cervical manipulation

TABLE 11.2 *Lesions Affecting Oculosympathetic Pathways*

First-order lesions (hypothalamus to C8-T2)	Meningitis
	Basal skull tumors, pituitary tumor
	Brain stem vascular malformation
	Cerebrovascular accident
	Demyelinating disease
	Intrapontine hemorrhage
	Neck trauma/cervical disk disease
Second-order lesions (preganglionic T1 to SCG)	Neuroblastoma
	Lymphadenopathy (reactive or malignant)
	Apical lung tumors
	Metastases
	Mandibular tooth abscess
	Lesions of the middle ear (e.g., acute otitis media)
	Thyroid adenoma
	Thoracic aorta, subclavian or common carotid artery aneurysm
	Trauma/surgical injury/chest tube/central venous catheter
Third-order lesions (postganglionic)	Internal carotid dissection/aneurysm/vasopasm
	Extension of cavernous sinus tumor, nasopharyngeal tumor
	Carotid cavernous fistula
	Cluster/migraine headaches
	Herpes zoster
	Otitis media
	Neck trauma/tumor (i.e., rhabdomyosarcoma)/inflammation

in patients <45 years of age was approximately 1.3 per 100,000 within one week of manipulative therapy. With regard to ischemic events, carotid artery dissections account for approximately 2% of ischemic strokes. The proportion is greater among younger patients, in whom carotid dissections may account for 10% to 15% of ischemic strokes. As discussed earlier, dissection of the intracranial part of the internal carotid artery is rare at any age because the intracranial carotid artery is less mobile and the skull absorbs most of the force of trauma. Spontaneous dissection of the vertebral artery usually occurs in the tortuous distal extracranial segment (segment III) but may extend into the intracranial portion or segment IV.

The clinical presentation of cervical artery dissections is broad. Some patients develop sudden debilitating neurological symptoms, but the typical presentation involves pain on one side of the head or neck, accompanied by the Horner's syndrome. After these warning symptoms occur, cerebral or retinal ischemia develops in 50% to 95% of cases of carotid

TABLE 11.3 *Predisposing Factors for Arterial Dissections*

Trauma	Motor vehicle accidents, falls, airbag or seatbelt accidents, cervical manipulation, physical abuse, bouts of violent coughing
Head position	Dental procedures, ceiling painting
Sports activities	Wrestling, judo, treadmill running, tennis, yoga
Fibromuscular dysplasia (15%)	Danlos syndrome
Connective tissue disorders	Ehlers-Danlos syndrome type IV, Marfan's syndrome, hyperhomocysteinemia, osteogenesis imperfect Type 1
Migraine	
Hypertension	In young patients, causes such as autosomal dominant polycystic kidney disease, pheochromocytoma
Bicuspid aortic valve (1%–5%)	
Oral contraceptive use	

artery dissections. Patients with a vertebral artery dissection may present with headache, posterior neck and occipital pain, vertigo, nausea, visual disturbances, or syncope. Sometimes, patients with dissections describe feeling or hearing a "pop" at the onset. In carotid dissections, patients may hear a turbulent sound with each heartbeat and have pain over the ipsilateral eye. TIAs or infarcts that can occur in the anterior or posterior circulation as a result of thromboembolization can present with a delay of hours to weeks between the onset of a dissection and ischemic events.

MRA remains the non-invasive way of detecting VA or ICA dissections. The neuroimaging characteristics include

- Luminal narrowing
- Occlusion
- Thrombus appearing as high signal on T1-weighted imaging
- Increased external diameter of the vessel
- Aneurysms

Diagnosis is made by MRI/MRA, CTA, or catheter-based contrast angiography of the neck showing vessel irregularity, narrowing, and sometimes appearance of a false lumen in the vessel wall adjacent to the true lumen.

The optimum management of whether to use anticoagulation or antiplatelets agents in treating cervical artery dissections is unclear, as there have been no placebo-controlled or randomized trials comparing anticoagulant and antiplatelet therapy. In one study, the annual rate of recurrent stroke, TIA, or death was 12.4% among patients treated with aspirin versus 8.3% in those given anticoagulants. Anticoagulation may also cause a higher risk of subarachnoid hemorrhage in the event of intracranial extension of a cervical artery dissection.

Recent guidelines regarding the management of cervical artery dissections issued by a consortium of organizations, recommend either anticoagulation with intravenous heparin followed by warfarin (target INR of 2.5), or low-molecular-weight heparin followed by warfarin, or oral anticoagulation without antecedent heparin for 3 to 6 months, followed by antiplatelet therapy with aspirin (81 to 325 mg daily) or clopidogrel (75 mg daily), for patients with symptomatic cervical artery dissections. Regardless of initial antithrombotic therapy during the acute phase, antiplatelet therapy may replace anticoagulation once symptoms resolve, but no uniform approach has been developed regarding the timing of this transition, and no antithrombotic regimen has been established as the standard of care. Additionally, endovascular methods such as carotid angioplasty and/or stenting might be considered when ischemic neurological symptoms have not responded to antithrombotic therapy after acute carotid dissections. While endovascular stent angioplasty has been effective in some patients, it has also been associated with complications in other cases. Other surgical revascularization techniques include direct carotid repair and resection with vein graft replacement. If the dissection is discovered early, patients have an excellent prognosis for recovery, thus preventing embolic and hemorrhagic events.

Based on the initial symptoms and clinical features of the case, other differential diagnoses would have included ischemia involving the lateral medulla (vertebral artery or PICA), lateral caudal pons (AICA), lateral hypothalamus, apical lung tumor, or cluster headache. Other less likely diagnoses would include hemorrhage into a vascular malformation, abscess, or demyelinating disease.

AICA infarcts involve mainly the caudal lateral pons, resulting in lateral brain stem tegmentum syndrome that can resemble the lateral medullary syndrome that is caused by thrombus of the vertebral artery or PICA. Both syndromes can have ipsilateral ataxia (middle cerebellar peduncle), vertigo, nystagmus (vestibular nuclei), pain and sensory loss in the ipsilateral face (trigeminal nucleus and tract) and contralateral body (spinothalamic tract), and an ipsilateral Horner's syndrome (descending sympathetic fibers) as prominent features. AICA infarcts, however, can cause unilateral hearing loss as a result of vascular compromise of the labyrinth artery supplying the inner ear that most commonly is a branch of the AICA (occasionally it can come off the basilar artery). Sometimes, patients with disease of the AICA or stenosis of the basilar artery experience TIAs that include a roaring sound in their ears. Lateral medullary syndrome on the other hand often has voice changes (i.e., hoarseness) or loss of taste associated with it. Additionally, sometimes a superior cerebellar syndrome as a result of infarction involving the superior cerebellar artery can also variably involve the lateral tegmental structures and produce similar clinical symptoms as aforementioned, but with ipsilateral ataxia (from infarction of the superior cerebellar peduncle and cerebellum) being the most prominent clinical feature.

Horner's syndrome can also be associated with cluster headaches, which are characterized by episodes of piercing sensations behind one eye, lasting 30 to 90 minutes, accompanied by autonomic symptoms such as tearing, eye redness, unilateral flushing, sweating, and nasal congestion. These episodes occur in recurrent patterns, from once to several times per day, every day over few weeks, with months of symptom-free periods.

In Pancoast's syndrome, an apical lung tumor, typically non-small cell carcinoma, invades the lower brachial plexus and T1 nerve root, resulting in a Horner's syndrome. Occasionally, the recurrent laryngeal nerve can also be involved producing hoarseness. If left untreated, the entire brachial plexus may be involved producing a flaccid upper extremity with loss of sensation. This patient had a normal chest X-ray with no other constitutional symptoms suggestive of such pathology.

Other etiologies, including abscess and demyelinating disease, were effectively ruled out in this case given the temporal association of sudden onset of symptoms and head/neck pain, lack of constitutional symptoms, and unremarkable intraparenchymal regions noted on MRI.

SUGGESTED READING

Blumenfeld H. *Neuroanatomy Through Clinical Cases*. 2nd ed. Sunderland: Sinauer Associates; 2010.

Campellone JV. Medical encyclopedia: Stroke secondary to carotid dissection. *Medline Plus*. 2004. http://www.nlm.nih.gov/medlineplus/ency/article/000732.htm. Accessed October 26, 2006.

Caplan LR, Zarins CK, Hemmati M. Spontaneous dissection of the extracranial vertebral arteries. *Stroke*. 1985;16(6):1030–1038.

Norris JW, Beletsky V, Nadareishvili ZG. Sudden neck movement and cervical artery dissection. *Can Med Assoc J*. 2000;163(1):38–40.

Saeed AB, Shuaib A, Al-Sulaiti G, Emery, D. Vertebral artery dissection: Warning symptoms, clinical features, and prognosis in 26 patients. *Can J Neurol Sci*. 2000;27:292–296.

CHIEF COMPLAINT: **Muscle stiffness and difficulty holding tools.**

HISTORY OF PRESENT ILLNESS

A 39-year-old butcher complained of severe muscle stiffness, for example, he had difficulty getting up in the morning from the bed. He also noticed difficulty using his hands at work. More than a year ago, he started to feel generalized morning stiffness of his muscles on waking up. He would get some relief with hot baths. About 9 months ago, he started noticing stiffness of his hands; he would be unable to move them, especially after getting meat from the freezer. He has difficulty buttoning clothes and opening door knobs and jars. About 1½ months prior to visit, he noted stiffness, pain, and spasms of his leg muscles. It is especially worse during the cold weather and after prolonged rest but improves when he starts moving around. He used to be able to walk a mile but for the past 3 months, he can only walk about six blocks. He has a tendency to trip on his feet on walking. His tongue occasionally gets "stuck" in his mouth causing difficulty speaking. He has some difficulty swallowing thin liquids. He complains of fatigue and increased daytime sleepiness. He does not have numbness or tingling sensations in his extremities. He did not complain of neck or back pain. He denied any bowel or bladder problems. He did not have any vision problems.

PAST MEDICAL HISTORY

As above.

PAST SURGICAL HISTORY

Unremarkable.

MEDICATIONS

None.

ALLERGIES

None.

PERSONAL HISTORY

He denied use of alcohol, tobacco, or drugs.

FAMILY HISTORY

His 67-year-old father had cataracts diagnosed when he was 40 years old but his 64-year-old mother is fine. He has three sisters (34, 32, and 25 years old) who are fine.

His father had two brothers (one died of MI) and five sisters (three of whom passed away from cardiac causes). One of his paternal aunts has two children: a 26-year-old girl who is "slow" and toe walked and a 19-year-old boy with severe neuromuscular disease since birth. He required tube feeding and oxygen support in the newborn period.

REVIEW OF SYSTEMS

Remarkable for mild headaches, fatigue, and excessive daytime sleepiness. He has mild dysphagia, frequent diarrhea three to four times a day, rare constipation, and occasional palpitations without chest pains.

PHYSICAL EXAMINATION

Vital signs: Blood pressure, 120/80; heart rate, 88/min, regular rhythm, respiratory rate, 16/min; temperature, 98.6°F.

He is dull appearing with decreased facial expression, a long thin face with premature frontal balding, temporal wasting, and mild ptosis.

NEUROLOGICAL EXAMINATION

Higher mental functions reveal an alert, coherent, oriented male, somewhat apathetic with nasal quality in his speech.

CNs II–XII: Is remarkable for mild ptosis, eyelid myotonia with difficulty opening eyes after forced closure for a few seconds, mild facial diparesis with difficulty puffing out cheeks and whistling.

Motor exam reveals mild neck flexor weakness and distal > proximal limb weakness without muscle atrophy. Strength in his shoulder abductors, elbow extensors, and flexors is British Medical Research Council (MRC) scale for muscle strength score of 5/5 with wrist flexors/extensors, finger flexors, and grip strength of grade 4/5. He has action myotonia with hand grip and also percussion myotonia.

In the lower extremities, hip flexors, knee extensors/flexors, ankle plantar flexors, and invertors are strong, grade 5/5 but ankle dorsiflexors and evertors are grade 4/5.

Sensory examination: Is intact to light touch, pin prick, vibration, and position sense.

Reflexes: DTRs are hypoactive.

Plantar: Bilateral flexor responses.

Gait: Mild steppage gait with inability to walk on heels, could walk better on toes. He was able to do tandem walk.

Coordination: He has no dysmetria on finger-to-nose test, no dysdiadochokinesia.

Romberg's sign: Negative and he is able to tandem walk.

STOP AND THINK QUESTIONS

➢ What diagnoses are unlikely with this clinical presentation: pain, spasms, and muscle weakness without any subjective sensory symptoms?

➢ Does the pattern of muscle weakness (distal more than proximal) help you think of certain myopathies?

➢ What is the clinical significance of finding action and percussion myotonia on examination?

➢ What other diagnostic tests should be done to confirm the clinical suspicion?

DIAGNOSTIC TEST RESULTS

CBC and SMA 20: Normal.

EMG-NCS of all four extremities: Nerve conduction studies of motor and sensory nerves showed normal conduction velocities and latencies. Abundant myotonic discharges are noted with low amplitude short duration voluntary MUAPs with early recruitment pattern.

CK: 125 (normal).

DNA testing: (+) CTG trinucleotide repeat size of 550 in allele 1 of DMPK gene and five CTG repeats in allele 2 of DMPK gene.

DIAGNOSIS: **Myotonic dystrophy type 1 (classic phenotype).**

DISCUSSION

Myotonic dystrophy type 1 (DM1) or Steinert's disease is the most common adult onset muscular dystrophy with incidence of 13.5 per 100,000 and prevalence of 3 to 5 per 100,000. It is autosomal dominant in inheritance. Unlike most muscle disorders that present with proximal muscle weakness, DM1 manifests with distal extremity weakness. It is a multisystemic disease with early development of cataracts. Aside from skeletal muscles, the respiratory, cardiac and smooth muscles, endocrine system as well as CNS can also be affected.

Molecular defect in DM1 is the CTG repeat expansion in the 3′ untranslated region of *DMPK* gene *on chromosome 19q.* The size of the expansion correlates with disease severity. The normal number of CTG trinucleotide repeat in an individual is 5 to 36. A repeat length >36 is unstable and leads to increased expansion during meiosis and mitosis. An individual with a repeat length of 37 to 50 may be asymptomatic but his or her offspring is at risk of developing the disease due to the larger expansion inherited. This is called permutation or mutable allele.

Myotonic dystrophy has variable phenotypes with onset of symptoms from birth to adulthood. There is a correlation between the size of the CTG repeat expansion and the onset and severity of the disease, but this correlation is more significant if expansion is below 400 CTG repeats. There is a considerable overlap of CTG repeat sizes for each phenotype, so it is not advisable to make predictions on disease severity based on the CTG repeats alone.

Mild type of DM1 is seen with CTG repeat sizes from 50 to 200. In one study, the presence of cataracts is the sole manifestation in 38% of 102 otherwise asymptomatic DM1 patients with CTG repeat size between 50 and 99. CTG repeat expansion from 100 to 200 present with mild myotonia, weakness, and excessive daytime sleepiness, but life span is normal.

Classic type of adult onset DM1 is the most common phenotype with symptom onset from 20 to 30 years of age. Common CTG repeat expansion is between 100 and 1000. Fatigue is a frequent initial complaint. Difficulty in relaxation interferes with daily activities, especially if it requires hand dexterity like using tools or household equipments, opening jars, or turning door knobs. Symptoms are worse with inactivity and exposure to cold, but improves with activity—the so-called "warm-up phenomenon." Early gait disturbance is due to weakness of ankle dorsiflexors, but weakness is gradually progressive with wheelchair confinement seen in advanced cases. Patients have distinctive facial features of premature frontal balding (in males), temporal atrophy, and long myopathic facies, often described as "hatchet" appearance, with ptosis, and weakness of the facial and jaw muscles. Iridescent posterior subcapsular cataracts may present early on. Weakness of pharyngeal and lingual muscles leads to hypernasal speech quality, and tongue myotonia leads to slurring of speech. Respiratory difficulties are frequent due to weakness/myotonia of intercostal muscles and diaphragm and aspiration may be a complication in advanced cases.

Involvement of the smooth muscles like the GI tract may present with constipation and intestinal pseudo-obstruction due to decreased peristalsis, but patient can have diarrhea as well as cholecystitis and gallstones due to increased gall bladder sphincter tone. About 28% of patients have GI complaints prior to diagnosis of DM1. During the 123rd ENMC International Workshop on Management and Therapy in Myotonic Dystrophy in 2004, it was suggested that use of cholestyramine may improve diarrhea, incontinence, and pain, and norfloxacin may be tried if cholestyramine is ineffective. Slow gastric emptying time may respond to erythromycin or metoclopramide.

Cardiac conduction defects are very frequent in DM1 (90%) whereas cardiomyopathy is less common. They vary from tachyarrhythmias; bradyarrhythmias; prolonged PR, QT, and QRS intervals on EKG or electrocardiogram; 1st degree AV block; bundle branch blocks; sustained and paroxysmal atrial fibrillation; premature ventricular contractions; and ventricular tachycardia. Malignant tachyarrhythmias lead to higher risk of sudden death and are a significant cause of early mortality. Patients may benefit from a cardiac pacemaker or defibrillator. It is more common in older patients with longer disease duration and in male patients, but younger patients have been reported to have this complication. Severity of cardiac conduction abnormalities and sudden death is not correlated with severity of skeletal muscle weakness or with size of mutation.

The CNS is also involved. Neuropsychological issues are frequent in DM1. Minor intellectual deficits present as difficulties in memory and spatial orientation. Personality disorder (avoidant, obsessive-compulsive, or passive-aggressive personality), apathy, anxiety, and depression are common. Excessive daytime sleepiness is a usual complaint and sleep apnea (primary central or obstructive) should be considered. The neuropathologic finding of loss of serotonergic neurons in the central raphe and superior central nucleus of the brain stem is thought to be the cause of daytime somnolence.

DM1 patients are at risk for endocrinopathies affecting the thyroid, pancreas, hypothalamus, and gonads. Hypothyroidism, insulin resistance (although overt diabetes mellitus is not increased compared to the general population), testicular atrophy, and infertility in male patients, as well as growth hormone secretion abnormality are seen.

Benign calcifying tumors of the hair matrix cells, called pilomatrixomatas, may be found in the scalp, head, and neck. These may be confused with sebaceous cysts.

Women with DM1 have high-risk pregnancies since they are at risk for spontaneous abortion, prolonged labor, retained placenta, and postpartum hemorrhage. If the fetus is affected, polyhydramnios and/or decreased fetal movement may be present.

Patients are surgical risks with anesthetic complication in 10%, prolonged respiratory depression and postoperative pneumonia, especially after cholecystectomy or upper abdominal surgery.

The lifespan of patient with classic DM1 is shortened due to respiratory compromise as well as sudden death from malignant tachyarrhythmias. The clinical features of Classic DM1 are summarized for the readers in Table 12.1.

Congenital DM1 is usually maternally inherited, with larger repeat size (usually >2000 CTG repeats) seen because of genetic anticipation. In utero, polyhydramnios is present, and fetal movements are decreased leading to positional malformation of the extremities, such as clubfoot or arthrogryposis (multiple joint contractures found at birth). Infants are born floppy with severe generalized weakness and hypotonia. Respiration is compromised, and mortality rate is increased (about 25%). Myopathic facies is noted with a typical "tented" or "fish"-shaped upper lip due to significant facial diplegia. This makes sucking and feeding very difficult resulting in failure to thrive. Infants who survive the first 6 months of life actually improve. About 75% of cases have psychomotor retardation with mental retardation in 50% to 60%. Cerebral atrophy and ventricular dilation is often evident on neuroimaging studies at birth, but it is unclear if this is due to early respiratory failure, a direct effect of the *DMPK* mutation on the brain or both. Although motor delays are seen, gradual improvement in milestones is expected and patients are eventually able to walk. Progressive myopathy and classic features of DM1 develop in early adulthood. Lifespan is shortened due to cardiorespiratory complications in the third to fourth decades of life.

In childhood onset or juvenile form of DM1, neuropsychological issues are prominent, as noted in about two third of children. This includes learning disabilities, mental retardation, attention deficit disorders, psychomotor slowing, visuo-spatial impairments, and

TABLE 12.1 *Clinical Features of Classic DM1*

System Involvement	Manifestations	Intervention/Management
Facial features	Premature frontal balding Temporal atrophy Long lean facies Ptosis Nasal speech	Blepharoplasty for severe ptosis if vision is impaired
Ophthalmologic	Posterior subcapsular cataracts	Excision of cataract if vision is impaired

Skeletal muscles	Myotonia—action/percussion
	Distal limb weakness
	a. Decreased hand dexterity
	b. Gait difficulty (weak ankle dorsiflexors)
	Proximal weakness sets in later
		Anti myotonia drugs like mexiletine,
		  carbamazepine, phenytoin, calcium channel
		  blockers, tricyclic antidepressants
		Rehabilitation: Orthotics, OT/PT
		Assistive devices for mobility

Cardiac muscles	Conduction defects (90%) (prolonged PR/QT/QRS intervals, AV block, atrial fibrillation/flutter, PVC, ventricular tachycardia) Cardiomyopathy	EKG, Holter monitoring Echocardiogram Pacemaker, cardiac defibrillators
Pulmonary	Respiratory difficulties Aspiration pneumonia	Overnight Polysomnography OSA: CPAP Central sleep apnea: BiPAP +/− Modafinil
GI	Dysphagia Constipation/Intestinal pseudo-obstruction Diarrhea Cholecystitis/Gallstones	GI consult Erythromycin/metoclopramide Cholestyramine/norfloxacin
Endocrinopathies	Thyroid disorders Insulin resistance Testicular atrophy and infertility in males Growth hormone abnormalities	Replacement of hormones as needed Treatment of diabetes
CNS	Cognitive limitation, ADD Personality disorder (avoidant, obsessive- compulsive, or passive-aggressive personality) apathy, anxiety and depression Excessive daytime sleepiness	Referral to Psychiatry/Psychology CNS stimulants like Atomoxetine Antianxiety medications Tricyclic antidepressants BiPAP/Modafinil

OB-GYN	Risk for spontaneous abortion, prolonged labor,
	  retained placenta, and postpartum hemorrhage;
	  if carrying an affected fetus, polyhydramnios and
	  decreased fetal movements
		High risk pregnancy clinic follow-up

Surgery	Increased anesthetic risk and perioperative
	  pulmonary complications—prolonged
	  respiratory depression and post-op pneumonia
		Chest physiotherapy
		Incentive spirometry
		Ventilatory assistance

Dermatologic	Pilomatrixomata, Epitheliomas	Excision of benign tumors

anxiety disorders. Motor development may be normal or mildly delayed. Mild facial and neck weakness, dysarthria, mild myotonia, and distal extremity weakness of foot/ankle dorsiflexors and hands may be present. Cardiac conduction abnormalities are seen early on; with the onset of severe heart involvement between 10 and 18 years of age. Therefore, annual EKGs should be undertaken from age 10 onwards. As patients get older, classic symptoms and gradual worsening of adult onset DM1 may develop.

DIAGNOSTIC WORK-UP

DNA testing using targeted mutation looking for CTG repeat expansion of the *DMPK* gene is the gold standard for diagnosis of DM1. It is indicated if index of suspicion is high such as the presence of typical features, distal weakness, and myotonia. If another diagnosis is being entertained, a CK level and EMG and NCV studies may be undertaken. CK levels are normal or mildly increased in DM. Motor and sensory nerve conduction studies are normal, but EMG reveals classic myotonic discharges with "dive bomber" or "motorcycle" sound, fibrillation potentials, positive sharp waves, and myopathic motor unit potentials (low amplitude short duration discharges with early recruitment pattern). A muscle biopsy is not necessary since it shows nonspecific findings of increased internal nuclei, type 1 fiber predominance and atrophy, hypertrophic type 2, ring fibers, small angulated fibers, atrophic fibers, and pyknotic nuclear clumps. Unlike other muscular dystrophies, there is not much increase in necrotic fibers or connective tissues noted.

MANAGEMENT

Management at this time is mainly supportive. Avoidance of exposure to cold temperatures may help with myotonia. Use of orthotics provides ankle support and stability to make walking easier. Assistive devices, including wheelchairs, help with mobility and maintaining independence. Working with various specialists is of utmost importance. Sleep study or polysomnography can differentiate between central and obstructive sleep apnea and management can be determined based on the results. Assisted ventilation such as CPAP is recommended for obstructive apnea and BiPAP for nocturnal hypoventilation and/or central sleep apnea. CNS stimulants such as modafinil can also be used. Because of increased incidence of cardiac conduction defects and high risk of sudden death due to malignant arrhythmias, annual EKG and 24-hour Holter monitoring is recommended with referral to cardiology, especially if patient is symptomatic or if EKG shows evidence of arrhythmia. Annual/biannual ophthalmologic evaluation is suggested and cataracts extracted if it impairs vision. Management of pain, treatment of hypothyroidism, or hormone replacement therapy is provided as needed. Fasting serum glucose, hemoglobin A1C, and nutritional status should be monitored. Avoid statins in the treatment of hyperlipidemia because it can increase muscle weakness. If surgery is indicated, careful monitoring in the perioperative period decreases pulmonary complications (acute ventilatory failure, atelectasis, and pneumonia), which are common especially after upper abdominal surgery in patients with severe muscular disability. Protection of the upper airways, chest physiotherapy, and incentive spirometry should be undertaken early on.

Myotonic dystrophy type 2 or PROMM is also autosomal dominant in inheritance with similar multisystem involvement: myotonia (90%), muscle dysfunction (82%), iridescent posterior subcapsular cataracts (36%–78%), endocrinopathies (insulin insensitivity (25%–75%), and testicular failure (29%–65%) and cardiac conduction defects (19%). The age of onset is typically in the third decade of life. Myotonia may be seen during the first decade and intermittent muscle pain, stiffness and fatigue may be prominent. Hip flexors are usually involved early. Proximal lower extremity weakness without distal hand or feet weakness has been reported in 21 out of 27 patients in one study but the characteristic pattern of weakness includes neck flexors, elbow extensors, thumb and deep finger flexors, hip flexors, and extensors of the legs. Cognitive symptoms are milder—like problems with organization, concentration, word finding, and excessive daytime sleepiness. Cardiac conduction defects are not as common as in DM1 but still needs to be monitored. The clinical course of DM2 is milder than DM1. Patients are less likely to need assistive devices, although they progressively have difficulty negotiating the stairs. The molecular defect in DM2 is the expansion of CCTG repeat in intron 1 of *ZNF9* gene on *chromosome 3q*. The size of the repeat expansion is much larger than for DM1 and ranges from 75 to over 11,000 repeats, but unlike DM1, the size of DNA repeats does not affect the age of onset or disease severity.

PATHOGENESIS

DM1 and DM2 have very similar phenotypes with multisystemic involvement but their genotypes are very different and their encoded proteins are not functionally related. In DM1, the expanded CTG repeat of *DMPK* gene encodes a serine/threonine protein kinase, whereas DM2 has expanded CCTG repeat of ZNF9, which encodes a nucleic acid binding protein. It is now known that the pathology is due to their parallel RNA toxicity. DM is an RNA-mediated muscle disease. Their protein products play no major role in pathogenesis. The RNA repeats form hairpin-like structures of nuclear ribonuclear inclusions in muscle cells, which recruit antagonistic RNA binding proteins such as MBNL1 and CUGBP1. The decreased MBNL1 and increased CUGBP1 lead to abnormal splicing of following specific "at risk" targets:

- Chloride channel (causing myotonia)
- Insulin receptor (causing insulin resistance)
- Cardiac troponin T (possible etiology of cardiac abnormalities)
- RYR1 and MTMR1 (muscle weakness and wasting)
- N-methyl-D-aspartate (NMDA) receptor 1 or tau Amyloid precursor protein (CNS effects).

TREATMENT

No specific drug is available to treat myotonic dystrophy. Antimyotonia medications such as sodium channel blockers (phenytoin, carbamazepine, gabapentin, procainamide, and tocainide), quinine, calcium channel blockers, tricyclic antidepressants (amitriptyline, clomipramine, imipramine), and benzodiazepines have been tried but treatment should only be undertaken if symptoms are severe or cause pain. Mexiletine has been recommended as an off-label drug to decrease severe painful myotonia. Its safety and efficacy has been shown in two small trials but a bigger randomized placebo-controlled study should be performed. Cardiology consultation can be very helpful because it is prudent to avoid drugs that cause cardiac arrhythmias. Patients with intractable pain may be referred to a comprehensive pain management program.

Various treatment strategies are currently being investigated to treat myotonic dystrophy. These include reduction of myotonia, reversal of muscle wasting, correction of spliceopathy by upregulation of MBNL1 or downregulation of CUGBP1, neutralization, and elimination of mutant RNA.

Muscle wasting in DM1 is postulated to be due to defect in muscle anabolism. Use of anabolic steroids has been tried. Trials of testosterone and creatine have not been effective. DHEA has been shown to improve strength in 11 DM patients in a pilot study, but randomized double blind placebo control trial (phase II/III) of 75 patients showed no improvement when studied over 12 weeks. A Phase II randomized placebo control double blind multicenter trial is currently underway to determine the safety and efficacy of recombinant human insulin like growth factor 1 complexed with recombinant human insulin like growth factor binding protein 3. The report of an open-label dose escalation trial of 15 moderately affected genetically confirmed DM1 showed that it is generally well tolerated but showed no significant changes in muscle strength or functional outcomes. Some metabolic benefits were noted such as increased lean body mass and improvement in metabolism (decrease in triglyceride levels, increase in HDL levels, and decrease in hemoglobin A1C levels and increase in testosterone level).

Other strategies currently being considered or investigated include (a) inhibition of myostatin function either by gene deletion, antibodies against myostatin using MYO-029, morpholino antisense oligonucleotides to block translation or skip exon 3 of myostatin, deacetylase inhibitors to block myostatin receptors and upregulate follistatin levels, (b) reduction of RNA-mediated toxicity include antisense oligonucleotide-induced exon 7a skipping of ClC 1 to reverse myotonia, (c) upregulation of MBNL1 activity by injections of adeno-associated virus, (d) downregulation of CUGBP1 activity using protein kinase C inhibitors, and (e) neutralization or elimination of mutant RNA using antisense gene therapy, ribozymes or siRNA (short interfering RNA).

SUGGESTED READING

Amato A, Russell JA. *Neuromuscular Disorders.* McGraw Hill Co. Inc., New York; 2008.

International Myotonic Dystrophy Consortium (IDMC). New nomenclature and DNA testing guidelines for myotonic dystrophy type 1 (DM1). *Neurology.* 2000;54:1218–1221.

Machuca-Tzili L, Brook D, Hilton-Jones D. Clinical and molecular aspects of the myotonic dystrophy: A review. *Muscle Nerve.* 2005;32:1–18.

Turner C and Hilton-Jones D. The myotonic dystrophies: Diagnosis and management. *J Neurol Neurosurg Psychiatry.* 2010;81:358–367.

van Engelena B, Eynard B, Wilcox D. Workshop report: 123rd ENMC International Workshop: Management and therapy in myotonic dystrophy, 6–8 February 2004, Naarden. The Netherlands. *Neuromuscul Disord.* 2005;15:389–394.

Wheeler TM. Myotonic dystrophy: Therapeutic strategies for the future. *Neurotherapeutics.* 2008;5(4):502–600.

Wheeler TM, Thornton CA. Myotonic dystrophy: RNA mediated muscle disease. *Curr Opin Neurol.* 20:572–576;2007.

New Onset First Unprovoked Seizure

Anuradha Singh, Phillip Paul Amodeo, and Christina Coyle

CHIEF COMPLAINT: **Had a seizure at work.**

HISTORY OF PRESENT ILLNESS

A patient was presented to the emergency room after a witnessed seizure at his job as a mechanic. He did not have any preceding aura but witnesses described the event as characterized by stiffening, frothing, loud screaming, and a wide stare. His eyes rolled back, and he had convulsions for 2 to 3 minutes. He was confused, disoriented, and combative after the seizure, and he bit his tongue. He reported a bad headache and a feeling of extreme exhaustion. He also reported headaches the week prior to the seizure. These headaches were 4/10, band-like, and dull in nature. He further described intermittent episodes of right arm and leg numbness associated with headaches that would resolve with time. During these episodes, he had never lost consciousness. In the past, he had experienced similar episodes of weakness on the right side of his face that would resolve within several hours of their onset. The patient stated that he had not had seizures or headaches previously. He denied any nausea, vomiting, photophobia, phonophobia, or visual symptoms. In addition, he did not have any fever, night sweats, joint pains, head trauma, history of travel, or exposure to toxins.

He denied any history of febrile seizures, meningitis, encephalitis, family history of seizures or migraines, or other common neurological symptoms.

PAST MEDICAL HISTORY

As above.

PAST SURGICAL HISTORY

None.

MEDICATIONS

None.

ALLERGIES

NKDA.

PERSONAL HISTORY

The patient was from El Salvador and moved to the United States in 1998. He grew up in a rural area on a farm where there were free-ranging pigs. He does not smoke, drink, or use any recreational drugs. He lived in an apartment with his wife and family.

FAMILY HISTORY

His first cousin has seizures.

PHYSICAL EXAMINATION

Vital signs: Temperature, 97.4°F; pulse, 76; blood pressure, 110/78 mm Hg; respiratory rate, 18/min.
General: Left side of his tongue bitten, no other physical injuries noted.

NEUROLOGICAL EXAMINATION

Mental status: Awake and alert, normal attention and concentration and normal affect, spoke fluent Spanish with intact comprehension, naming, repetition, reading, and writing. 3/3 recall.

CNs II–XII: Normal conjugate eye movements, OU 20/25, no visual fields deficits, facial sensations intact, face symmetric, hearing normal, palate elevates symmetrically, tongue midline, shoulder shrug equal on both sides.

Motor: 5/5 both upper and lower extremities, no pronator drift.

Sensory: Intact to light touch, pain, temperature, vibration, proprioception in all four extremities.

Reflexes: 1+ B/L biceps, brachioradialis, triceps, patellar, Achilles.

Coordination: No FNF or heel-to-shin dysmetria. Rapid alternating movements normal. No tremors.

Romberg: Absent.

Gait: Independent and able to walk on heals, toes; could tandem walk well.

STOP AND THINK QUESTIONS

➤ What basic tests would you get in a patient with new onset seizures?

➤ What could cause this patient's complaints of intermittent episodes of right arm and leg numbness and right facial weakness? (seizures, TIAs, complicated migraines)

➤ What element of his history requires special considerations when developing a differential diagnosis for this patient?

DIAGNOSTIC TEST RESULTS

CBC, BMP, Hepatic, and coagulation profile: Normal.

Noncontrast CT brain: Numerous fluid containing lesions with a central focus of increased density scattered throughout the brain (Figure 13.1). MRI brain showed multiple hyperintense neurocysticerci lesions in the right frontal, left parietal lesion, left occipital and another lesion on the left abutting the splenium of the corpus callosum. Postgadolinium MRI showed ring enhancement around the lesions (see Figure 13.2).

DIAGNOSIS: Neurocysticercosis (NCC).

DISCUSSION

NCC is the leading cause of adult onset epilepsy in the developing world especially Latin America, Asia, and Africa. This could be attributed to poor sanitation, free-ranging pigs, and contamination of the soil by human feces. Reports of NCC in the United States have been increasing over the past 50 years, and these reports reflect disease in Hispanic immigrants.

The infection is acquired by ingesting eggs from the adult tapeworm, *Taenia solium.* Man is the definitive host; pig serves as an intermediate host. The carrier sheds eggs in the feces and due to poor hygiene, the host acquires the infection through the oral–fecal route. Eggs are sticky and can be found under the fingernails of tapeworm carriers. Human cysticercosis follows ingestion of ova from a tapeworm carrier. Close personal contact with a tapeworm carrier is noted in most cases. The eggs hatch in the upper intestines, releasing the *oncospheres* (invasive larvae) that penetrate the intestinal mucosa, enter the bloodstream, and migrate to the tissues, where they mature into cysticerci. Cysticerci have been

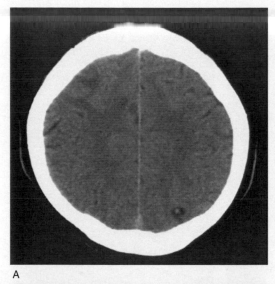
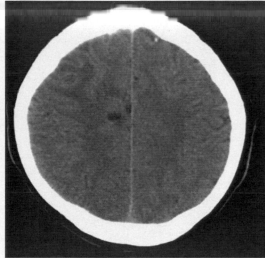
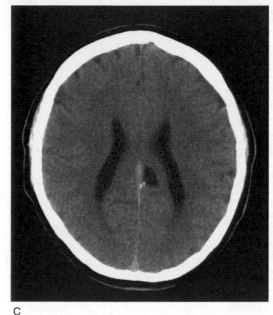

FIGURE 13.1 *Noncontrast CT axial images of the brain. (A) Ill-defined multiple lesions in the right frontal convexity with mild surrounding vasogenic edema; another well-defined cystic lesion in the left parietal cortex with hyperdense signal representing scolex. (B) Calcified lesion seen as punctuate calcification in the left frontal convexity and multiple (at least) 3 lesions in the right mesial frontal and another lesion in the right frontal region at the gray–white junction with surrounding vasogenic edema. (C) Isointense lesion seen medially in the left hemisphere at the level of lateral ventricles with punctate calcifications.*

identified in skeletal, cardiac muscle, and subcutaneous tissue. In these locations, they are normally clinically silent. Cysticerci may remain in the dormant stage for several years. It is not very clear what mechanisms play a role in the development of immune tolerance.

Once the cysticerci have reached the parenchyma of the brain, it undergoes four stages of involution. The first is the *vesicular stage* characterized by a cyst with a translucent vesicular wall, transparent fluid, and a viable invaginated scolex. During this stage, there is little host inflammatory reaction. The cyst then develops a thick vesicular wall, the fluid becomes turbid and the scolex degenerates during the next stage, which is termed the *colloidal stage*. An intense inflammatory host response is seen and is reflected in the pathology, which reveals varying degrees of acute and chronic inflammation. Radiographic examination

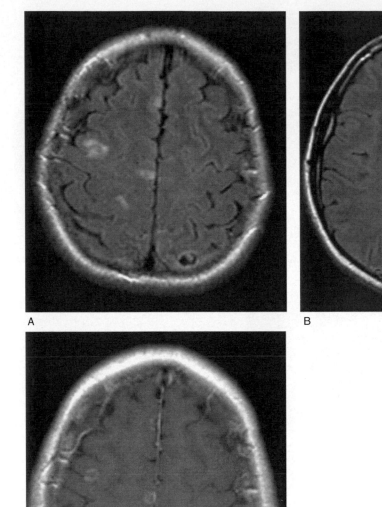

FIGURE 13.2 *MRI brain axial images, FLAIR sequences showing multiple hyperintense neurocysticerci lesions in the right frontal and left parietal lesion (A) left occipital and another lesion on the left abutting the splenium of the corpus callosum (B) MRI brain axial T1 with gadolinium showing ring enhancement around the lesions (C).*

reveals cystic lesions with edema and enhancement at this stage, and seizures are common as seen in this patient. The cysts continues to degenerate as it moves into the *granular stage,* which is characterized by a thick vesicular wall, degenerated scolex, gliosis, and little inflammatory response. Ultimately, the parasite transforms into a coarse calcified nodule, the *calcific stage.* Clinical features and neuroimaging characteristics of the four stages of NCC are listed in Table 13.1.

Many cysts in the parenchyma remain clinically silent until they begin to degenerate eliciting an inflammatory host response. Many patients with epilepsy and NCC from

TABLE 13.1 *Four Different Stages of NCC*

Stages I to IV	Clinical Features	Neuroimaging
I. Vesicular	New onset seizures	Hypodense, minimal mass effect, non-enhancing lesions, and scolex
II. Colloidal	Most epileptogenic phase	Hypodense and isodense lesion, loss of scolex, perilesional edema and mass effect, peripheral enhancement
III. Nodular or granular	Chronic epilepsy	Mural nodule with diffuse enhancement, no cystic component, some mass effect
IV. Calcified or degenerating cyst	Chronic epilepsy	Punctate calcifications, no mass effect, at times better seen on the CT and missed on the MRI brain

endemic regions have calcified NCC. Many of these patients have perilesional edema around the calcified lesion. The pathogenesis and natural history are not well known, and further studies are required.

About 80% of infections are asymptomatic. Most common symptoms include seizures, focal neurological signs, and intracranial hypertension. The peak of onset of symptoms occurs 3 to 5 years after the initial infection. Seizures are commonly associated with degenerating lesions and lesions surrounded by inflammatory lesion.

Most disease results from cysticerci in the CNS, including the brain, cerebral ventricles, or eye. Cysticercosis involving the nervous system is termed as NCC. Extraneural cysticercosis can involve other organs such as eye, muscle, or subcutaneous tissue.

NCC can also occur in the extraparenchymal space of the brain and the spine. Giant cysts in the Sylvian fissure have been reported and can cause mass effect. At times, NCC in the subarachnoid space can become an aberrant proliferating cestode larva rather than a single cyst, consisting of several bladders that "bud" exogenously to form a multilocular cyst usually devoid of scolices. This is referred to as *racemose subarachnoid NCC*. This form of disease can proliferate in the subarachnoid space in a manner similar to a tumor and elicits an exuberant inflammatory host response. This form of NCC carries a high morbidity and can result in obstructive hydrocephalus, mass effect, and stroke.

NCC can also involve the ventricles. Hydrocephalus can result from cysts lodging in the ventricles blocking CSF flow mechanically and/or secondary to inflammation and fibrosis. Sudden death has been described, as patients may present with symptoms of sudden increased intracranial pressure. The symptoms of NCC are pleomorphic and are dependent upon the location of the cyst and the host response. Seizures and headache are the most common symptom in most series, but headache, focal neurologic deficits, and symptoms related to increased hypertension have been well described. About 1% to 3% of cases of NCC involve the spinal cord, more so in the thoracic spinal regions.

NCC is diagnosed by neuroimaging. CT and magnetic resonance imaging (MRI) brain can diagnose various stages of the disease. Punctate calcifications is the most frequent finding on neuroimaging. The pathognomonic lesion is "scolex," a mural module within a cyst. MRI can miss calcifications but is superior to CT in detecting small, brain stem or intraventricular lesions, scloex. Degenerative changes in the parasite and perilesional edema around the calcific lesion can be better identified on the CT. Patients with perilesional edema have enhancement on a T2-weighted MRI and have recurrences around a subset of lesions.

ELISA, complement fixation, radioimmunoassay, and EITB are the common serologic tests employed to diagnose NCC. EITB is the test of choice to detect anticysticercal antibodies in the serum or CSF. It is an immunoblot assay employing semipurified membrane antigens. EITB is 100% specific, but sensitivity drops between 30% and 70% in the setting of a single lesion or calcified diease. Serum EITB is more sensitive than CSF.

There are a variety of antigen assays that are useful in patients with extraparenchymal disease. These assays have been proven useful when following patients with NCC patients with extraparenchymal disease to evaluate response to therapy. Lumbar punctures in patients with parenchymal disease are not helpful, but examing CSF is useful in patients with subarachnoid disease. It can also help follow the response to therapy.

Asymptomatic patients with nonviable NCC do not need to be treated. The treatment for parenchymal disease in the vesicular or colloidal stage is albendazole under the cover of steroids. A double-blind placebo randomized controlled study showed a decrease in generalized seizures in the group treated with albendazole compared to a placebo. The length of treatment ranges from 10 days to a month. Albendazole destroys 75% to 90% of parenchymal brain cysts. Patients with subarachnoid disease, especially the racemose form, may need to be treated for months with albendazole and steroids. PPD and a strongyloides serology should be performed before initiating steroids treatment. Ophthalmology consultation must be obtained to exclude ocular involvement. Praziquantel, is considered a second-line drug; it has decreased efficacy compared to albendazole and is decreased in the setting of steroids. Antiepileptics should be initiated in patients who present with seizures and should be continued in patients with recurrent seizures. Antiepileptics should be considered in patients with multiple cysts even in the absence of history of seizures. Methotrexate has been suggested as a steroid sparing agent in patients who cannot tolerate steroids. Endoscopic removal has emerged as the treatment for patients with the intraventricular disease. Shunting is necessary in patients with hydrocephalus and may need revisions. Surgical intervention may be recommended for cysts located in the fourth ventricle or the spinal areas.

SUGGESTED READING

Garcia, HH, Evans CAW, Nash, TE, Osvaldo. Current consensus guidelines for treatment of neurocysticercosis. *Clinical Microbiology Reviews*. Oct. 2002;15(4):747–756.

Garcia, HH, Pretell, EJ, Robert H. A trial of antiparasitic treatment to reduce the rate of seizures due to cerebral cysticercosis. *N Engl J Med*. 2004;350(3):249–258.

Nash, TE, Singh, G, White, AC. Treatment of neurocysticercosis: Current status and future research needs. *Neurology*. 2006;67:1120–1127.

Nash, TE, Pretell, EJ, Lescano, AG, Bustos, JA. Perilesional brain oedema and seizure activity in patients with calcified neurocysticercosis: A prospective cohort and nested case–control study. For The Cysticercosis Working Group in Peru. *Lancet Neurol*. 2008;7:1099–1105.

Rapidly Deteriorating Visual Problems, Confusion, and Cognitive Decline

Lara V. Marcuse and Martin J. Sadowski

CHIEF COMPLAINT: **Progressive confusion and cognitive decline for the past 3 months.**

HISTORY OF PRESENT ILLNESS

A 68-year-old woman's family describes her as being in perfect health up until 3 months before presentation. Her initial presenting symptom was fatigue. Her family noticed a change in her personality. Before the onset of illness, she used to enjoy grocery shopping, exercising, and spending time gardening. She was no longer interested in doing those chores. She started experiencing visual problems interfering with her driving skills. She was unable to see the road signs and kept asking for directions at obvious intersections. She had difficulty recognizing ordinary objects and would sometimes turn the lights on in a well-lit room. At this point, her family took her for an eye examination and was told that "everything was fine." She remains distractible, confused, and seems to lack insight. Her speech started getting more and more slurred. About 6 weeks prior to presentation, she stopped speaking altogether and did not seem to understand what others were saying to her. The family reported intermittent frequent rapid jerking movements that would affect both arms and her trunk. She could no longer walk and became wheelchair bound within the past 2 months.

PAST MEDICAL HISTORY AND PAST SURGICAL HISTORY

None.

MEDICATIONS

None.

ALLERGIES

None.

PERSONAL HISTORY

No history of alcohol, drug, or tobacco use.

FAMILY HISTORY

Noncontributory.

PHYSICAL EXAMINATION

Blood pressure, 128/88 mmHg; pulse, 78/min; respiratory rate, 14/min; temperature, 97.4.
She was able to breathe spontaneously with no mechanical assistance but required frequent suctioning for secretions. Her cardiovascular, abdominal, and skin examination was unremarkable. She had no meningeal signs.

NEUROLOGICAL EXAMINATION

Her neurological examination was limited. She was nonverbal and unresponsive to all commands. She opened her eyes spontaneously but did not track objects or faces. Pupils were equal and reactive. Oculocephalic reflexes were present. She had bilateral corneal and gag reflex. She withdrew to pain symmetrically in all four extremities. Reflexes were brisk throughout with five to six beats of clonus at the ankles bilaterally. Toes were downgoing. Frequent whole-body myoclonic jerks occurring once every few seconds were noted during the interview.

STOP AND THINK QUESTIONS

➢ What is your differential diagnosis for such a rapidly progressive decline in her condition?

➢ What test(s) would you perform to confirm your clinical suspicion?

➢ What treatment can you offer her?

DIAGNOSTIC TEST RESULTS

CBC, chemistry, LFTs, TFTs, B_{12}, RPR, antithyroid antibodies were all normal.

Brain MRI (Figure 14.1): Diffusion positive lesions in the basal ganglia (particularly the caudate and putamen b/l with sparing of globus pallidus) and ribbon-like appearance of the insular cortex.

EEG (Figure 14.2) showed slow and low voltage background and frequent generalized PSW at a frequency of 2–3 Hertz. The discharges were often but not always accompanied by a myoclonic jerk.

Brain biopsy (Figure 14.3) of the right frontal cortex demonstrated no gross pathology. Microscopic pathology showed vacuolization/spongiform degeneration through the thickness of the cortical neuropil. Western blot performed on the brain biopsy material showed presence of the PK-resistant PrP^{Sc} with a type one banding pattern. Analysis of the codon 129 polymorphism revealed that she was methionine homozygote.

DIAGNOSIS: **Sporadic Creutzfeldt-Jakob disease (sCJD) (Heidenhain variant).**

DISCUSSION

Prion diseases are fatal degenerative diseases of the nervous system caused by a pathogenic form of the prion protein (PrP^{C}; C-cellular). PrP^{C} is a normal constituent of cell membranes, particularly in neurons. The pathogenic forms of the prion protein called PrP^{Sc} (Sc=scrapie) and PrP^{C} have identical amino acid sequence but different tertiary structure. This conformational change makes PrP^{Sc} resistant to standard disinfecting agents, including, formaldehyde, ethanol, standard autoclaving, and ionizing radiation. PrP^{Sc} shows partial resistance to proteolytic degradation by PK digestion. This hardiness of PrP^{Sc} is conferred by a change in the protein with increased β-sheet content. The infectivity of PrP_{Sc} rests with its ability to cause neighboring PrP^{C} to shift conformation to the abnormal scrapie form PrP^{Sc}. PrP^{Sc} accumulates in cell membranes, disrupting normal neuronal activity.

sCJD is the most common form of the disease, which has an incidence of about 1 in 1 million of general population. The cause of sCJD is not known. It occurs in all climates and seasons and affects men and woman equally. It occurs most frequently in people in their 60s (5 in 1 million), but the disease spectrum ranges from 17 to 83 years.

Given its lack of proclivity for a particular type of person (e.g., abattoir worker), season, or geography, an infective source is unlikely. It is postulated that the disease is caused by a random conformation change in the normal cellular prion protein to the scrapie version, which then causes a cascade of conformation changes. Another possibility is that a somatic mutation of the gene occurs that encodes the prion protein.

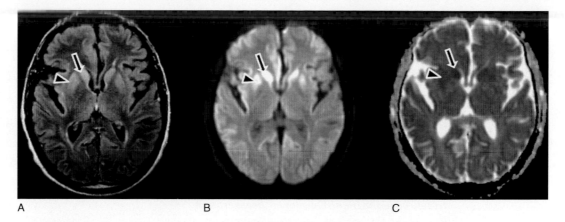

FIGURE 14.1 *MRI FLAIR (A); diffusion (B); and bilateral caudate (arrow) and putamen (carrot) hyperintensities with corresponding hypointensities seen on the ADC (C).*

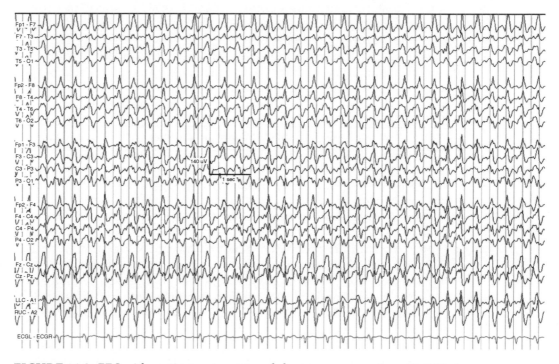

FIGURE 14.2 *EEG with continuous paroxysmal sharp waves occurring at 2–3 Hertz.*

The gene encoding PrP^C (PRNP) has been mapped to the short arm of chromosome 20. In humans, this gene shows little polymorphism; however, if they do occur, they can have clinical significance. In particular, the 129 codon MV polymorphism in its homozygote state seems to have an increased risk for sCJD. Specifically, 72% of people with sCJD are MM homozygotes, 17% are VV homozygotes, and 12% are MV heterozygotes.

Clinically, the most common presenting symptom is fatigue followed by a rapidly progressive dementia. Aphasia, apraxia, motor deficits, ataxia, oculomotor difficulties, behavioral disturbances, and cognitive decline in various domains can all be presenting features of the disease.

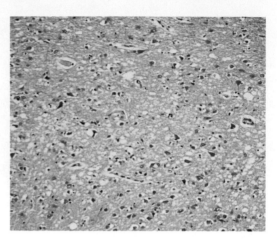

FIGURE 14.3 *Frontal cortical specimen demonstrates vacuolization/spongiform degeneration through the thickness of the cortical neuropil.*

Classic sCJD is the most common subtype of sCJD where the prominent clinical features are rapidly progressive dementia and myoclonus. For this subtype, the EEG shows PSW that occur at a rate of about 1 Hz, and patients typically die within 3 to 4 months. Classic sCJD accounts for 70% of sCJD cases. *Heidenhain variant sCJD,* which is still classified under Classic sCJD, is characterized by visual disturbances (cortical blindness, which dominates the clinical picture during early stage of the disease) is credited to A. Heidenhain, and bears his name. Patients typically die between 2 and 18 months of disease onset. Our case is classified as classic sCJD (Heidenhain variant); with myoclonus, PSW on EEG, and the MM polymorphism with banding pattern type one.

Cerebellar or ataxic variant is the next most common variant with ataxia as the presenting symptom. PSW are only present in 10% of the EEGs of these patients. The EEG often shows nonspecific generalized slowing. Myoclonus is not a prominent feature. These patients live longer, typically 3 to 18 months following disease onset.

Clinical differences in subtypes of sCJD are linked to the polymorphism present at codon 129 (MM, VV, or MV) in the host's cellular prion protein and the banding pattern (Type 1 or 2) of PrP^{Sc} on Western blot following PK digestion (refer to Table 14.1). Both PrP^{C} and PrP^{Sc} are simultaneously present in the brain in three isoforms: nonglycosylated, monoglycosylated, and diglycosylated. While PK digestion degrades PrP^{C} completely, the nonglycosylated band of PrP^{Sc} can be truncated to either 21 kDa or 19 kDa, what defines type 1 and 2 banding pattern, respectively. Combining codon 129 polymorphism and the banding pattern allow identifying six molecular variants of CJD: MM1, MM2, MV1, MV2, VV1, and VV2, which appear to vary in prevalence and are associated with distinct clinical phenotypes. Specifically, the MM and MV polymorphisms with banding pattern type 1 correlate with the classic CJD phenotype. The Heidenhain variant is included in this category. The MM1 and MV1 variants combined constitute 70% of sCJD cases. The ataxic variant correlates with the molecular variant VV2 and is present in 16% of sCJD patients. The MV2 variant is present in 9% of sCJD, and its clinical picture is somewhat similar to that of VV2 variant with protracted clinical course. VV2 and MM2 clinical variants are rare.

Familial prion diseases all have autosomal dominant modes of inheritance of the mutated *prion protein gene* (PRNP) and account for 10% to 15% of human prion diseases. In general, fCJD has an earlier age of onset and longer clinical course than sCJD. There are a number of mutations known to cause fCJD; all linked to either octapeptide insertions or missense mutations. The most common mutation occurs at codon 200 of

TABLE 14.1 *Sporadic CJD Phenotypes*

Codon 129 Polymorphism and PrP^Sc Banding Type	Phenotype	Myoclonus	EEG	Disease Duration	Pathology
MM 1 MV 1	Classic sCJD Rapidly progressive dementia, prominent myoclonus. 70% of cases.	Yes	PSW	3 to 4 months	Spongiform degeneration of the cerebral cortex, putamen, caudate, thalamus, and molecular layer of cerebellar cortex.
VV 2	Cerebellar or ataxic variant Presents with ataxia followed by cognitive impairment and oculomotor signs. 16% of cases.	Much less prominent at presentation	PSW present only in 10% of cases	3 to 18 months	Spongiform degeneration of the cerebral cortex, putamen, caudate, thalamus, and molecular layer of cerebellar cortex.
MV 2	Similar clinically to VV2 but with longer survival. 9% of cases.	Much less prominent at presentation	PSW present only in 10% of cases	Average survival 17 months	Prominent "Kuru" plaques in the cerebellem, consisting of amyloid based sphericals with spicules.

M, methionine; V, valine; PSW, periodic sharp waves; sCJD, sporadic CJD. Clinical differences in the course of sporadic CJD are secondary to the polymorphism present at codon 129 (MM, VV, or MV) and the banding pattern (Type 1 or 2) of PrPSc on Western blot following PK K digestion.

the PRNP, and the phenotype is very similar to sCJD. Two unique forms of fCJD, GSS and FFI are further detailed in Table 14.2.

Transmission from human to human is of tremendous concern; however, only a few cases have been reported worldwide. Iatrogenic CJD has occurred with corneal transplants, hormones extracted from pituitary glands such as human growth hormone, contaminated neurosurgical instruments and EEG depth electrodes, and dural grafts (Lyodura). There are no reported cases of transmission from household contact, sexual transmission, or nosocomial transmission. There are anecdotal cases of blood transfusion causing the new variant CJD but not sCJD.

Another area of tremendous concern is the transmission of prion disease among species. The first documented prion disease occurred in sheep over 250 years ago, with ataxic sheep that would scrape against fencing, hence the name for the scrapie form of the prion protein. There is no clinical or experimental evidence of scrapie in sheep and goats to be transmissible to humans. However, sheep scrapie is readily transmissible to cattle. It is what gave rise to an epidemic-scale proportion of the BSE in the United Kingdom and to a lesser extent in other Western European countries, when cattle feed became enhanced with sheep offal (entrails and internal organs of a butchered animals). Subsequently, BSE, more colorfully referred to in the news as mad cow disease, appeared to be transmissible to humans and gave raise to a new form of CJD termed nvCJD. The first case of nvCJD was recorded in 1994. Unlike sCJD, which occurs in patients in their 60s, nvCJD affects mainly young individuals (Table 14.3). The most frequent presenting symptoms are psychiatric

TABLE 14.2 *Familial Prion Diseases*

Familial CJD Type	Clinical Features	Prognosis	Genetics	Pathology
GSS	Cerebellar ataxia and dysarthria; can have parkinsonism with masked facies, rigidity, and tremor; dementia	5 to 12 years after disease onset	Point mutation at codon 102 or 107 of PRNP (most frequently)	Severe amyloidosis with amyloid plaques composed of truncated versions of the PrP peptide. Present in the cerebellar cortex, cerebral cortex and in the basal ganglia. Minimal spongiform degeneration. There can be severe neuronal loss throughout the brain.
FFI	Progressive insomnia, sympathetic system hyperactivity, and dementia	2 to 6 years after disease onset	Caused by a combination of PRNP mutation at codon 178 with MM homozygosity at codon 129, can be sporadic	Severe neuronal loss and atrophy of anteroventral and mediodorsal nuclei of the thalamus.

GSS, Gertsmann Straussler Scheinker syndrome; FFI, Fatal familial insomnia; PRNP, prion protein gene.

TABLE 14.3 *Transmissible CJD*

	Presenting Symptoms	Prognosis	EEG	CSF	Polymorphism at Codon 129	Pathology	MRI
Iatrogenic CJD	Dementia	12 months	PSW	Over 90% with elevated 14-3-3	Varies	Spongiform degeneration (similar to sCJD)	Diffusion positive lesions in basal ganglia (similar to sCJD)
New Variant CJD (nvCJD)	Psychiatric disturbances and sensory dysfunctions	14 months	Nonspecific slowing	50% with elevated 14-3-3	All M/M homozygotes	Florid amyloidosis (similar to GSS)	"Pulvinar sign" with hyperintense lesions in the pulvinar
Kuru	Cerebellar ataxia	12 months	Unknown	Unknown	Unknown	Kuru plaques in cerebellum	Unknown

in nature and include anxiety, depression and, more rarely, psychosis. Cognitive impairment, ataxia, chorea, sensory symptoms, and dystonia follow the psychiatric complaints by several months. The median survival time is 14 months from diagnosis. Typical autopsy picture of nvCJD brain reveals vast amyloid plaque deposits containing PrP^{Sc}. Spongiform degeneration and neuronal loss are found in highest intensity in the thalamus and basal ganglia followed by cerebral and cerebellar cortices. Interestingly, most of the cases tested have been homozygous for MM at codon 129. The salient distinguishing feature of acquired form of prion diseases including iatrogenic CJD and nvCJD is the presence of PrP^{Sc} in the lymphatic organs. Familial prion diseases and sCJD do not possess PrP^{Sc} in the lymphatic organs. Following extracerebral infection, PrP^{Sc} harbors and replicates within various cell lines of the lymphatic system for months to years prior to entering the brain and causing neurological symptoms. Therefore, histopathological examination of the lymphatic tissue including anti-PrP immunostaining can be used to distinguish acquired cases of prion disease from those that are sporadic or genetically defined. Furthermore, tonsil biopsy has been often utilized to confirm diagnosis of nvCJD in live subjects.

Kuru is a form of transmissible CJD that is now mainly of historical interest, as the cessation of cannibalism has ended the disease. It was a disease of the Fore people in New Guinea, affecting predominantly women and children, who would preferentially eat the brain. Upon the death of a family member, maternal kin were responsible for the dismemberment of the corpse. The epidemic peaked in the 1960s with 1,000 deaths caused by Kuru in 10 years. The word "Kuru" means "trembling with cold and fear." The initial symptoms of the disease were ataxia with dsyarthria and tremor followed by loss of the ability to ambulate and progressive dementia. The clinical course is about 12 months. Rare cases of Kuru have been reported within the past years in older Fore subjects, who performed cannibalism in their youth. It is estimated that the incubation period in these cases could be as long as 50 years, what provides a vivid example of protracted incubation period characteristic for prion diseases.

There is not one test that can be used to diagnose prion disease. Rather, it is the constellation of a rapidly progressive dementia with characteristic imaging, EEG, and CSF data that support the diagnosis. Definite CJD requires pathologic confirmation by brain biopsy or autopsy. Tonsilar biopsy can be used to confirm nvCJD in live subjects. There are surgical risks of bleeding and infection, therefore, it should only be done when nvCJD is being suspected. This approach, however, is not recommended to be routinely performed in older subjects as a part of workup for suspected sCJD, since age-related tonsilar atrophy predisposes to a high rate of iatrogenic complication resulting from the biopsy itself.

CSF studies show elevation of 14-3-3 protein in over 90% of patients with sCJD. However, 14-3-3 protein is a nonspecific marker of neuronal damage and can be elevated in advanced stages of many neurodegenerative diseases including Alzheimer's disease and frontotemporal dementia as well as in a number of more acute processes such as MS exacerbation, stroke, or encephalitis. Therefore, validity of 14-3-3 protein in supporting diagnosis of sCJD can be considered only when rapidly progressive dementia lasts not more than 12 months (as opposed to Alzheimer's disease and frontotemporal dementia, where clinical course is more protracted) and when brain imaging rules out aforementioned acute brain pathologies. The CSF level of 14-3-3 protein is known to increase during the symptomatic course of CJD; therefore, repeated spinal taps and measures of 14-3-3 have been demonstrated to be helpful in cases where the value of 14-3-3 during the initial assessment was within normal range or it was equivocally elevated. 14-3-3 protein is less sensitive in iatrogenically transmitted CJD and nvCJD groups with about 70% showing an elevation. The 14-3-3 protein is elevated in most familial forms of CJD but not in familial fatal insomnia or GSS. To determine 14-3-3 protein level, CSF samples can be shipped to the National Prion Disease Pathology Surveillance Center located in Cleveland Ohio, by following the instructions posted on line at http://www.cjdsurveillance.com.

Tau protein is similarly elevated in the CSF of patients with CJD and may precede the elevation of 14-3-3. Unlike Alzheimer's disease and frontotemporal dementia, CJD is characterized by elevation of the total tau level with phosphorylated tau fraction remaining grossly in physiological ratio to the total tau. The level of total CSF tau in CJD may rise three to fourfold above normal levels. Therefore, in rapidly progressive cognitive decline with clinical course under 12 months, CSF tau measurements may contribute to substantiation of CJD diagnosis.

The characteristic EEG pattern of PSW occurring at 1 H is seen in sCJD in about 65% to 85% of cases. Often, it is not present at presentation but develops at later stages of the disease. Initially, there are sporadic and sometimes asymmetric biphasic or triphasic discharges. As the disease advances, the pattern changes to more synchronous and generalized 200 to 400 ms sharp waves occurring every 0.5 to 1.0 seconds. This pattern is less frequently seen in familial cases but not in nvCJD. Another condition called SSPE and associated with measles is also known to be associated with PSW. In SSPE, PSW are usually of high voltage (300–1500 µV) that may last 0.5 to 2 seconds and recur every 4 to 15 seconds. Rarely, the complexes of SSPE can occur at intervals of 1 to 5 minutes but the interval between complexes may shorten with disease progression.

MRI is increasingly being used as a diagnostic test for CJD. Typically, increased signal on T2-weigthed sequence and diffusion restriction in the caudate and the putamen ("the puck and hockey stick" sign), the neocortex (the "cortical ribbon" sign) and in the posterior and medial thalamus (the "pulvinar" sign), are found. Unilateral involvement of basal nuclei and segmental involvement of the cortical ribbon are common. Over time, the restricted diffusion does not resolve, as it would in stroke, but it spreads to involve the other caudate and then moves posteriorly to involve the putamen bilaterally. The globus pallidus is most often spared. fCJD tends to show a similar pattern with the possible exception of GSS, which can also show lesions in the white matter. The MRI lesions of nvCJD are similar but more posterior with diffusion restriction occurring in the posterior region of the thalamus, causing the pulvinar sign. The DWI hyperintensity correlates with the degree of spongiform change on pathology.

Genetic testing should be undergone if there is a family history of rapidly progressive dementia and neurological deterioration. However, as many as 50% of patients with known genetic mutation do not have a positive family history. These have been ascribed to poor family histories, varying penetrance, or unknown paternity.

One of the most important parts of evaluating a person with suspected CJD is ruling out potentially treatable causes of dementia. An LP should be done to exclude subacute meningitis and viral encephalitis. Antithyroid antibodies should be checked because steroid-responsive autoimmune encephalitis can cause myoclonus and a rapidly declining mental status. Vitamin B_{12} levels and RPR should also be checked. Some of the Parkinson's plus disorders like olivopontine cerebellar atrophy and corticobasal ganglionic degeneration can resemble CJD. A paraneoplastic work-up should be considered as paraneoplastic encephalitis can resemble CJD. This work-up consists of a scanning CT of the chest, abdomen, and pelvis and performing the paraneoplastic antibody panel. Table 14.4 highlights the individual sensitivity and specificity of individual test performed to confirm the diagnosis.

TREATMENT

Unfortunately, there is no current treatment that can halt or even ameliorate the progression of CJD. Treatment consists of supportive and symptomatic care. If psychosis is a prominent feature, low-dose antipsychotics may be helpful. The myoclonus can be treated

TABLE 14.4 *Diagnostic Tests for CJD*

Diagnostic Test Results	Sensitivity (%)	Specificity (%)
MRI brain: Diffusion restriction in the caudate, putamen, and cerebral cortex	91	95
EEG: PSW	70	Unknown
CSF: elevation of 14-3-3 protein	94	93
CSF: elevation of Tau protein	94	90

with benzodiazepines, valproic acid, or levetiracetam. It should be kept in mind that the myoclonus should be treated only in so far as it bothers the patient. There is no utility in aggressive treatment of the myoclonus or the EEG in terms of the patient's overall mental status or prognosis.

A number of experimental treatments are under investigation. Quinacrine, an anti-malaria agent was found to be an efficient inhibitor of PrP^{Sc} propagation in infected cells, and given its fairly low side effect profile, it is currently in a phase II trial in CJD patients. However, a report of off-label use of quinacrine in CJD failed to show any clear benefits.

SUGGESTED READING

Information on National Prion Disease Pathology Surveillance Center (NPDPSC). www.cjdsurveillance.com

Johnson RT. Prion diseases. *Lancet Neurol.* 2005 Oct;4(10):635–642.

Trevitt CR, Collinge J. A systematic review of prior therapeutics in experimental models. *Brain.* 2006 Sep;129(Pt 9):2241–2265.

Young GS, Geschwind MD, Fischbein NJ, et al. Diffusion-weighted and fluid-attenuated inversion recovery imaging in Creutzfeldt-Jakob disease: High sensitivity and specificity for diagnosis. *AJNR Am J Neuroradiol.* 2005 Jun–Jul;26(6):1551–1562.

Winfred Peiyi Wu, Benjamin Gu, Mushuy Nawood Khawaja, and Anuradha Singh

CHIEF COMPLAINT: **Hands are losing all muscle strength, and now the right leg is also weak.**

HISTORY OF PRESENT ILLNESS

A 37-year-old, right-handed Chinese cook presented to the neurology clinic with increasing weakness and clumsiness in his arms and right leg. The patient's complaints began 4 months prior to being referred to a neurologist. He initially experienced neck and shoulder pain of increasing severity while working in the kitchen. He also described feeling clumsy while using the spatula and wok, and had difficulty lifting heavy pots and pans. The weakness and clumsiness gradually progressed over the next few months, and he began to notice a significant decrease in the muscle mass of his arms and hands, more so in his right hand. The progressive weakness forced him to quit his job. He began to experience small "fast twitches" in both his arms. In the past few weeks, he developed significant weakness of his right leg.

There was no prior history of trauma. He denied any weakness in his left leg, and he denied any bowel or bladder problems. He did not suffer from neck pain, back pain, or shooting pains on bending his neck forward. He denied having slurred speech or having trouble breathing or swallowing. Prior to being referred to a neurologist, he sought the care of a primary care physician, who placed the patient on a muscle relaxant and a nonsteroidal anti-inflammatory drug, which did not alleviate his symptoms.

PAST MEDICAL HISTORY AND PAST SURGICAL HISTORY

Hepatitis B diagnosed 3 years ago.

MEDICATIONS

Epivir-HBV 100 mg once daily, Motrin 600 mg tid PRN, Cyclobenzaprine 5 mg tid PRN.

ALLERGIES

No known allergies.

PERSONAL HISTORY

Denies tobacco, drug, or alcohol consumption. Married, with two healthy children.

FAMILY HISTORY

No known history of any neurological disorders.

PHYSICAL EXAMINATION

Vital signs: Pulse, 72/min; respiratory rate, 14/min; blood pressure, 110/65 mm Hg; O_2 saturation, 100% on room air. No acute distress. The remainder of his general exam was unremarkable.

NEUROLOGICAL EXAMINATION

Mental status: Consolidates appropriately. Fluent in Mandarin. Knowledge of current events, affect, language (comprehension, expression, naming, repetition, reading, and writing), judgment, abstraction, memory, calculation, and praxis were normal.

CNs II–XII: Full conjugate eye movements. Pupils equal and reactive to light. Visual fields were full. Face symmetrical, tongue midline. Muscles of mastication and facial sensation are normal. Soft palate elevates bilaterally symmetrically. No dysphonia, and no tongue atrophy or fasciculations are noted.

Motor: Significant atrophy of bilateral biceps and triceps, and of all the intrinsic hand muscles. Strength testing revealed 5-/5 in both deltoids, 4/5 in the biceps bilaterally and 5-/5 in the triceps bilaterally. Left wrist extension was 4/5, and right wrist extension was 5-/5. Wrist flexion was 5-/5 bilaterally. Intrinsic hand muscles were 3/5 bilaterally. Finger flexors were 4+/5 on the left and 5-/5 on the right. Fasciculations were seen in the bilateral arms, especially in the triceps. Significant muscle wasting of right leg is present: right thigh circumference 52.2 cm versus the left leg circumference of 58 cm, right leg proximally 4-/5 with right foot drop; left leg strength is full and 5/5.

Sensory: Normal throughout to light touch, pin prick, joint position sense, and vibration.

Reflexes: *Upper extremities:* Left biceps and triceps 3+, right biceps and triceps 3+ with spread, bilateral brachioradialis 2+. *Lower extremities:* Left patellar 3+, left ankle jerk 3+ with crossed hip adductors, right patellar and right ankle jerk 3+; Hoffman sign was present bilaterally. Five to six beats of ankle clonus are noted bilaterally.

Cerebellar: No nystagmus, ataxia, dysmetria, or dysdiadochokinesia.

Gait: Right steppage gait, with negative Romberg test.

STOP AND THINK QUESTIONS

➢ What do you make of UMN and LMN signs in this case?

➢ What is the differential diagnosis in the patient?

➢ What is the importance of fasciculations?

➢ What tests would you order to elucidate the diagnosis?

DIAGNOSTIC TEST RESULTS

Brain MRI with and without gadolinium: Hyperintense signal on both FLAIR and T2WI and hypointense signal on T1WI in the corticospinal tracts within the posterior limb of the left internal capsule and through the cerebral peduncle in comparison with the right (Figure 15.1). The hyperintense signal on FLAIR and T2WI extends superiorly through the corona radiata and centrum semiovale into the left precentral gyrus superomedially.

Cervical spine MRI: Small central herniated disc at C5 to C6 level with no cord compression, and with no significant neuroforaminal narrowing.

EMG and NCS all four extremities: Motor and sensory NCSs were unremarkable. The needle EMG exam of the bilateral upper extremities (deltoid, biceps brachii, first dorsal interossei) showed mild membrane instability, unstable motor unit action potentials with greatly increased amplitude and loss of motor units. Needle EMG examination of the lower extremities (tibialis anterior, gastrocnemius, vastus medialis) showed membrane instability and increased amplitude of motor unit action potential with loss of motor units on the right side. Examination of the tongue showed mild membrane instability and no loss of motor units. Examination of the T2 paraspinal muscles showed mild membrane instability.

Labs: CBC and BMP were within normal limits, CPK: normal; HIV negative; HTLV-Abs: negative; Lyme Ab: negative.

DIAGNOSIS: **Amyotrophic lateral sclerosis (ALS).**

DISCUSSION

ALS is a specific type of adult-onset rapidly progressive motor neuron disease character-ized by both upper and lower motor neuron signs. "Amyotrophic" refers to the muscle atrophy, weakness, and fasciculations signifying the degeneration of lower (spinal) motor neurons in the brain stem and spinal cord. "Lateral sclerosis" refers to the reactive gliosis of the lateral columns in the spinal cord as upper (corticospinal) motor neurons originating in the motor cortex degenerate and produce over active tendon reflexes, Hoffman signs, Babinski signs, and clonus.

The prevalence of ALS in the United States is estimated to be 5 cases per 100,000 with an average age of onset between the fourth and seventh decade. Whites are affected more than nonwhites (1.6:1) and males more than females (1.5:1). As a rapidly progressive motor neuron disease, death occurs in most cases within 5 years due to complications with respi-ratory failure. The disease with young age of onset is reported to be associated with pro-longed survival.

The incidence of ALS is fairly constant worldwide with the exception of a special vari-ant of parkinsonism-dementia-ALS unique to Guam. There are also reports of clusters of ALS in American war veterans of first Persian Gulf War and in Italian professional soccer players.

Monomelic form (affecting one extremity) of ALS is more common in Southern parts of India. The prevalence of ALS in Guam is 50 times the worldwide prevalence and can be attributed to consumption of neurotoxin in cycad seeds or giant fruit bats.

The onset is insidious over months with the first symptoms often presenting as UMN (spasticity, hyperreflexia, and clonus) and LMN (atrophy, weakness, and fasciculations) signs in a single limb. The muscular wasting may start in one group of muscles but in most patients with ALS, it spreads to the other parts of the body and sooner or later becomes generalized. More than 80% of patients with ALS with arm onset have ipsilateral or con-tralateral leg symptoms at 60 months after onset. Pain is not a typical feature of ALS.

Bulbar dysfunction such as dysarthria and dysphagia are poor prognostic factors that are uncommon when ALS presents in the third and fourth decades, but becomes more prevalent when ALS presents in the sixth and seventh decades. Atrophy and fasciculations of the tongue should strongly clue in the clinician to suspect ALS. When there is corticob-ulbar tract involvement, patients can also have emotional lability (pseudobulbar affect), manifested as crying or laughing in inappropriate circumstances. Cognitive and neuropsy-chological impairment in the form of a frontotemporal dementia can also manifest itself as the disease progresses.

While no test alone can provide a definitive diagnosis of ALS, the presence of isolated upper and lower motor neuron findings in a single limb strongly suggests the disease. The diagnosis of ALS and its progression are primarily based on the symptoms and signs elic-ited upon physical examination. There are typical and atypical forms of ALS as summa-rized in Table 15.1.

Classical ALS is a distinct syndrome characterized by symptoms and signs of upper and lower motor neurons and occurs in about two thirds of people with ALS.

PBP is a motor neuron disease that was originally described by Duchenne in 1860. In approximately 25% of people with ALS, the initial symptoms begin in muscles innervated by the lower brain stem that control articulation, chewing, and swallowing. Sometimes, the disease remains in this form for years, but it usually progresses to generalized muscle weakness and looks like typical motor neuron disease. When the disease is strictly lim-ited to the bulbar muscles clinically and electrodiagnostically, it is referred as PBP and

TABLE 15.1 *Types of Motor Neuron Diseases*

Typical	Atypical
UMN and LMN: ALS	Mills' hemiplegic variant
UMN signs only: Primary lateral sclerosis	Scapulohumeral form of ALS (Vulpian-Bernart's form of ALS)
LMN signs only: Spinal muscular atrophy	Monomelic ALS (Hirayama's disease)
Bulbar symptoms only: Progressive bulbar palsy	Wasted-leg syndrome
Familial ALS	Flail arm syndrome
Juvenile ALS	Unilateral leg hypertrophy

is associated with a poor prognosis. Video swallowing studies are required to assess the upper pharyngeal strength and function to determine the risk of aspiration. Pulmonary function tests must be done to assess forced vital capacity and inspiratory and expiratory volumes. It is hard to speculate whether the above two forms of sporadic ALS represent a spectrum of the same disease or distinct entities.

FAMILIAL AMYOTROPHIC LATERAL SCLEROSIS (FALS)

FALS cases comprise 5% to 10% of all cases of ALS. Almost 20% of people with FALS have a mutation in the gene that codes for the protein Cu/Zn SOD1 located on chromosome 21. FALS genetic testing is available commercially. The exact mutation in the same gene can cause different phenotypes. There are no differences between familial and sporadic ALS on neurological exam except for occasional sensory loss in people with FALS. Several mutations in genes have been identified on chromosomes 2, 9, 15, 18, and the X chromosome. Patients with A4V mutation usually present with LMN signs and progress rapidly. An H46R mutation in the same gene can cause different phenotypes. While there are multiple foci, most SOD1 mutations are believed to be autosomal dominant. We expect to find more genes that can modify disease through research and genetic studies in families and siblings of people with both sporadic and FALS.

PATHOPHYSIOLOGY

While the disease progression and prognosis have remained relatively unchanged since ALS was first described over a century ago, significant strides have been made in understanding its pathophysiology. Some leading hypotheses are described below.

Defective Glutamate Metabolism: To date, one of the most robust theories of pathogenesis of ALS is excito-toxicity of glutamate. Glutamate is a neurotransmitter in the nervous system used for signaling between neurons. While it is important for normal nerve cell function, a surplus of glutamate can be neurotoxic. There is evidence of increased glutamate levels in the CSF of ALS patients. The increased glutamate may result from either abnormal transport of glutamate out of the nerve cell environment or increased release of glutamate from nerve cells. To date, there is some evidence that the transporter responsible for removing glutamate from the nervous system may be altered and/or damaged.

SOD1 Mutation: One of the most studied pathophysiologic causes of ALS is the SOD1 mutation of chromosome 21. The mutation is believed to be a gain of function type resulting in toxic accumulation of SOD1 resulting in excessive oxidative stress. Unfortunately, the discovery of the SOD1 linkage has not yet translated into an effective therapy for ALS.

Aside from the SOD1 model, other pathophysiologic mechanisms are implicated in the pathophysiology of ALS (see Table 15.2). These include excitotoxicity by overactivation of excitatory synapses, immune and inflammatory reactions, and defects in axonal transport, mitochondrial dysfunction, and accumulation of toxic metabolites, growth factor dysregulation, and premature apoptosis.

TABLE 15-2. Possible Causes of ALS

Defective glutamate metabolism
Free radical injury
Mitochondrial dysfunction
Gene defects
Programmed cell death or apoptosis
Cytoskeletal protein defects
Autoimmune and inflammatory mechanisms
Accumulation of protein aggregates (clumps)
Viral infections

Autoimmunity may have a role in the pathogenesis of ALS as well, since activated microglia and T cells have been found in the spinal cords of patients with IgG antibodies against motor neurons. However, immunotherapy has not been effective in patients with ALS. Corticosteroids, plasmapharesis, intravenous immunoglobulin, cyclophosphamide, and whole body radiation have not been proven to show any benefit.

A definitive diagnosis under the strictest guidelines of the El Escorial diagnostic criteria of the World Federation of Neurology Research Group on Motor Neuron Disease requires the presence of the following:

- evidence of LMN degeneration by clinical, electrophysiological, or neuropathologic examination
- evidence of UMN degeneration by clinical examination
- progressive spread of symptoms or signs within a region or to other regions, as determined by history or examination

Together with the absence of:

- electrophysiological and pathological evidence of other disease processes that might explain the signs of LMN and/or UMN degeneration, and
- neuroimaging evidence of other disease processes that might explain the observed clinical and electrophysiological signs

According to these criteria, electrophysiological features should include evidence of both active and chronic denervation. The signs of active denervation are:

- Positive sharp waves
- Fibrillation potentials

Signs of chronic denervation are:

- Large motor unit potentials of increased amplitude and duration with an increased polyphasia
- Reduced interference pattern with firing rates higher than 10 Hz unless there is a significant UMN component, in which case the firing rate may be lower than 10 Hz
- Unstable motor unit potentials

Fasciculation potentials are another characteristic feature of ALS. Their presence in EMG is helpful in the diagnosis of ALS, particularly if they are of long duration and polyphonic, and when they are present in muscles in which there is evidence of active or chronic partial denervation and reinnervation.

The EMG signs of LMN dysfunction required to support a diagnosis of ALS should be found in at least two of the four CNS regions: brain stem (bulbar/cranial motor neurons), cervical, thoracic, or lumbosacral spinal cord (anterior horn motor neurons).

NCSs are required for the diagnosis principally to define and exclude other disorders of the peripheral nerves, neuromuscular junction and muscles that may mimic or confound the diagnosis of ALS. These studies should generally be normal or near normal.

MRI of the brain or spinal cord may be normal, or in some cases, MRI brain may demonstrate hyperintense signals on T2W and FLAIR images along the corticospinal tracts. Muscle biopsy should only be done when the presentation is atypical and to confirm the presence of neurogenic atrophy (denervation) and fiber-type grouping (reinnervation).

DIFFERENTIAL DIAGNOSIS

A variety of tests that can be done to assess for ALS and to rule out other conditions that may present with similar presentations (Table 15.3). Because there is no curative therapy for ALS, it is important to rule out treatable pathologies. For example, multifocal motor neuropathy, which can present like ALS would respond to cyclophosphamide or intravenous immunoglobulin. Cervical pathologies (herniated disk, spondylitic myelopathy, and syringomyelia), spinal cord tumors, Guillain-Barré, and multiple sclerosis are treatable pathologies that can imitate some of the clinical symptoms of ALS. Based on the patient's history and physical examination, the physician can also order blood and urine tests to rule infectious and environmental causes. For example, HIV, HTLV, Lyme disease, and lead toxicity have been known to mimic ALS.

The differential diagnoses of ALS by region and by pathology at or below the level of the brain stem include the following:

LMN signs with bulbar involvement: PBP, cranial nerve palsies

LMN signs with limb involvement: PMA, radiculopathy, plexopathy, neuropathy, chronic inflammatory demyelinating polyneuropathy, multifocal motor neuropathy, mononeuropathy multiplex, vasculitic neuropathy, toxic neuropathy (lead, mercury), metabolic or endocrine (thyrotoxicosis or hyperparathyroidism) neuropathies, myopathies

LMN signs with bulbar and/or limb involvement: Myasthenia gravis, GBS

UMN signs with bulbar involvement: Pseudobulbar palsy, brain stem lesions, including syrinx, mass, stroke, demyelinating and neurodegenerative diseases, Foramen magnum tumors

UMN signs with bulbar involvement: PLS, cervical myelopathy, syrinx, hereditary spastic paraparesis, transverse myelopathy and myelitis, HIV-related myelopathy, syrinx, other cord tumors or lesions, postradiation, infectious (HTLV1, Lyme, CMV)

Both LMN and UMN Signs: Amyotrophic lateral sclerosis, spinal muscular atrophy and spinobulbar muscular atrophy. These entities typically involve both bulbar and limb dysfunction.

TREATMENT

While there is no cure for ALS, the fields of gene therapy and stem cell research are promising. The mainstay of treatment is generally symptomatic (see Table 15.4).

The mainstay of all treatment regimens is palliative care. A multidisciplinary team of health care professionals provides individualized relief of symptoms and aims to improve the quality of life for patients. Drugs are available to reduce fatigue, control spasticity and cramping, as well as reduce oral secretions. Physical, occupational, and speech therapy help maintain the patient's independence and ability to communicate. As the patient's

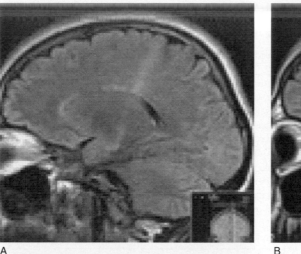
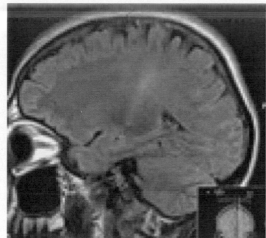

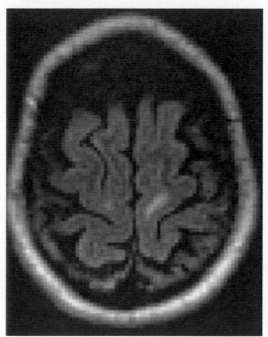

FIGURE 15.1 *(A) Sagittal FLAIR MRI brain showing hyperintensity of corticospinal tract extending through corona radiata. (B) Sagittal FLAIR MRI brain showing hyperintensity of corticospinal tract extending through corona radiata and internal capsule. (C) Axial FLAIR MRI brain showing hyperintensity of corticospinal tracts, left more than right.*

Table 15.3 *Some of the Diagnostic Tests That Can Help Narrow Down the Long Differential List*

Labs	CBC, ESR, BMP, LFT,CK, TFT, Calcium, PTH, ACE, Lyme, ANA, B12, folate, HIV testing, GM1 and MAG antibodies, quantitative immunoglobulins, immunofixation electrophoresis, latex fixation, serum hexosaminidase levels
Neuroimaging	MRI brain, MRI spine
Electrodiagnostic studies	EMG/NCS can differentiate myopathies, neuropathies, CIDP, multifocal motor neuropathies; SFEMG/RNS can help confirm the diagnosis of MG
Spinal tap	Can r/o CIDP, HTLV-1, Lyme, sarcoidosis, infectious or other inflammatory neurological conditions (oligocloncal bands and myelin basic protein)
Muscle biopsy	Can be done to exclude inflammatory myopathies
Genetic testing	Tay Sach's (Hex A gene mutation), Kennedy's disease (CAG triple repeat expansion in the androgen receptor gene), SOD1 mutation

TABLE 15.4 *Drugs and Non-Drug Therapies for Patients With ALS*

Symptoms	Commonly Used Drug and Non-Drug Therapies
Spasticity	Baclofen, Flexeril, Tizanidine, Dantrolene, Diazepam, Botox A injection, Levetiracetam, Physical therapy, Hydrotherapy
Sialorrhea (drooling)	Amitriptyline, Scopolamine patch, Botox A injection, Low-dose radiation to parotid glands, Atropine, Benztropine, Glycopyrrolate
Bronchial Secretions	Guaifenesin, N-acetylcysteine, Metoprolol or Inderal, Ipratropium, Nebulizer, Portable suction devices, Cricopharyngeal myotomy
Constipation	Hydration, increased fiber intake, increased physical activity, Colace, senna, miralax, dulcolax, milk of magnesia, lactulose, dulcolax suppository, enema
Depression	TCAs, SSRIs, counseling, psychotherapy
Anxiety	Inderal, Klonopin, BuSpar, Ativan, Wellbutrin, Diazepam, SSRI, Psychotherapy
Fatigue	Balancing rest and activity, Sleep hygiene, Modafinil, Nuvigil, Ritalin, Cylert, Dexedrine
Pseudobulbar affect (PBA)	Dextromethorphan and quinidine (Nuedexta), amitryptiline and Fluvoxamine, psychosocial support to caregivers
Cramps	Massage, Physiotherapy, Hydrotherapy, Carbamazepine, Levetiractam, Gabapentin, Verapamil

symptoms worsen, care should be focused on maintaining a patent airway, ensuring proper nutrition, and controlling the patient's pain. Sleep-disordered breathing disorders and confusion can indicate impending respiratory failure. End-of-life issues, including the question of assisted ventilation and PEG placement should be addressed with the patient and the family.

For the past decade, the only drug approved to treat ALS is Riluzole, which prolongs median survival by 2 to 3 months but has little effect on the rate of functional deterioration. The drug is believed to reduce damage to motor neurons by slowing the release of the excitotoxic neurotransmitter glutamate but has little effect on reversing previously damaged neurons. The prolonged survival has been attributed to Riluzole's ability to delay the onset of bulbar deficits (ventilation, swallowing, etc.). Several current and future ALS drug trials will elucidate if drugs such as ceftiaxone or dexpramipexole may confer additional neuroprotective effects on cases of ALS, or whether therapies such as ISIS-SOD1 (an antisense oligonucleotide drug for SOD1-related ALS) may be effective. A list of these, and other current ongoing clinical trials in ALS is available online at http://www.alsa.org/research/clinical-trials.

Medications for the symptomatic treatment of ALS include baclofen and tizanidine for spasticity, SSRIs and tricyclic antidepressants for emotional lability, and botox injections or amitryptiline for increased salivation.

Current research places a heavy emphasis on gene therapy and presymptomatic treatment. On the gene therapy front, the replacement of defective genes and the activation and insertion of neuroprotective genes are being explored. Presymptomatic treatment has proven effective in some animal models, but has yet to translate into benefit for humans.

SUGGESTED READING

Bensimon G, Lacomblez L, Meninger V. ALS/Riluzole Study Group. A controlled trial of riluzle in amyotrophic lateral sclerosis. *N Engl J Med.* 1994;330:585–591.

Bradley, W, Daroff, R, Fenichel, G, Jankovic, J. *Neurology in Clinical Practice.* 4th ed. Philadelphia: Butterworth Heinemann, 2004.

Brooks BR, Shodis KA, Lewis DH, et al. Natural history of amyotrophic lateral sclerosis. Quantification of symptoms, signs, strength, and function. In: Serratrice J, Munsat TL, eds. *Pathogenesis Therapy of Amyotrophic Lateral Sclerosis. Advances in Neurology.* Philadelphia: Lippincott-Raven; 1995:68:163–184.

Carvalho, M. et al. Brief communications. *Neurology.* 2004;63:721–723.

Charcot JM, Joffroy A. Deux cas d'atrophie musculaire progressive avec des lésions de la substance gris et des faisceaux antéro-latéraux de la moelle épinière. *Arch Physiol Norm Path.* 1869;2:54–367, 745–760.

Emery AEH, Holloway S. Familial motor neuron disease. In: Rowland LP, ed. *Human Motor Neuron Disease. Advances in Neurology.* Vol. 36. New York: Raven Press; 1982:139–147.

Gilmore N, O'Neill MB, et al. Case 22-2006: A 77-year-old man with a rapidly progressive gait disorder. *N Engl J Med.* 2006;355:296–304.

Ikeda M, et al. A novel point mutation in Cu/Zn SOD mutation in a patient with familial ALS. *Hum Mol Genet.* 1995;4(3):491–492.

Miller RG, Rosenberg JA, Gelinas D, et al. Practice parameter: The care of the patient with amyotrophic lateral sclerosis (an evidence based review): Report of the Quality Standards Subcommittee of the American Academy of Neurology. *Neurology.* 1999;52(7):1311–1323.

Orell, R. Understanding the causes of amyotrophic lateral sclerosis. *N Engl J Med.* 2007;357:822–823.

Rabin BA, Griffin JW, Crain BJ. Autosomal dominant juvenile amyotrophic lateral sclerosis. *Brain.* 1999;122:1539–1550.

Revised El Escorial Criteria for the Diagnosis of Amyotrophic Lateral Sclerosis: http://www.wfnals.org/guidelines/1998elescorial/elescorial1998.htm

Ropper A, Brown R. *Principles of Neurology.* 8th ed.. New York: McGraw Hill; 2005.

Rowland L, Shneider N. Amyotrophic lateral sclerosis. *N Engl J Med.* 2001;344:1688–1700.

Strong MJ, Grace GM, Orange JB, Leeper HA, Menon RS, Aere C. A prospective study of cognitive impairment in ALS. *Neurology.* 1999;53:1665–1670.

Insidious Right Leg Weakness

Thomas J. Kaley and Lauren E. Abrey

CHIEF COMPLAINT: **Right leg is getting weaker.**

HISTORY OF PRESENT ILLNESS

A 47-year-old female was seen in the neurology clinic for frequent falls. She stated that she had been tripping while climbing stairs and near the curbs in the street. This came on insidiously, and she noticed difficulty bending the right foot toward her face. She denied any trauma, fever, travel history, or tick bite. She reported new low back pain but denied any neck pain, numbness, pins and needles, or bowel/bladder disturbances. The pain did not radiate and was not exacerbated by coughing or straining. Upon questioning, she informed us that she was experiencing dull headaches starting about 1 month ago. The headaches were described as shock-like shooting pains on the left side of the face and behind the eye, occurring 10 to 20 times per day. She denied any nausea, vomiting, fever, or trouble with light or sounds. She had no visual complaints or any other common neurological symptoms.

PAST MEDICAL HISTORY

Hypertension; prior myocardial infarction.

PAST SURGICAL HISTORY

Heart angioplasty

ALLERGY

NKDA.

PERSONAL HISTORY

She smoked in her early 20s for about 5 years. She denied significant alcohol use. She currently lives alone and independently, requiring no assistance for her activities of daily living.

FAMILY HISTORY

Noncontributory.

PHYSICAL EXAMINATION

Vital signs were all normal.

NEUROLOGICAL EXAMINATION

Mental status examination was normal.
CN II-XII: Revealed pupillary asymmetry with the left pupil larger than the right; impaired left eye adduction and decreased pin prick sensation along the left V2 distribution.
Motor: 3/5 weakness of the right foot on dorsiflexion, eversion, and inversion.
Sensory: Intact for all modalities of sensation.
Reflexes: Symmetrical.
Plantars: Flexors.
Gait: Right steppage gait.

DIAGNOSTIC TEST RESULTS

Basic labs including CBC, metabolic profile, and hepatic function were normal.

MRI of the LS spine demonstrated nodular enhancement at the L5 level (see pre- and postgadolinium spine images, Figure 16.1A and 16.1B).

MRI of the brain reveals diffuse enhancement in the subarachnoid space (refer Figure 16.2A and 16.2B). CSF analysis demonstrated no WBCs or RBCs, glucose of 31, and protein of 98; CSF ACE level negative, VDRL negative, and viral PCRs were negative; cytology was positive for malignant cells.

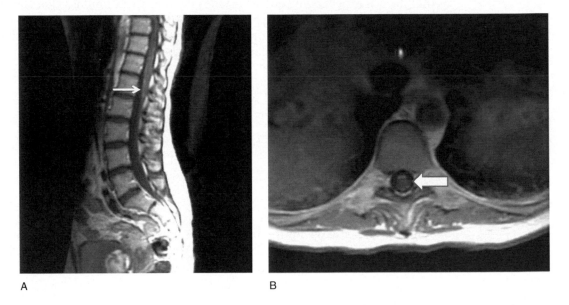

A   B

FIGURE 16.1 *Sagittal T1 postcontrast (A) and axial T1 postcontrast (B) showing meningeal enhancement.*

DIAGNOSIS: Cavernous malformation (CM); leptomeningeal metastases.

DISCUSSION

CM occurs when cancer cells spread to the CSF. CM usually represents a late stage of disease in patients with known cancer, but less commonly can be an initial presenting symptom. As the CSF space is large and bathes many neural structures, the presenting signs and symptoms can be highly variable. However, this leads to the cardinal feature of CM—multifocal neurologic deficits involving cranial nerves and/or peripheral nerves and/or nonspecific symptoms.

Theoretically, any systemic cancer or primary CNS tumor can invade the leptomeninges. However, a number of solid cancers invade the leptomeninges more frequently, especially

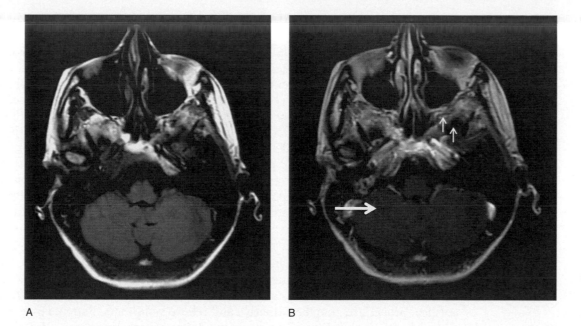

FIGURE 16.2 *Axial MRI brain T1 precontrast (A) and T1 postcontrast (B) showing enhancement in the cerebellar folia, a common place where leptomeningeal metastases can be seen.*

breast or lung cancer, or hematologic malignancies. Therefore, in a patient without a cancer diagnosis, breast or lung cancer should be seriously considered. The incidence of CM appears to be increasing. However, this is due in part to better detection techniques, especially the MRI techniques. Also, as systemic treatment improves, if these therapies do not penetrate the CNS, it may act as a sanctuary in which these cells can survive. The signs and symptoms of CM can be either nonspecific or specific.

Nonspecific symptoms include headache, nausea and/or vomiting, and lethargy (often arise due to hydrocephalus caused by CM), or back or neck pain (mimic pain due to degenerative spinal disease).

Specific symptoms can result from involvement of cranial nerves, peripheral nerves, or parenchymal invasion. The most common pattern is mononeuropathy, mononeuropathy multiplex, radiculopathy, and/or symptoms of hydrocephalus. Neurologic examination can help narrow down the list of differential diagnoses.

The diagnosis of CM can be difficult to establish. The two most common techniques for detecting CM are contrast-enhanced MRI and CSF analysis. The more definitive examination is CSF analysis; however, contrast-enhanced MRI of the involved location (either brain or spine) should be performed first. MRI will also allow determination of safety for spinal tap, to ensure there are no large masses that would put the patient at risk for herniation. CM on MRI can be

- focal or multifocal
- thin and linear or lumpy and nodular

Often, imaging is sought of both the brain and the spine. The contrast-enhanced T1 sequence will demonstrate enhancement following a sulcal pattern in the brain or enhancement along cranial or peripheral nerves, the brain stem, or spinal cord.

In a small percentage of patients, MRI will be negative, and in those patients, CSF analysis needs to be performed. Although more specific than MRI, CSF analysis is often less positive. CSF analysis can help exclude other diagnostic possibilities such as infections or inflammatory conditions. Often, repeat spinal taps need to be performed. CSF should be tested for cells, glucose, protein, cytology, and cancer-specific markers. The examination of CSF may reveal a lymphocytic pleocytosis, hypoglycorrhachia (low glucose in the CSF), elevated protein, and malignant cells. Although not all of these abnormalities are usually seen together, the CSF is often abnormal in some respect. Some tumor-specific markers may be present, for example β-HcG in a germinoma patient.

An even smaller number of patients will have a normal MRI and normal CSF. In these patients, if CM is suspected, repeat spinal tap should be performed. In addition, other processes that may involve the leptomeningeal compartment should be investigated, including infectious, autoimmune, inflammatory, or vasculitic diseases, or other multifocal processes.

TREATMENT

The treatment of CM involves both symptomatic (nonsteroidal and narcotic analgesics) and disease-specific treatment. One of the most important management issues may arise with hydrocephalus. Patients may need shunt placement for hydrocephalus, which although a surgical procedure, may be palliative and relieve symptoms. Patients may need pain control and antiemetics. Dexamethasone, in addition to treating any edema or inflammatory response associated with the CM, may also help as an antiemetic.

The treatment of CM itself involves both radiotherapy and chemotherapy. Focal radiation to bulky or symptomatic areas may provide palliation and is the treatment of choice in these scenarios. Chemotherapy is also sometimes used, either initially or after RT failure.

Theoretically, as the CSF space is the compartment involved in CM, delivering chemotherapy directly into that space should be helpful. However, in reality, this is often only helpful when there is no bulky disease and the patient has mild or no symptoms after RT. Intrathecal chemotherapy can be given via Ommaya reservoir or lumbar puncture. Caution must be given to patients with abnormal CSF flow, which can be determined via flow study, as this will impair drug distribution in the CSF. The two most commonly used agents for intrathecal therapy are methotrexate and cytarabine.

Systemic chemotherapies may be beneficial in some patients. Systemic high-dose intravenous methotrexate has been used; however, this requires patients to receive treatment on an inpatient basis, which itself may impact quality of life. Other drugs such as capecitabine (breast) or gemcitabine (lung) may be helpful. Hopefully, in the future, newer targeted therapies, such as antiangiogenic therapies, will improve survival.

PROGNOSIS

Despite current treatments, the prognosis remains dismal, with an average overall survival of approximately 2 to 3 months. One treatment option that should be discussed, especially if palliative radiotherapy fails, is stopping treatment. It is important to remember that not pursuing further treatment may be the "treatment" of choice for some patients.

SUGGESTED READING

DeAngelis LM, Posner JB. *Neurologic Complications of Cancer.* New York: Oxford University Press; 2009.

Drappatz J, Batchelor TT. Leptomeningeal and peripheral nerve metastases. *Continuum.* 2005;11(5): 47–68.

Lassman AB, Abrey LE, Shah GG, et al. Systemic high-dose intravenous methotrexate for central nervous system metastases. *J Neurooncol.* 2006;78:255–260.

Rikki Racela, Varendra Gosein, and Anuradha Singh

CHIEF COMPLAINT: **Face is all paralyzed for the last 3 days.**

HISTORY OF PRESENT ILLNES

Patient was a 42-year-old, right-handed man who complained of weakness of the left side of his face for the last 3 days. He woke up with a "funny feeling" on the left side of his face. He did not feel any numbness or tingling but it just "felt weird." His left lip seemed droopy and he found it was hard to move the left side of his face. His friends commented that his speech was not very clear. By the end of the day, he noticed that the droopiness progressed from his lip to his entire left cheek and some of his left eyelid. Two days prior to admission, his entire left face was not moving, and he could not lift the left side of his mouth to speak clearly. He had never experienced similar symptoms in the past. Patient denied any fever or chills, recent illnesses, or headache. He denied any visual or hearing problems. He did not notice any weakness of his arms, hands, or legs. He had mild aches and pains in his arms, legs, and back for the past month and was prescribed Percocet. He had noticed a rash on his back a month ago that had completely dissipated.

PAST MEDICAL HISTORY

None.

PAST SURGICAL HISTORY

Appendectomy.

MEDICATIONS

Percocet 5/325 mg 1 to 2 tabs qid PRN.

ALLERGIES

NKDA.

PERSONAL HISTORY

Denied smoking or using illicit drugs, drinks alcohol occasionally.

FAMILY HISTORY

Not significant.

PHYSICAL EXAMINATION

Vitals: Blood pressure, 132/78; pulse, 66; R 12, pulse oximetry: 99% on room air. Patient had diffuse, slight joint and muscle tenderness. His skin had no rashes. Other systems showed no abnormal findings on examination.

NEUROLOGICAL EXAMINATION

Mental status: Awake, alert, and oriented × 3. He had knowledge of current events, normal affect, and normal language comprehension and expression and could recall three objects.

CNs II–XII: All normal except CN VII examination showed bilateral lower motor neuron facial paresis, left worse than right; patient could not smile on left; slight smile on right; could not wrinkle forehead on left; could slightly wrinkle forehead on the right.
Motor: Normal muscle bulk and tone, strength 5/5 arms and legs bilaterally.
Sensory: Normal to all modalities.
Reflexes: 2+ and symmetrical.
Coordination: normal.
Romberg: negative.
Gait: normal.

STOP AND THINK QUESTIONS

➢ Has he had a stroke?

➢ How do you differentiate between a central versus a peripheral facial lesion?

➢ Can VII nerve paralysis be bilateral?

DIAGNOSTIC TEST RESULTS

ESR 48; CRP 27; Chest X-ray: Normal
EKG: normal sinus rhythm.
CT head without contrast: Normal.
MRI head with and without gadolinium: Abnormal enhancement of the VII nerve bilaterally and of the left V nerve (see Figure 17.1).
CSF: Clear and colorless, glucose: 53, protein 203. Cell count: RBCs 365, WBCs 185 (89% lymphs, 4% polys, atypical lymphocytes present), Gram stain and culture negative.
CSF Lyme Western blot: IgM 3/3 bands positive (need two for positive result).
IgG 7/11 bands positive (need 5 for positive result).

DIAGNOSIS: **CNS Lyme disease.**

DISCUSSION

This patient had bilateral Bell's palsy. Bell's palsy is the most common cranial neuropathy.
Anatomy of Cranial Nerve VII (Facial Nerve): The facial nerve is one of a pair of nerves arising between the pons and medulla. The motor fibers of CN VII arise from its nucleus

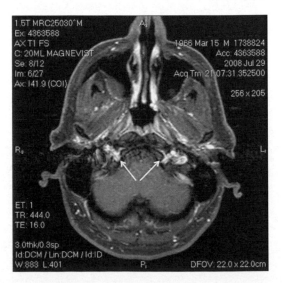

FIGURE 17.1 *Abnormal enhancement of cranial nerve VII.*

located in the lower one third of the pons. Supranuclear part refers to fibers above the level of the nucleus. Facial motor areas reside in the precentral and postcentral gyri of the cerebral cortex. Facial fibers descend through the corticobulbar areas and go through the internal capsule, midbrain, and the pons. The corticobulbar tracts from the lower face cross once, but fibers from the upper face cross and recross on their way to the pons. The *efferent* pathway stimulates the muscles of facial expression. The afferent pathways carry taste sensations from the anterior two thirds of the tongue, some pain sensations and comprises of secretomotor fibers from lacrimal, submandibular, sublingual glands, mucus membranes of the nasopharynx, and the hard and soft palates (see Figure 17.2). The facial nerve consists of both motor and sensory fibers, with motor and sensory tracts arising from and synapsing at different locations in the brain stem. Emotional facial expression is thought to originate in the thalamus and globus pallidus and seems to be spared in supranuclear lesions.

The sensory portion begins at the superior salivatory nucleus and courses through the nervus intermedius or nerve of Wrisberg. The sensory and motor tracts meet and exit the

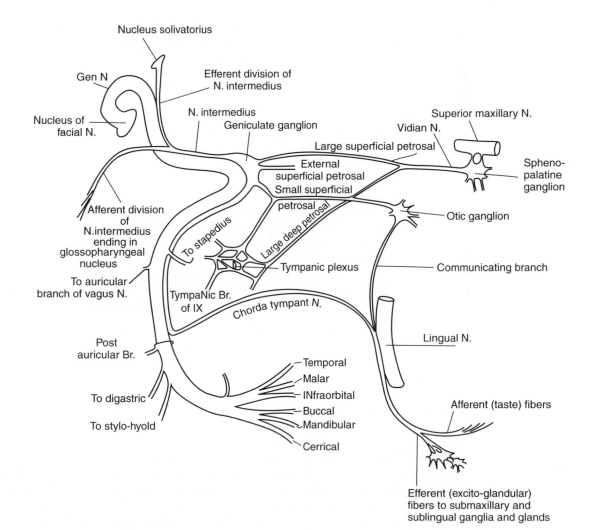

FIGURE 17.2 *Anatomy of the facial nerve.*

brain stem together as the facial nerve to enter the internal auditory meatus. It then passes through the facial canal in the temporal bone. Facial nerve carries motor, sensory, and parasympathetic innervations to different areas as described below.

1. **General sensations:** General sensory information from the concha of the external ear and behind the earlobe courses with the motor fibers through the stylomastoid foramen to synapse at the geniculate ganglion. It then exits the internal auditory meatus as part of the nervus intermedius and synapses in the spinal nucleus of the trigeminal nerve.

2. **Parasympathetic innervation:** The parasympathetic innervation begins at the superior salivatory nucleus in the pons. Fibers from this nucleus help form the nervus intermedius. Through its course in the facial canal, these fibers branch to form two nerves, the greater petrosal nerve and the chorda tympani. The greater petrosal nerve exits the facial canal through the petrosal foramen. It then joins with sympathetic fibers of the deep petrosal nerve and forms the *vidian nerve* (also known as the nerve of the pterygoid canal). The parasympathetic fibers from this nerve then synapse at the pterygopalatine ganglion in the pterygopalatine fossa and subsequently innervate the lacrimal gland and the mucus membranes of the nasopharynx. The fibers of the chorda tympani serve two distinct functions. Upon exiting the base of the skull, the parasympathetic fibers join the lingual branch of CN V3, synapse at the submandibular ganglion, and then innervate the sublingual gland. The second function of the chorda tympani is to carry taste sensation from the anterior two third of the tongue, hard, and soft palates. Taste sensation from these areas is carried from the lingual nerve to the chorda tympani, to the nervus intermedius. Fibers synapse at the geniculate ganglion, then join the tractus solitarius and eventually synapse in the gustatory nucleus.

3. **Motor innervation:** The motor fibers of the facial nerve pass through the geniculate ganglion without synapsing, and exit through the stylomastoid foramen. Before it exits, however, the nerve to the stapedius muscle emerges. Then, upon exiting the stylomastoid foramen, three motor nerves emerge. These are the posterior auricular nerve, the nerve to the posterior belly of the digastric, and the nerve to the stylomastoid muscle. The remaining fibers pass through the parotid gland without innervating it, and give off five branches. These include the temporal branch, the zygomatic branch, the buccal branch, the mandibular branch, and the cervical branch. These branches innervate the muscles of facial expression.

Central Versus Peripheral Facial Nerve Lesion: A peripheral facial nerve (also known as LMN) lesion results in a Bell's palsy. This results in upper and lower facial weakness on the same side of the lesion. This occurs because the motor neurons that innervate muscles of the upper face receive input from the motor cortex of both cerebral hemispheres. However, the lower facial muscles receive input from the contralateral motor cortex. Therefore, a lesion of the facial nerve or its nucleus will result in ipsilateral upper and lower facial weakness. A lesion to the upper motor neuron of a facial nerve (also known as central lesion) will result in weakness of contralateral lower facial weakness.

Bell's palsy is an acute unilateral paralysis of the face thought to be from inflammation of CN VII. It is named after Sir Charles Bell (1774–1842) who studied facial nerve and its anatomy extensively during the Battle of Waterloo. Onset is usually abrupt. Occasionally, a patient identifies a preceding viral illness, and also about 50% of patients will complain of pain in the mastoid area. Patients frequently notice trouble tolerating the typical levels of noise called *hyperacusis* due to paralysis of the stapedius muscle. The patient may also have ipsilateral loss of taste in the anterior two thirds of the tongue called "dysgeusia." The House-Brackmann grading (see Table 17.1) system has been widely used to grade the degree of facial nerve involvement. In this scale, grade I is considered as normal function, and grade VI refers to complete paralysis. About 85% of patients will have close to or total recovery from the deficit.

Most cases of Bell's palsy are idiopathic, although there are numerous treatable causes that should be worked up. For example, vesicles noted in the auditory canal should raise suspicion of Ramsay Hunt syndrome (Table 17.2), a herpes zoster infection of the facial nerve. Complicated otitis media can cause injury to the VII nerve. A patient with an associated hearing deficit and/or CN V deficit may have an acoustic neuroma or other pontocerebellar neoplasm. If the patient had lung disease, uveitis, parotitis, or bilateral hilar lymphadenopathy on chest X-ray, this would suggest neurosarcoidosis. Incidence of Bell's is 29% higher in patients with diabetes. Women with pregnancy in their third trimester are more likely to get Bell's palsy. Blacks and the Japanese race may have a slightly higher incidence.

Our patient is interesting in that he has bilateral Bell's palsy, which can be caused by neurosarcoidosis, myasthenia gravis, and Lyme disease. The patient gives a good history indicative of CNS Lyme disease. The patient says he walks in the park all the time with his son, and 1 month ago had a rash on his back. He was unable to describe the rash but the typical rash in Lyme is called "erythema migrans," which describes a bull's eye rash, with redness and an area of central clearing. This rash is pathognomonic and warrants instant treatment for Lyme disease until proven otherwise. The patient describes fatigue, diffuse muscle and joint pain after the rash along with lymphadenopathy, and headache, which can be a manifestation of Lyme disease. After resolution of the rash the bacteria that cause Lyme, *Borrelia burgdoferi*, can spread to the heart, joints, and CNS. On physical examination, the patient had bilateral Bell's without vesicles in the auditory canals.

TABLE 17.1 *House-Brackmann Score for Bell's Palsy*

Grade	Description	Measurement	Function (%)	Estimated Function (%)
I	Normal	8/8	100	100
II	Slight	7/8	76–99	80
III	Moderate	5/8–6/8	51–75	60
IV	Moderately Severe	3/8–4/8	26–50	40
V	Severe	1/8–2/8	1–25	20
VI	Total	0/8	0	0

TABLE 17.2 *Pathogenesis of Bell's Palsy*

Infectious	HSV (first most common cause), herpes zoster oticus (Ramsay Hunt syndrome), CMV, Lyme, EBV, syphilis, acute mastoiditis, acute parotitis
Physiological	Pregnancy (threefold risk)
Endocrine disorders	Diabetes (account for 5%–10% of cases), hypothyroidism
Immunological disorders	Sarcoidosis, lupus, Sjogren's, MCTD
Vasular/Ischemic	Benign intracranial hypertension
Hereditary	
Congenital	Mobius syndrome, Treacher Collins syndrome
Neoplasm	Facial neuroma, acoustic neuroma
Iatrogenic	Neurosurgical interventions/radiation therapy such as acoustic neuroma surgery or parotid gland surgery or brain stem tumors
Trauma	Temporal bone fracture, barotrauma

TABLE 17.3 *Treatment of Bell's Palsy*

Prednisolone (tapering doses) + Valacycloovir	Prednisolone 20 mg tid ×5 days
	Prednisolone 10 mg tid ×3 days
	Prednisolone 10 mg once daily ×2 days
	500 mg bid for 5 days
Ophthalmic care	Taping/eye patch, artificial tears, lacrilube, tarsorraphy (gold weight to upper eyelid to facilitate eye closure) sunglasses
	Avoid wearing contact lenses
Surgical decompression	Middle fossa approach, transmastoid, retrolabyrinthine, retrosignoid, translabyrinthine

Diagnostic studies included an MRI, which ruled out possible tumor involvement, as well as demonstrated inflammation of the facial nerves, supportive of a diagnosis of Lyme. Finally, CSF studies showed aseptic meningitis and were positive for Lyme disease by Western blot.

TREATMENT

Management of Bell's palsy is conservative but surgical decompression may be required under rare circumstances (refer to Table 17.3). Medical treatment includes steroids and antiviral agents. High- to low-dose steroids have been used in the treatment of Bell's palsy. Facial reconstructive surgery may be offered to patients with significant facial asymmetry.

Patient's age, comorbid conditions, and return of muscle function should be evaluated against the risks of surgical intervention. EMG studies can be helpful to prognosticate the spontaneous recovery. The presence of active voluntary motor units action potentials (VMUAP) suggests intact motor axon. Complete absence of VMUAP is indicative of complete nerve degeneration. However, presence of polyphasic VMUAP suggests regeneration of the facial nerve.

SUGGESTED READING

Brazis et al. *Localization in Clinical Neurology.* 5th ed. Lippincott Williams and Wilkins, New York 2007:287–306.

Gantz B. Surgical management of Bell's palsy. *Laryngoscope.* August 1999;109(8):1177–1188.

Steere A. Medical progress: Lyme disease. *NEJM.* July 12, 2001;345(2):115–125.

Anuradha Singh, John Engler, and Ramesh P. Babu

CHIEF COMPLAINT: **Right leg pain for the past 2 years.**

HISTORY OF PRESENT ILLNESS

Patient is a 34-year-old, right-handed female from Pakistan who was referred to a neurology clinic for severe pain in her right leg and back pain for the past 2 years. At the onset, she recalls experiencing severe pain in the back upon awakening. Since last year, pain has been progressively getting worse. Any kind of physical activity or prolonged standing makes the pain worse. Pain can be 8 to 9/10 at times. There has been slight improvement in her pain after she had an ESI. She has had at least 3 or 4 ESI in the past. Pain is described both as deep and sharp over the lower back and right thigh (front and back). She cannot stand for a long time. She has been using a walker for the past couple of months. Pain would radiate to the front and back of her right thigh and occasionally to the top of the right foot. She has no weakness or loss of sensations but pain does not allow her to walk or perform her daily chores. She denies any history of falls or trauma. She did not give any history of fever or generalized malaise. She denies any bladder or bowel problems. She denies any neck pain and weakness or numbness in the arms or over the body.

PAST MEDICAL HISTORY

As above; otherwise, in good health.

PAST SURGICAL HISTORY

Cholecystectomy.

MEDICATIONS

Tramadol 100 mg bid
Flexeril 10 mg bid
Gabapentin 300 mg tid

ALLERGIES

None.

PERSONAL HISTORY

No smoking, drugs, or alcohol. She lives in Brooklyn with her husband and her family. She has had several miscarriages. She has one alive and healthy child from a triplet pregnancy; other two were stillbirths.

PHYSICAL EXAMINATION

Mildly obese; blood pressure, 120/82 mm Hg, pulse, 84/min, Afebrile, respiratory rate, 14/min.

DIAGNOSTIC TEST RESULTS

MRI LS spine showed mild to moderate scoliosis, straightening of the lumbar spine, moderate chronic endplate signal change at L5/S1, L4/L5, and L5/S1 disc desiccation, annular tear at L4/L5, posterior disc changes, small to moderate posterolateral/right paracentral protrusion at L1/L2, mild to moderate bulge with posterolateral bilateral paracentral protrusion at L4/L5. Moderate to large right paracentral, posterocentral, and posterolateral protrusion at L5/S1 (see Figure 18.1A and 18.1B). There is inferior extrusion component at this level, maximal inferior extension from superior S1 endplate of about 7 mm, no sign of sequestered fragment. PLL appears intact. Mild to moderate bilateral L4/L5 degenerative changes and central canal stenosis at L4/L5 and L5/S1, right lateral recess stenosis at L5 and S1 and mild right L5 and S1 neuroforaminal narrowing. There are bilateral facet joint degenerative hypertrophy noted at L4/L5 and L5 and S1.

EMG/NCS lower extremities at Upstate—does not know the results.

NEUROLOGICAL EXAMINATION

Higher mental functions: Alert and oriented to time, place and person, speech fluent, normal comprehension and expression, affect normal, memory 3/3 at 1 and 5 minutes.

CNs II–XII: PERRL, EOMI, no nystagmus, facial sensation intact, no facial asymmetry, hearing normal by whispering method, SCM and trapezii intact, tongue midline, no atrophy.

Motor: Full strength against resistance in arm flexion/extension, arm abduction/adduction; hip flexion/extension, leg flexion/extension, foot dorsiflexion/plantar flexion; no pronator drift; Extensor hallucis longus and gluteus medii normal strength 5/5.

STOP AND THINK QUESTIONS

➢ What is the etiology of this patient's one-sided lower extremity pain?

➢ Which neuroimaging of the spine will be most helpful to see any nerve root compression?

➢ When will you refer this patient to a neurosurgeon?

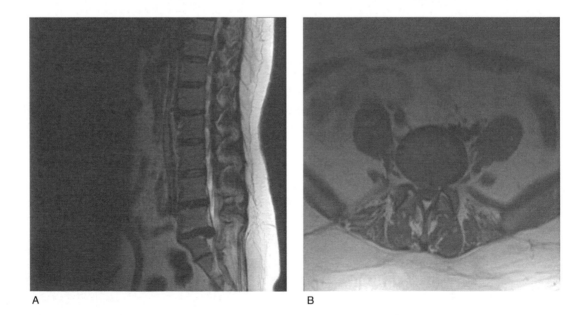

A   B

FIGURE 18.1 *Moderate to large right paracentral, posterocentral, and posterolateral protrusion at L5/S1 on Sagittal (A) and Axial (B) MRI Lumbosacral spine.*

Sensory: Vibration, soft touch, pin prick, temperature intact bilaterally.
Reflexes: 2+ symmetrical biceps, triceps, brachioradialis, patellar, achillis both sides.
Plantars: Down.
Coordination: Finger-to-nose, heel-to-shin, rapid alternating hand movements intact.
Gait: Antalgic, broad based, walks with a walker, right lower extremity everted and lordotic.
Romberg test: Negative.
Straight Leg Raise Test: Positive.
Femoral Stretch Test: Positive.

DIAGNOSIS: Right L5-S1 intervertebral disc herniation.

DISCUSSION

Lower back pain is one of the most common problems seen in neurology outpatient clinics and is the major cause of work disability worldwide. Congenital, traumatic, and degenerative causes are common causes of back pain. Back pain cases are on the rise with increasing obesity rates, sedentary lifestyle, and prolonged hours of sitting in front of the computers and sports-related injuries in the United States. Other etiologies include myofascial syndrome, infectious, inflammatory, metabolic, metastases, and psychological. Referred pain from retroperitoneal or pelvic inflammatory disease should not be forgotten in the differential diagnosis.

Lumbar disc herniation affects people in middle age (30–50 years), males more than females. The nerve is compressed showing first pain, then tingling, then numbness, last loss of movement (drop foot). Herniation at L4-5 affects L5 nerve root, which will weaken the extensor of the leg (dorsiflex foot; extend toes). Herniation at L5-S1 affects S1 nerve root, which causes weakness of leg flexors (plantar flex foot; flex toes). If the lumbar disc is herniated, its corresponding vertebra has an obvious tender area. When the area is pressed, pain occurs along the sciatic nerve distribution. Nerve root tension can be elicited by performing, beside clinical examination:

Lasegue's Test: It is performed in a supine position. If there is pain in the lumbar area and lateral leg on performing a straight leg raise up to 70° and dorsiflexing the foot, the test is positive.

Kernig's Test: Severe stiffness of the hamstrings causes an inability to straighten the leg when the hip is flexed to 90 degrees.

Wasserman's Test: (Prone) The hip joint is overextended. If pain presents at the anterior border of the thigh, the test is positive.

Lindner's Test: The patient's neck is passively flexed, gradually bringing the chin to the chest. If pain occurs at the lower back and leg, the test is positive, because of meningeal irritation.

Anatomy: The intervertebral discs are made of fibrocartilage that connects the vertebral bodies. These act like shock absorbers. The thickness of a lumbar disc is about 12.7 mm. The central part of the disc is made of collagen and proteoglycans with high water-retaining capacity called nucleus pulposus and the peripheral fibrous part is called annulus fibrosus. T2WI of normal discs show brighter signal of nucleus pulposus while annulus fibrosus and cortical bone appear darker. Hyaline cartilage of the superior and inferior surfaces of the vertebral body helps bear the weight and protects the nucleus pulposus. Ligamental support is provided anteriorly by ALL and posteriorly by PLL. The PLL extends from axis to the sacrum and gets thinned out caudally. L5-S1 is the most common site of disc herniation in the lumbosacral region. It is believed that annular tear leading to disc herniation is the result of repetitive torsional stress in a degenerative disc. The disc can herniate anteriorly through the ALL or the nucleus pulposus may drill through the hyaline cartilage into vertebral body forming "Schmorl's nodes."

DEGENERATIVE CHANGES IN THE DISC

With aging, several changes can be seen, such as:

- Loss of height of disc
- Disc signal becomes darker and more homogeneous (black discs)
- Increased fatty bone marrow infiltration resulting in brighter vertebral signal
- Vacuum phenomenon: the presence of a linear radiolucency in the disc space as a result of nitrogen gas, most commonly seen in L4-L5-S1.
- End plate changes: The signal intensity changes in vertebral body marrow adjacent to the endplates of degenerative discs were first described by Michael T. Modic in 1988. These have been classified into three main types: Modic Type I-III (see Table 18.1).
- Disc bulge: Annular fibers are intact.
- Disc protrusion: Damage of some annular fibers with focal bulging.
- Disc extrusion: Loss of all annular fibers with extended bulge.
- Disc sequestration: Part of the disc breaks off from the nucleus pulposus, losing its connection with the mother disc; these can wander both caudally or cranially. The extruded disc material may shrink slowly over couple of years. It can reside in the neuroforamen or lateral recess and compress dorsal root ganglion or penetrate the dura.

TREATMENT

Conservative: Most of the cases with lumbar disc herniation and radicular symptoms resolve on their own within about 2 weeks. Non-steroidal anti-inflammatory drugs, oral steroids (prednisone or methylprednisone),

Translaminar lumbar epidural steroid injections can be performed under fluoroscopic guidance. Triamcinolone 40 to 80 mg or methylprednisolone 40 to 80 mg with local anesthetic is injected by 20 gauge Touhy needle on the right or left side based on patient's pain location. Local anesthetic provides immediate relief, while steroids anti-inflammatory response takes about 12 to 48 hours.

Transforamainal ESI is another alternative approach when translaminar ESI fails to relieve the symptoms or when there is a correlating lesion on the MR with radiculopathy. 22 G spinal needle is directed under fluoroscopy into foramen of affect nerve root and

TABLE 18.1 *Modic Classification of Endplate Degenerative Changes*

Modic Type	T1WI	T2WI	Histological Changes
I	Hypointense	Hyperintense	Marrow edema; disruption and fissuring of the endplate, granulation tissue within subchondral bone
II	Hyperintense	Iso or slightly hyperintense	Endplate disruption with yellow marrow replacement in the adjacent vertebral body, Fatty degeneration of subchondral marrow
III	Hypointense	Hypointense	No marrow left to produce MRI signal, dense woven bone and extensive bony sclerosis

contrast is injected to confirm entry into the epidural space. This approach requires less dose of steroid/local anesthetic.

Risks of ESI include bleeding, infection, localized tenderness, postdural puncture headache, and paresthesias. Selected nerve root block can be helpful in radicular pains. A 22G needle is inserted lateral to spinous process, directly medially to lower border of root of transverse process.

Surgical intervention for disc herniation: Dandy (1) first reported a case of intervertebral disc herniation in 1929, but it was not until 1934 when Mixter and Barr (2) compiled the evidence from several case reports, as well as their own series of 11 patients, that the link between intervertebral disc herniations and sciatica became elucidated. The surgery was initially performed using an extensive lumbar laminectomy and transdural disc removal. This procedure remained largely unchanged until the 1960s when the advent of microsurgical techniques allowed for less extensive exposure and bony removal. Yasargil (3) and Caspar (4) first described using the operative microscope in 1977 and Williams (5) popularized the procedure in the United States the following year. The use of the operating microscope and newer microsurgical techniques allowed for the development of the hemilaminotomy as an exposure for microdiscectomy. The original laminectomy and facetectomy used by Mixter and Barr involved complete removal of the lamina at the offending level with wide disruption of the facets. Over time, this extensive bony removal leads to spinal instability with associated kyphosis and scoliosis. The improved lighting and visualization of the microscope permits the surgeon to safely access the disc space through a hemilaminotomy, that is, removal of one half of the lamina, without significant disruption of the bony facets, thereby preserving spinal stability. More recently, minimally invasive approaches have been developed, which allow for the creation of the hemilaminotomy and disc removal to be performed through a three-quarter-inch tube with either the help of the microscope or endoscope for visualization.

Approximately 250 to 300,000 procedures are performed in the United States annually for low back pain, and lumbar microdiscectomy has become the most common neurosurgical procedure in the United States. Despite the large volume of surgeries performed annually in the United States, the surgical morbidity and mortality are low. Surgical technique must be soundly maintained to prevent temporary or even permanent neurologic injury from overzealous nerve root retraction, and to prevent dural tears that can lead to wound healing problems as well as a potential route for the introduction of postoperative wound infection and meningitis (see Table 18.2).

The current goal standard for unilateral disc herniations is the hemilaminotomy and medial facetectomy (see Table 18.3). The addition of the medial facetectomy allows for better visualization of the disc space, while limiting nerve root retraction. Structural integrity of the lumbar spine is maintained by limiting the medial facetectomy to less than one third of the facet. The procedure is typically done as an outpatient surgery with a typical hospital stay of less than 24 hours. The decision to operate on disc herniations is made by correlating the level of the patient's disc herniation on MRI with the appropriate symptomatology. The operation is done under general endotracheal anesthesia. The patient will be placed in a prone position on a variety of frames. If the frames are not available, gel rolls may be substituted with the goal of preventing pressure on the abdomen, which would cause epidural venous engorgement and increases the blood loss and difficulty of surgery. After positioning the patient prone, careful attention is taken to pad all pressure points so as to protect the patient from developing pressure ulcers and postoperative peripheral nerve palsies due to positioning-related compression. Once the back of the lumbar area is sterilely prepped and draped, an X-ray is done to identify the levels of the surgery and minimize the extent of the incision. The incision is made in the midline with lateral retraction of the paraspinal muscles.

After the level is again confirmed using intraoperative X-ray, the microscope is brought in and under high-power magnification; a high-speed air drill is used to create a hemilaminotomy at the appropriate level. The hemilaminotomy involves removal of the inferior portion of the lamina directly superior to the disc herniation as well as the superior aspect of the lamina directly inferior to the disc herniation. As previously stated, a medial facetectomy encompassing up to one third of the width of the facet may also be performed to aid in exposure and limit nerve root retraction. Once drilling is completed the ligamentum flavum is visualized, which is cleared from its attachments from the superior and inferior lamina and is removed as a single piece. This brings the nerve root and the dural tube into the view and allows for identification of the disc herniation. If the patient symptoms result from an extruded disc fragment, the fragment can often be removed without entering into the disc space. The annular tear through which the extruded disc fragment migrated will spontaneously heal without further surgical manipulation. However, if the annulus is intact and posterior longitude ligament is intact, an incision must be made into the annulus to allow exploration of the disc space and removal of any herniated intervertebral discs. In these cases, once the accomplishment of herniated disc material has been removed the wounds will be closed in a routine manner.

With this approach, no additional lumbar stabilization is required and patients are typically ambulatory on the same day of surgery and discharged within 24 hours of surgery. The most common complications from surgery include postoperative infection and dural tears resulting in a cerebrospinal fluid leak. Postoperative infections can usually be treated with a course of intravenous antibiotics, with the rare cases requiring reoperation for wound revision and debridement. Intraoperative dural tears can be repaired primarily by suturing the dural defect closed with a nonabsorbable suture, bolstered by an onlay of biodegradable glue. Persistent or recurrent CSF leaks may be treated by a trial of lumbar drainage, which diverts the CSF through an external catheter placed in the lumbar subarachnoid space via a lumbar puncture. The diversion of fluid through the catheter allows the dural tear to heal by reducing fluid tensions at the site of the defect. Postoperative incisional pain is managed with narcotics, and postoperative radicular pain from intraoperative nerve root manipulation is treated with a trial of steroids. Patients with severe preoperative radicular pain respond quickly after surgery with near complete resolution of their pain, whereas weakness and numbness can take months to several years to recover.

Other techniques include percutaneous lumbar microdiscectomy and percutaneous laser decompression. These are mainly done by pain management specialists to decrease the intradiscal pressure and allow for regression of the herniated fragment back into the disc space. These procedures are not indicated for extruded disc fragments. The patient with back pain and only with minimal radicular pain would respond to this kind of a procedure. The chemonucleolysis, which is an injection of chymopapain, has been used and because of the allergic reactions, it has been given up in the neurosurgical community. Cauda equina syndrome is an absolute indication for surgery. Severe and progressive motor deficits of recent onset also warrant neurosurgical intervention. Some of the relative indications for surgery are listed in Table 18.4.

Absence of lower back pain, nonwork-related injury, minimal psychosocial stressors, radicular pain with positive tension signs and higher socioeconomic status have been associated with better outcomes.

There is lack of optimal timing of the surgery. Cauda equina is a neurosurgical emergency. Surgery should rarely be done in less than 6 weeks after the onset of symptoms because spontaneous resolution of symptoms is more likely. The chances of improvement

TABLE 18.2 *Complications of Surgery for Disc Herniation*

Recurrent herniation (5%–15%)
Durotomy (0.8%–7.2%)
Nerve root damage (0.2%)
Infection (2%–3%)
Epidural hematoma
Epidural fibrosis
Iatrogenic instability
Wrong level (1.2%–3.3%)
Cauda equina syndrome

TABLE 18.3 *Surgical Interventions for Lumbar Radiculopathy*

Open Discectomy

Microdiscectomy	Shorter hospital stay
	No difference versus open discectomy after 8 to 12 weeks
	Faster return to sedentary work
Chemonucleolysis with Chympopapain	
Manual percutaneous discectomy	
Automated percutaneous nucleotomy	
Percutaneous endoscopic discectomy	
Endoscopic or percutaneous laser discectomy	

TABLE 18.4 *Absolute and Relative Indications for Surgery*

Absolute	Relative
Cauda equina syndrome	Failure of nonoperative treatment of radicular pain Severe intractable radicular pain
Recent onset, progressive motor deficits	Severe intractable radicular pain
	Large extruded discs
	Significant motor deficits
	Recurrent radicular pain
	Herniation into an already stenotic nerve root or stenotic canal
	Presence of positive nerve root tension signs

in radicular pain are slight and decrease further in patients with symptoms lasting more than 6 months.

Exogenous growth factors (promoting discal proteoglycans synthesis), gene therapy (reversing degeneration by increasing the metabolic activites of the disc cells), cell-based therapy (transforming marrow stromal cells into disc cells) are still under experimental stage.

REFERENCES

1. Dandy WE. Loose cartilage from intervertebral disk simulating tumor of the spinal cord. *Arch Surg.* 1929;19:660–672 (reference unverified).
2. Mixter WJ, Barr JS. Rupture of the intervertebral disc with involvement of the spinal canal. *N Engl J Med.* 1934;211:210–215.

3. Yasargil MG. Microsurgical operations for herniated lumbar disc. *Adv Neurosurg.* 1977;4:81–82 (reference unverified).
4. Caspar W. A new surgical procedure for lumbar disc herniation causing less tissue damage through a microsurgical approach. *Adv Neurosurg.* 1977;4:74–80.
5. Williams RW. Microlumbar discectomy: A conservative surgical approach to the virgin herniated lumbar disc. *Spine.* 1978;3:175–182.

New Onset Memory Difficulties and Episodes of Unresponsiveness

Rachel Brandstadter, Betty Mintz, and Lara V. Marcuse

CHIEF COMPLAINT: **There's something wrong with my mom's memory.**

HISTORY OF PRESENT ILLNESS

A 68-year-old woman was brought to the emergency room by her daughter with concern for a change in her behavior and memory. One month prior to the emergency room visit, her daughter noticed she would repeat things frequently, often asking the same question 4 to 5 times. Rarely, she would appear to be unresponsive for 30 seconds with her eyes open. The patient had no prior history of cognitive impairment and was celebrated throughout the family as being particularly smart and organized. Four days prior to admission, the patient began to have frequent brief episodes of unresponsiveness, now with right arm flexion and at times a right head turn. She became increasingly confused and disoriented and had frequent lapses of time and spatial disorientation.

Family denied any fever, night sweats, chronic cough, weight loss, change in bladder or bowel habits, or changes in appetite. Family did not report any skin rash. There was no history of travel.

PAST MEDICAL HISTORY

Emphysema and hypertension.

MEDICATIONS

Lisinopril 10 mg PO daily.

ALLERGIES

None.

PERSONAL HISTORY

No history of alcohol, drug, or tobacco use.

FAMILY HISTORY

Noncontributory.

PHYSICAL EXAMINATION

Blood pressure, 130/90; pulse, 76 bpm; respiratory rate, 14/min; temperatutue, 98.4°F. General examination was unremarkable.

NEUROLOGICAL EXAMINATION

She was alert and oriented to year and month but not to place or exact date. She was well groomed and her affect was normal. She was able to spell the word "WORLD" backwards and forwards. She performed serial sevens with no errors. Her immediate memory was 0/3 at 5 minutes. She was not the least bit disturbed or aware of her memory problems. She was able to repeat a ten-digit number back without errors. She could name eight animals in 1 minute. She was unable to consolidate the date or the name of the examiner. She asked the examiner on two occasions where she was. She was euthymic. The rest of the neurological exam was unremarkable. No episodes of unresponsiveness were observed in the emergency room.

STOP AND THINK QUESTIONS

➢ What is your differential diagnosis for subacute onset of behavioral changes, memory deficits, and episodes of decreased responsiveness?

➢ What test(s) would you perform to narrow your differential?

➢ What treatment can you offer her?

DIAGNOSTIC TESTS RESULTS

CBC, chemistry, LFTs, TFTs, and tumor markers were all within normal limits.

EEG: An EEG was done in the emergency room and demonstrated two 30-second left temporal seizures (Figure 19.1). The background was well organized but there was mild left temporal slowing. She was admitted to the epilepsy monitoring unit for video EEG monitoring. Thirty-nine left temporal seizures were captured. These were mostly subclinical though often there was decreased responsiveness and rarely right arm flexion. These were controlled with levetiracetam and oxcarbazepine.

Lumbar puncture: CSF was normal, with 0 RBC, 2 WBC, and normal protein and glucose. No organisms were seen on culture or Gram stain.

Brain MRI: Abnormal signal intensity in the right hippocampus, amyglada, and adjacent temporal lobe (Figure 19.2).

MR spectroscopy demonstrated an elevated choline peak.

CT chest/abdomen/pelvis with contrast: Normal.

Paraneoplastic/autoimmune antibody tests: VGKC antibodies were found in the serum. Upon further testing, LGI1 antibodies were detected in the serum and CSF.

DIAGNOSIS: Limbic encephalitis caused by antibodies to LGI1.

DISCUSSION

The patient improved for a short period of time on levetiracetam and oxcarbazepine but then deteriorated with increased confusion and difficulty consolidating. After confirmation of

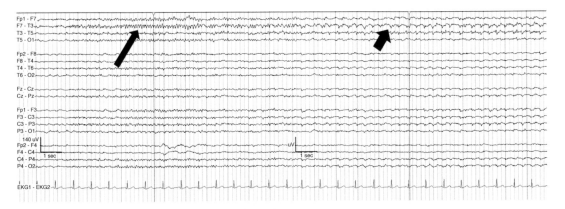

FIGURE 19.1 *EEG shows a left temporal seizure with left temporal rhythmic 9 Hz activity (long arrow) that evolves to slower 2 to 3 Hz activity (short arrow).*

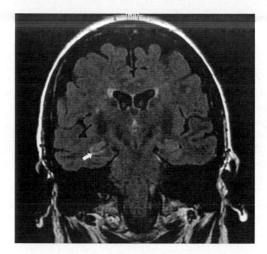

FIGURE 19.2 *Coronal T2 FLAIR MRI with increased signal in the right hippocampus (arrow).*

the LGI1 antibodies, the patient received five treatments of plasma exchange with improvement in her anterograde memory. She was discharged to a rehabilitation facility and ultimately left the hospital 10 days later.

Autoimmune encephalitides cause subacute onset of behavioral and cognitive decline that may present similarly to a wide variety of other disorders including psychiatric disorders, infectious encephalitides, metabolic imbalances, toxic exposures, dementia, prion diseases, thyroid disease, systemic autoimmune disorders, and epilepsy. Modalities that aid in diagnosis for these disorders include LP, EEG, MRI, CT, and the presence of certain serum or CSF autoantibodies. Recognition of these syndromes is critical, as they may be the initial presentation of an undiagnosed underlying malignancy that warrants treatment. However, these disorders are not always associated with malignancy. Timely diagnosis is vital because these syndromes can be very responsive to immunomodulatory treatment.

This patient's inability to consolidate new information was indicative of bitemporal cerebral dysfunction. It was initially confounding that her MRI showed *right* hippocampal hyperintensity, and her EEG showed *left* temporal seizures. This made the diagnosis of simply a seizure disorder less likely. In fact, it was the LGI1 autoantibodies manifesting differently in both temporal lobes.

Commonly encountered *antibodies to synaptic antigens* have been summarized in Table 19.1.

LGI1 Antibodies: The clinical picture of limbic encephalitis (LE) due to LGI1 antibodies involves neuropsychiatric symptoms (including anxiety, depression, confusion, delirium, and hallucinations), temporal lobe seizures, anterograde memory impairment, and sometimes, dementia. These patients may demonstrate lymphocytic pleocytosis in the CSF and often have mesial temporal signal intensity on T2/fluid–attenuated inversion-recovery (FLAIR) MRI. EEG may reveal epileptic discharges from one or both temporal lobes in the context of slow background activity. Other distinguishing features of this form of LE are associations with hyponatremia, rapid eye movement sleep behavior disorders, and male predominance.

Initially, the LGI-1 autoantibodies in the sera and CSF of patients with limbic encephalitis were falsely attributed to VGKC. LGI1 is a neuronal secreted protein that interacts to connect presynaptic disintegrin and metalloproteinase domain-containing protein 23 (ADAM 23) with postsynaptic ADAM22. Interestingly, a defect in the LGI1 gene is known to cause autosomal dominant partial epilepsy with auditory hallucinations.

TABLE 19.1 *Overview of Antibodies to Synaptic Antigens*

Antibodies	Syndrome	Most Common Associated Malignancy	% Associated With Tumor
LGI1	Limbic encephalitis	SCLC, thymoma	20
Caspr-2	Encephalitis, peripheral nerve dysfunction, Morvan syndrome	Thymoma	Not yet determined
NMDA receptor	Encephalitis, autonomic instability, movement disorder, catatonia	Ovarian teratoma	9–56
AMPA receptor	Limbic encephalitis	SCLC, breast, thymoma	70
GABA$_B$ receptor	Limbic encephalitis with high prevalence of seizures	SCLC	47

LGI1 (Leucine-rich glioma inactivated-1); NMDA (N-methyl D-aspartate); GABA (gamms-aminobutyric acid); AMPA (2-amino-3-(5-methyl-3-oxo-1, 2-oxazol-4-yl) propanoic acid); Caspr2 (contactin-associated protein like 2); SCLC (small cell lung carcinoma).

Limbic encephalitis can be paraneoplastic but only 20% of cases attributed to LGI antibodies are associated with cancer. The most common associated neoplasms are thymoma and small cell lung cancer.

Caspr2 Antibodies: Antibodies against Caspr2 are now recognized to cause clinical syndromes that were also previously ascribed to VGKCs. These syndromes include encephalitis, peripheral nerve dysfunction, and Morvan syndrome (both CNS and PNS dysfunction). These disorders may present with the following symptoms: cognitive impairment, memory loss, psychiatric symptoms (hallucinations, delusions), seizures, peripheral nerve hyperexcitability, and axonal sensorimotor neuropathy. Caspr2 antibodies can be paraneoplastic or nonparaneoplastic. The most recognized associated tumor is thymoma.

The proposed function of Caspr2 involves a role in concentrating VGKCs at the juxtaparanodal region of myelinated axons located in both the PNS and CNS. A patient with homozygous deletion of the gene that encodes Caspr2 displayed a history of seizures with progressive painful peripheral neuropathy and neuromyotonia. A genetic knockout mouse model illuminated that the peripheral neuropathy seen in patients with genetic or autoimmune Caspr2 dysfunction likely requires dysregulation of other Caspr2-related proteins as well.

NMDA Receptor Antibodies: Patients with anti-NMDA receptor antibodies experience a prodromal illness with headache and fever and then develop a variety of neuropsychiatric symptoms including perturbations in memory and behavior. Patients often initially present to a psychiatric service. These patients can have seizures, psychosis, and dyskinesias of the face, limbs, and trunk. They can also show signs of dystonia, choreoathetoid movements of the limbs, opisthotonic postures, and catatonia. Furthermore, they exhibit autonomic instability with changes in blood pressure, fluctuation in cardiac rhythm, hyperthermia, and central hypoventilation that may require long-term mechanical ventilation. The differential diagnosis should include other autoimmune encephalitides, viral encephalitides, toxic-metabolic disorders (e.g., drug ingestion, porphyria, and mitochondrial disorders), neuroleptic malignant syndrome, lethal catatonia, and even serotonin syndrome.

CSF findings of these patients can include a lymphocytic pleocytosis, increased protein, and oligoclonal bands. Increased signal on FLAIR or T2 sequences in the cerebral or cerebellar cortex or in the medial temporal lobes are common MRI findings.

Over half of patients with anti-NMDA-receptor encephalitis have a malignancy, largely an ovarian teratoma. There are case reports of anti-NMDA-receptor encephalitis associated with teratoma of the mediastinum, SCLC, Hodgkin's lymphoma, neuroblastoma, breast cancer, and germ-cell tumor of the testes. This disorder is often cured by removal of the teratoma.

AMPA Receptor Antibodies: Limbic encephalitis can occur as a result of anti-AMPA-receptor antibodies, and 70% of patients have an associated malignancy. The most common tumors are in the lung, breast, and thymus. The vast majority of patients with syndrome are females. Similar to anti-NMDA-receptor encephalitis, there is a lymphocytic pleocytosis in the CSF and abnormal signal on FLAIR MRI images in the medial temporal lobes. These patients require treatment of their underlying malignancy as well as immunotherapy.

$GABA_B$ Receptor Antibodies: These antibodies also cause a clinical picture of limbic encephalitis but with significant seizure activity. Approximately half of patients have SCLC or a neuroendocrine tumor of the lung. It is proposed that these patients often have other autoimmune syndromes, as it has been shown that they have other autoantibodies (TPO, GAD65, SOX1, and N-type voltage-gated calcium channels) present. CSF and MRI findings are similar to those described above for limbic encephalitis.

Antibodies to Intracellular Antigens causing well-described paraneoplastic neurological disorders are listed in Table 19.2.

PCD: The cerebellum is a common target for paraneoplastic syndromes. The malignancies most often associated with PCD are SCLC, breast and other gynecological cancers, and Hodgkin's lymphoma. Typical symptoms include ataxia, diplopia, oscillopsia, opsoclonus, dysarthria, and dysphagia. In some patients, the neurological symptoms follow a viral-like prodromal illness. Often, the syndrome is diagnosed before discovery of the malignancy. The syndrome progresses quickly, over a matter of days to weeks. Imaging findings may be normal initially or may demonstrate enlargement of the cerebellar hemispheres with contrast enhancement of the cerebellar meninges. These MRI findings proceed to cerebellar atrophy.

The best-known antibodies causing PCD are anti-Yo antibodies, which are associated with ovarian, breast, or other gynecological cancer. Other possible antibodies include

TABLE 19.2 *Overview of Common Paraneoplastic Neurological Disorders and Associated Antibodies*

Paraneoplastic Syndrome	Associated Antibodies	Associated Malignancy
Paraneoplastic cerebellar degeneration (PCD)	Anti-Yo	Ovarian, breast
	Anti-Hu	SCLC, others
	Anti-CV2/CRMP5	SCLC, thymoma
	Anti-Tr	Hodgkin lymphoma
Paraneoplastic encephalomyelitis (PEM)	Anti-Hu	SCLC, others
	Anti-Ma	Germ-cell tumors of the testis and other solid tumors
	Anti-amphiphysin	Breast
Opsoclonus-myoclonus	Anti-Ri	Breast, ovarian
	Anti-Hu	SCLC, others
Stiff-person syndrome	Anti-amphiphysin	Breast
	Anti-GAD	None
Paraneoplastic sensory neuronopathy (PSN)	Anti-Hu	SCLC, others

anti-Hu antibodies, anti-mGluR1, anti-Ri (ANNA-2), anti-Tr, anti-CV2/CRMP5, and less commonly anti-Ma proteins (associated with germ-cell tumors of the testes).

PEM: This syndrome has broad effects on the CNS and is caused by inflammatory infiltrates and neuronal death. Clinically, both features of limbic encephalitis and cerebellar degeneration can be present in patients with PEM. The most common antibodies associated with PEM include anti-Hu, anti-CV2/CRMP, anti-Ma2, and amphiphysin antibodies. There is significant brain stem involvement in some manifestations of PEM. For example, Hu antibodies tend to affect the lower brain stem and present with symptoms of dysphagia, dysarthria, and central hypoventilation. These patients can also manifest with pontine symptoms such as vertical nystagmus and ataxia. Nonconvulsive status epilepticus has been reported as the presenting symptom in some patients with Hu antibodies. Anti-Ma2 antibodies, on the other hand, largely affect the upper brain stem.

Furthermore, movement disorders are sometimes included in the constellation of symptoms seen with PEM, as the basal ganglia can be affected. This is illustrated in patients with anti-Ma2 antibodies, who may have a syndrome in which they are severely hypokinetic often with vertical gaze paresis. Other complications include jaw dystonia and blepharospasm. Chorea is seen in patients with CV2/CRMP5 antibodies.

The spinal cord is another site of damage in PEM and can produce symptoms of lower motor neuron disease. Dysfunction can also stem from disruption of the corticospinal tracts.

Paraneoplastic Opsoclonus-Myoclonus: This syndrome includes opsoclonus (chaotic, oscillating eye movements), myoclonus, and severe ataxia. In adults the most commonly associated tumors are SCLC, breast, and ovarian cancers. The most commonly detected antibodies are anti-Ri antibodies, though others have been found as well. In children, neuroblastoma is the most notable associated malignancy. Treatment for this syndrome is immunomodulatory but also is heavily dependent on tumor control.

Stiff-person Syndrome: Stiff-person syndrome is characterized by progressive muscle stiffness of the trunk and upper leg muscles with spasm. If paraneoplastic in origin, it is most commonly associated with anti-amphiphysin antibodies but if nonparaneoplastic, anti-GAD can be found. The mainstay of therapy for this condition is IVIG.

PSN: This presentation is commonly seen in conjunction with PEM and largely with Hu antibodies. PSN is characterized by pain and numbness in the extremities and trunk. It also causes sensory deficits that may involve cranial nerves. Multiple sites can be involved, resulting in an asymmetric sensory deficit. Patients may even have decreased or absent reflexes. Nerve conduction studies demonstrate diminished or absent sensory nerve action potentials.

TREATMENT

Treatment for autoimmune encephalopathies is mainly immunomodulatory. Corticosteroids are often used in combination with other techniques such as plasma exchange or IVIg. Immunosuppressive therapy such as cyclophosphamide and rituximab can be utilized. Treatment for autoimmune encephalopathies of paraneoplastic etiology is heavily dependent on treatment of the underlying malignancy itself. Prognosis varies with the type of antibodies present and also depends on the success of treatment of the malignancy.

Due to current lack of class I or II treatment data, Rosenfeld and Dalmau (2011) formulated treatment recommendations based off of a large series of patients with anti-NMDA-receptor encephalitis. They recommend a five-day course of concurrent IVIG (or plasma exchange) and methyprednisolone (1g IV/day) if no tumor is found or after tumor removal. They advise supportive care if clear improvement is seen within 10 days. If there is a blunted response or no response to treatment they recommend cyclophosphamide monthly and rituximab weekly for 4 weeks. In patients refractory to this regimen, other forms of immunosuppression can be instituted. Lastly, for patients without tumor, they propose yearly surveillance for 2 to 3 years and administration of mycophenolate mofetil or azathioprine for 1 year to prevent relapse. For patients with seizures, anti-epileptic drugs are an important component of the treatment routine.

Immunomodulatory therapies for many of these disorders have been successful, though the time course of treatment varies greatly. For example, for patients with limbic encephalitis caused by anti-NMDA receptor antibodies, clinical improvement is slow and these patients often require ICU monitoring due to their dysautonomia. The potential for reversal of the encephalopathy caused by autoantibodies stresses the importance of early detection of these disorders.

SUGGESTED READING

Lai M, Huibers, M GM, Lancaster E, et al. Investigation of LGI1 as the antigen in limbic encephalitis previously attributed to potassium channels: A case series. *Lancet Neurology.* 2010;9:776–785.

Lancaster E, Huijber MGM, Vered B, Boronat A, et al. Investigations of Caspr2, an autoantigen of encephalitis and neuromyotonia. *Ann Neurol.* 2011;69(2):303–311.

Rosenfeld MR, Dalmau J. Anti-NMDA-receptor encephalitis and other synaptic autoimmune disorders. *Curr Treat Options in Neurol.* 2011;13(3):324–332.

Rosenfeld MR, Dalmau J. Update on paraneoplastic and autoimmune disorders of the central nervous system. *SeminNeurol.* 2010;30:320–331.

Vincent A, Irani SR, Lang B. The growing recognition of immunotherapy-responsive seizure disorders with autoantibodies to specific neuronal proteins. *CurrOpin in Neurol.* 2010;23:144–150.

CHIEF COMPLAINT: **Pain on the right side of the face.**

HISTORY OF PRESENT ILLNESS

This is a 55-year-old, right-handed Caucasian female who comes with a history of pain on the right side of her face. The pain started 4 years ago which is described as electric-shock-like in nature. The patient has periods of pain-free intervals, but when the pain comes on, she gets pain attacks that can be as many as 10 to 15 times a day. The pain has been intermittent and lasts for a few seconds. During these attacks, the patient cannot talk or chew. She keeps her mouth closed. The patient also experiences pain with brushing her teeth. The pain involves the right cheek mainly and radiates occasionally to the jaw and teeth. Talking and chewing can precipitate an attack. She could not tell if she was experiencing pain in her teeth. She consulted a dentist who did not see anything wrong with her teeth. She denies any headaches, nausea, vomiting, or blurring of vision. She has no other common neurological symptoms.

PAST MEDICAL HISTORY

As above.

PAST SURGICAL HISTORY

Tubal ligation.

MEDICATIONS

Motrin 400 mg tid PRN.

ALLERGIES

None.

PERSONAL HISTORY

She denies any history of tobacco, alcohol, or drugs.

STOP AND THINK QUESTIONS

➤ What neurological condition(s) can cause stabbing and electric-shock-like pains in parts of the face?

➤ What pharmacotherapy can help alleviate the facial pain?

➤ What will you do if the patient fails to respond to medical therapy?

DIAGNOSTIC TEST RESULTS

Routine labs, ESR, CRP: Normal; Lyme negative, RPR negative.
MRI brain (first study): No evidence of any intracranial pathology.
She was started on Carbamazepine XR 200mg bid which was slowly increased to 600 mg bid. Patient reported significant but partial relief with tegretol monotherapy. Adjunctive

therapy with Neurontin at 900 mg tid and Elavil at 50 mg HS provided additional pain relief. About 6 months later, patient developed severe side effects from these medications including nausea, sleepiness, and ataxia. Her labs revealed hyponatremia, leucopenia, and slight elevation of liver enzymes, probably all related to the use of tegretol. Her pain became 10/10 as tegretol was slowly tapered. She tried Tylenol #3, and Percocet with partial relief in pain. At this point, the patient was referred to a neurosurgeon.

MRI brain was repeated with special attention to posterior fossa and DREZ of the fifth nerve. The study revealed an abnormal vascularity in the area of the fifth nerve DREZ (Figure 20.1).

The patient was informed about all the options including surgery, rhizotomy procedures, balloon compression, and gamma-knife radiation therapy. In view of her age, surgery was considered as the primary choice of treatment. She underwent a right retromastoid craniectomy and MVD of the fifth cranial nerve. At surgery, a superior cerebellar artery was found to be compressing the DREZ of the fifth cranial nerve which was gently mobilized, and Teflon felt was inserted between the nerve and the artery. The patient did well postoperatively and her medications were tapered off over a period of 4 to 12 weeks. She remains pain free and off medications.

DIAGNOSIS: Trigeminal neuralgia (TN).

DISCUSSION

TN is a syndrome of severe, recurrent episodes of pain in the distribution of one or multiple branches of the trigeminal nerve. The patient has a very classical history of TN (see Table 20.1). Trigger zones are most commonly located on the cheek, lip, nose, or buccal mucosa. Early in the disease course, the periods of exacerbation are shorter and periods of remission are longer in duration. As the disease progresses, the periods of exacerbation get more frequent. Later in the disease course, the pain may be continuous and unremitting. Pulsation of vessels upon the trigeminal nerve root does not visibly damage the nerve. The irritation from repeated pulsations may lead to changes of nerve function and delivery of abnormal signals to the trigeminal nerve nucleus. The chronicity of the condition results in hyperactivity of the trigeminal nerve nucleus, resulting in the generation of TN pain.

The syndrome of TN is broadly classified into two groups: Type I TN (typical) or Type II TN (atypical). The pain of typical TN is characterized by sharp, lancinating, or shock-

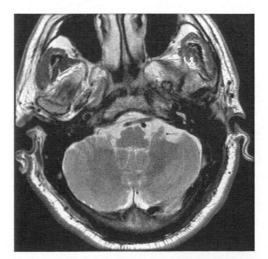

FIGURE 20.1 *MRI brain Axial T2 internal auditory canal-CP angle (attention to DREZ) of the fifth nerve revealing an abnormal vascularity in the area of the fifth nerve DREZ.*

TABLE 20.1 *Diagnostic Criteria for Classic Trigeminal Neuralgia*

- Paroxysmal attacks of pain lasting from a fraction of a second to 2 minutes that affect one or more divisions of the trigeminal nerve
- Pain has at least one of the following characteristics: intense, sharp, superficial or stabbing precipitated from trigger factors, or trigger areas
- Attacks are similar in individual patients
- Neurological examination is normal
- Symptoms cannot be explained by another disorder

like pain with intervals of spontaneous remission. Atypical TN is characterized more by periods of constant aching or burning pain with fewer periods of remission, and is associated with an overall decreased responsiveness to treatment across all treatment modalities. Zacest et al. (2) have suggested that these two subtypes are two points along a continuum of disease pathology with Type II TN representing more prolonged or severe trigeminal nerve injury. As such, the diagnosis is frequently made based upon clinical history alone.

The trigeminal nerve exits the brain stem from the ventrolateral pons as separate motor (portio minor) and sensory (portio major) roots. It then traverses the prepontine cistern and runs along the floor of the middle cranial fossa anterior to the petrous apex to enter Meckel's cave. The trigeminal ganglion is contained within Meckel's cave, which is posterolateral to the cavernous sinus. Three branches, the ophthalmic, maxillary, and mandibular, emerge from the trigeminal ganglion to provide sensation to the face, nasal mucosa, and supratentorial dura.

The first division of the trigeminal nerve (V_1), the ophthalmic nerve, passes forward in the lateral wall of the cavernous sinus. It courses anteriorly to enter the orbit through the superior orbital fissure. It supplies sensation to the eyeball, conjunctiva, lacrimal glands, part of the nasal mucosa, skin of the nose and forehead.

The second division of the trigeminal nerve (V_2) exits the cranium via the foramen rotundum inferolateral to the cavernous sinus. It enters into the pterygopalatine fossa. It then courses forward and divides into several branches. Its main trunk enters the floor of the orbit through the inferior orbital fissure, courses through the orbit and emerges onto the face via the infraorbital foramen to supply sensation to the midface and upper teeth.

The third division of the trigeminal nerve (V_3), the mandibular nerve, runs on the lateral aspect along the skull base. It exits the cranium through foramen ovale and enters the masticator space. The motor root of trigeminal unites the mandibular nerve in the foramen ovale. In the masticator space, the V_3 divides into several branches to supply sensation to the lower third of the face, tongue, jaw, and floor of the mouth. The motor branch provides motor innervations to the muscles of mastication: anterior belly of digastric, mylohyoid, tensor tympani, and tensor veli palatini.

The DREZ is the cisternal part of the V nerve as it enters the pons. It is the transition point between CNS myelin and peripheral nervous system myelin on the trigeminal nerve. DREZ is few millimeters from its exit from the pons.

The most common etiology involves direct neurovascular compression from closely apposed arterial or venous loops. Recent advances in imaging technologies have allowed improve visualization of the trigeminal nerve and its exit point from the pons. High resolution 3-T MR imaging helps to assess location and degree of vascular compression, as well as differentiation between arterial and venous compression (2,3).

Other less common etiologies include DREZ demyelinating lesions from multiple sclerosis or other primary demyelinating disorders, such as Charcot-Marie-Tooth disease and infiltrative or compressive lesions of the trigeminal nerve, including carcinomatous deposits within the trigeminal nerve, amyloidosis, and tumors of the CP angle.

Despite the wide range of etiologies of TN, the underlying pathophysiology remains relatively constant. Continued or recurrent compression of the trigeminal nerve DREZ causes focal, segmental areas of demyelination at the DREZ. Ultrastructural analysis of trigeminal nerves in patients with TN from neurovascular compression demonstrated these areas of focal demyelination limited to the immediate vicinity of the offending vascular loop, along with close apposition of demyelinated fibers in this location. Similarly, demyelination at the DREZ with close fiber apposition has been demonstrated in multiple sclerosis patients with TN and tumors of the CP angle resulting in TN-like symptoms. The prevailing theory is that the areas of close contact between demyelinated fibers result in spontaneous ectopic impulses from the demyelinated fibers with ephaptic transmission to adjacent fibers due to their close contact. Involvement of the DREZ is a critical factor in the pathogenesis of this disease as is the area of closest proximity between fibers involving light touch and those subserving the pain response (4).

The primary modality of treatment for TN is medical management with first line of drugs like tegretol and trileptal. Other first- and second-generation antiepileptics, muscle relaxants such as baclofen and klonopin have been used to treat TN (see Table 20.2).

However, a subset of the population will find the medications ineffectual, gradually become resistant, or be unable to tolerate them due to adverse side effects. In medically refractory TN, surgical intervention by either MVD or neurolysis is performed. MVD is designed to treat the most common etiology of TN—arterial or venous compression of the trigeminal nerve. Exposure of the trigeminal nerve is performed through a retrosigmoid craniotomy which exposes the CP angle and allows easy visualization from cranial nerve V to the foramen magnum. Once the trigeminal nerve is identified, the offending vessel, either artery or vein, is identified, and a piece of Teflon or felt is positioned between the vessel and the nerve, so as to prevent further vascular compression.

Either complete or partial immediate postoperative relief was demonstrated in 98% of patients in a large series of 1,166 patient undergoing this procedure. The same study demonstrates endurance of the treatment effect with a less than 2% annual recurrence rate for the first 5 years and less than 1% after 10 years (5). In patients where MVD is intended, but no offending vessel is identified at the time of surgery, a partial sensory rhizotomy of the trigeminal nerve may be performed. This procedure is similarly associated with a good outcome—88% initial relief, but decreased overall satisfaction compared with MVD due to a higher incidence of hypoesthesia or anesthesia postoperatively (6).

In patients with significant medical comorbidities or without obvious vascular compression on preoperative imaging, neurolysis through minimally invasive procedures becomes the treatment of choice (see Figure 20.2). Multiple modalities for neurolysis exist,

TABLE 20.2 *Commonly Used Drugs for the Treatment of Trigeminal Neuralgia*

First-Line Drugs	Second-Line Drugs	Others
Carbamazepine (Tegretol)	Gabapentin (Neurontin)	Phenytoin (Dilantin)
Oxcarbamazepine (Trileptal)	Lamotrigine (Lamictal)	Clonazepam (Klonopin)
	Lioresal (Baclofen)	Topiramate (Topamax)
		Evaporate (Depakote)
		Mexiletine (Mexitil)

including GKS, percutaneous glycerol rhizotomy, and percutaneous radiofrequency ther mocoagulation. Both percutaneous glycerol rhizotomy and radiofrequency thermocoagu-lation involve passing a stylet or probe through the tissues of the cheek, crossing through foramen ovale and ending within Meckel's cave, where the trigeminal ganglion resides. With glycerol rhizotomy, 0.3 to 0.5 of glycerol is injected into Meckel's cave under direct fluoroscopic guidance resulting in destruction of the unmyelinated and thinly myelinated pain fibers. Percutaneous radiofrequency thermocoagulation similarly involves introduc-tion of a probe through the foramen ovale into Meckel's cave with lesioning of the trigem-inal nerve by heat created from the electrode by radiofrequency waves. Both percutaneous radiofrequency thermocoagulation and glycerol rhizotomies are associated with lower overall complication rates, lower rates of initial pain relief, and higher rates of readmission for repeat procedures compared with MVD (7–9).

GKS offers the least invasive treatment for TN. It is suitable in elderly patients with other comorbidities and significant anesthesia risks or patients who have failed other treat-ment modalities including MVD or multiple percutaneous rhizotomies. In this procedure, 75 Gy radiation dose is applied to a 4 mm region at the DREZ with precautions taken to minimize brain stem radiation exposure. Unlike the other more invasive approaches, the

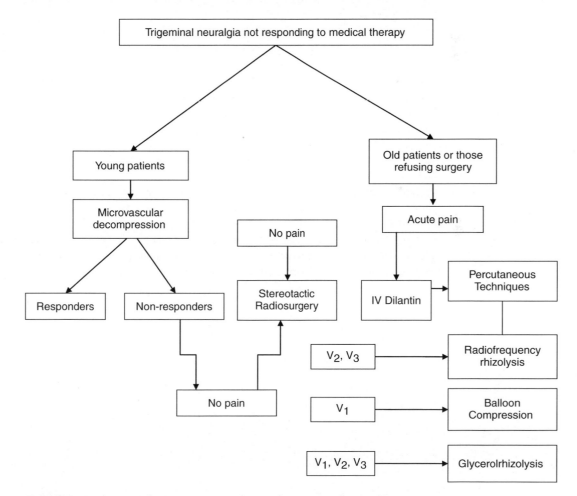

FIGURE 20.2 *Surgical options in a patient with trigeminal neuralgia.*

timing of postoperative pain relief varies, with published results of pain relief as early as 2 weeks to several months (10). Compared with the other methods, GKS is associated with fewer complications, but also a lower initial rate of response and higher rate of recurrence. GKS may be used as a salvage procedure for those that have had prior decompressions or rhizotomies with results similar to its use as a primary treatment modality, albeit with a slightly higher rate of facial sensory changes (11).

REFERENCES

1. Love S, Coakham HB. Trigeminal neuralgia: Pathology and pathogenesis. *Brain*. 2001;124:2347–2360.
2. Zacest AC, Magill ST, Miller J, Burchiel KJ. Preoperative magnetic resonance imaging in Type 2 trigeminal neuralgia. *J Neurosurg*. 2010;113(3):511–515.
3. Miller JP, Acar F, Burchiel KJ. Classification of trigeminal neuralgia: Clinical, therapeutic, and prognostic implications in a series of 144 patients undergoing microvascular decompression. *J Neurosurg*. 2009;111:1231–1234.
4. Barker FG, Janneta PJ, Bissonette DJ, Larkins MV, Dong Jho H. The long-term outcome of microvascular decompression for trigeminal neuralgia. *NEJM*. 1996;334(17):1077–1083.
5. Zakrzewska JM, Lopez BC, Kim SE, Coakham HB. Patient reports of satisfaction after microvascular decompression and partial sensory rhizotomy for trigeminal neuralgia. *Neurosurgery*. 2005;56(6):1304–1311.
6. Xu-Hui W, Chun Z, Guang-Jian S, Min-Hui X, Guang-Xin C, Yong-Wen Z, Lun-Shan X. Long-term outcomes of percutaneous retrogasserian glycerol rhizotomy in 3370 patients with trigeminal neuralgia. *Turk Neurosurg*. 2011;21(1):48–52.
7. Koopman JSHA, De Vries LM, Dieleman JP, Huygen FJ, Stricker BHCh, Sturkenboom MCJM. A nationwide study of three invasive treatments for trigeminal neuralgia. *Pain*. 2011;152:507–513.
8. Emril DR, Ho KY. Treatment of trigeminal neuralgia: Role of radiofrequency ablation. *J Pain Res*. 2010;3:249–254.
9. Dhople AA, Adams JR, Maggio WM, Naqvi SA, Regine WF, Kwok Y. Long-term outcomes of gamma knife radiosurgery for classical trigeminal neuralgia: Implications of treatment and critical review of the literature. *J Neurosurg*. 2009;111:351–358.
10. Park SY, Kim PJ, Chang WS, Kim HY, Park YG, Chang JW. Gamma knife radiosurgery for idiopathic trigeminal neuralgia as primar vs. secondary treatment option. *Clin Neurol Neurosurg*. 2011; 113(6):447–452.
11. Leal PR, Froment JC, Sindou M. MRI sequences for detection of neurovascular conflicts in patients with trigeminal neuralgia and predictive value for characterization of the conflict (particular degree of vascular compression). *Neurochirurgie*. 2010;56(1):43–49.

Involuntary Twitches and Vocalizations

Kristin M. Waldron

CHIEF COMPLAINT: **Body twitches.**

HISTORY OF PRESENT ILLNESS

A 19-year-old, right-handed male who complained of frequent twitches that began 6 years ago, at the age of 13. At that time, he reported feelings of "mosquitoes in my brain." He described "twitches" of his arm, legs, head and, at times, his full body. He would have intermittent vocalizations. He noticed drooling during these episodes. He would be seen to hop on one or both legs or would stomp his feet. He would chew on the collars of his shirts and make holes in them. He reported that his "mind would go blank." At times, his feet would turn inward and his knees would buckle. He had obsessive feelings that his "brain was rotting" and that his face was "swollen on both sides." He also had changes in his mood, was easily irritable, and was argumentative. He became easily distractible and reported difficulty concentrating. His grades dropped from As to Cs. He was the product of a normal pregnancy, labor, and delivery with normal developmental milestones. He had no history of head trauma or CNS infections.

PAST MEDICAL HISTORY

FS started during infancy; his last febrile seizure was at age 5. They are described as facial quivering, eyes rolling back, and "mild stiffening," in the setting of fever.

PAST SURGICAL HISTORY

None.

MEDICATIONS

None currently, but has used herbal medications from China, without improvement of his symptoms.

ALLERGIES

No known drug allergies.

PERSONAL HISTORY

He has lived in the United States for the past 9 years. Currently a sophomore in college, with poor grades. Used to play the piano, but is no longer able to do so secondary to incoordination.

PHYSICAL EXAMINATION

Vitals: Blood pressure, 121/77; heart rate, 89; respiratory rate, 14; temperature 98.3°F. Lungs clear, heart sounds within normal limits, abdomen soft, nontender, skin: warm and dry.

During the interview, intermittent clearing of his throat and motor tics of the head. Vocalizations were present throughout the exam. Red patches on lower cheeks (parents say due to vigorous wiping of drool).

NEUROLOGICAL EXAMINATION

Mental status: Alert, oriented to person and place but not date, speech is pressured, memory one out of three at 3 minutes, poor concentration, fixed ideas, poor judgment, mild impulsivity.
CN II–XII: Unremarkable.
Motor: Full strength to confrontation testing, normal bulk and tone.
Sensory: Intact to light touch and pin prick.
Reflexes: 2+ symmetric.
Plantars: Flexors bilaterally.
Gait: Steady and normal.
No tremors, rigidity, dystonia, no masked facies, good postural reflexes.

STOP AND THINK QUESTIONS

➢ What is the differential diagnosis of tics in an adolescent?

➢ Are there any substances/medications that might make tics worse?

DIAGNOSTIC TEST RESULTS

MRI brain: Normal.
VEEG: PDR 9Hz. No epileptiform discharges. Multiple events of tic like behavior not associated with any epileptiform discharges.
CBC, BMP, LFTs, PT/INR, TSH/T3/T4, ceruloplasmin, urine copper, PTH, lipoprotein electrophoresis: Normal.
ASO Ab: Negative.
CK: 309 (H).
Urine Arsenic: 66.2 (H).

DIAGNOSIS: Tourette syndrome (TS).

DISCUSSION

Tics are very common during childhood, some studies citing that 20% of children have a tic disorder at one time or another. A tic is defined as a sudden, brief, purposeless, repetitive, nonrhythmic, stereotyped movement or sound. Tics are involuntary or semi-involuntary. They can often be suppressed for minutes-hours, but when the patient is relaxed/distracted and no longer focused on suppressing them, they may have "tic flurries" lasting for several hours. Tics come out more when the patient is anxious, stressed, or tired, and tend to decrease when the patient is sleeping or is focused on something. There are many disorders whose symptom complex includes tics, but the most severe (and the most common) of the tic disorders is Tourette syndrome. Usually, the disease begins with simple tics and will progress to more complex tics. Tics wax and wane, with new tics replacing old tics, and often multiple tics are present at one time.

Tourette syndrome (TS) is more common in males (3:1). Prevalence is reported to be 2%. It is thought to be inherited, although no one gene has been identified as the culprit. Different theories of mode of inheritance include autosomal dominant with incomplete penetrance and variable expression, bilineal (inherited from both parents), and polygenic. Twin studies show concordance rates of 60% with monozygotic twins and 10% in dizygotic twins.

Mean age of onset is age 6 to 7. The disease usually peaks in severity at age 9 to 11. Eighty five percent of patients will eventually have remission or considerably improve, usually by early adulthood. Five percent to ten percent remain unchanged in severity, or worsen.

TOURETTE SYNDROME: DIAGNOSTIC CRITERIA

1. Multiple motor and one or more vocal tics present (they do not need to be present at the same time). Tics may be simple or complex. Common simple tics include eye blinking, shoulder jerking, picking, grunting, sniffing, and barking. Complex tics include grimacing, arm flapping, jumping, coprolalia (use of obscene language), palilalia (repeating one's own words), or echolalia (repeating someone else's words).

2. Tics occur multiple times per day, usually in clusters. It occurs for more than 1 year. There is no tic-free period greater than 3 months.

3. Tics cause marked distress or impairment in social, occupational, or other areas of daily functioning.

4. Onset before age 18.

5. Tics not due to substance abuse or medication use.

Etiology/Pathophysiology: It is thought to be related to dysfunction in the basal ganglia and frontal cortex. There is inappropriate regulation of dopamine: dopamine excess, increased sensitivity of the postsynaptic dopamine receptors, or alteration of the dopamine reuptake mechanisms. L-Dopa will exacerbate the syndrome.

Comorbidities: If comorbid conditions go undiagnosed, the child can be significantly impaired

1. ADHD (50%).

2. OCD (25%–40%). Patients may exhibit compulsive behaviors (30%–50%) involving arranging objects, touching things, smelling, licking, erasing, hand washes. They also often have obsessive thoughts (30%).

3. Learning disability (25%–30%). Some studies show that 65% of children with Tourette syndrome function below the expected level.

In general, 60% to 80% of patients with Tourette syndrome have behavioral problems, including having a short temper, mood swings, overreaction, exhibitionism, or negativism.

TREATMENT

Treatment is reserved for those patients who are significantly impaired/incapacitated by their disease. Tics are only treated if they interfere with functioning. Treatment is multifaceted, including behavioral modifications, pharmacologic, or surgical.

Behavioral modifications include positive reinforcement programs. Their aim is to improve skill deficiencies and decrease excess behaviors.

There are multiple medications used to treat motor tics. First-line treatment includes alpha adrenergic blockers including clonidine. They may also help the patients with irritability and impulsivity. Although they are the most effective for suppressing tics, D2 antagonists (including haldol and pimozide) are second-line therapy due to the side effects of sedation, weight gain, acute dystonia, and tardive dyskinesia. They should be used to treat multiple, complex tics. Other medications used to suppress tics include risperdal, klonopin, and botox. The lowest dose that effectively controls tics should be used.

Deep brain stimulation may be used for severely refractory cases.

Most patients only need pharmacologic therapy for 1 to 2 years. Fifteen percent will need to stay on them for long-term control. If tics have been well controlled for 4 to 6 months, medications can be gradually tapered off. They should be titrated to the lowest possible dose where tics are still well controlled, and not interfering significantly with the patient's life.

Comorbid conditions must be screened for and treated.

1. SSRIs for OCD.

2. Stimulants (i.e., methyphenidate) for ADHD. There is some controversy in this area, as it was previously thought that stimulants would worsen tics. This has been called into question, as recent studies show no significant increase in tics in most patients. In the end, severe ADHD must be treated regardless.

3. In addition, the patient should be screened for thyroid dysfunction (as tics may be present in hyperthyroidism), as well as Wilson's disease in certain cases.

4. Rule out drug abuse in adolescents who have the sudden onset of tics, as stimulants and cocaine may worsen tics.

SUGGESTED READING

Bagher MM, Kerbeshian J, Burd L. Recognition and management of Tourette's syndrome and tic disorders. *Am Fam Physician.* 1999 Apr 15;59(8):2263–2272, 2274.

Bradley W, Daroff R, Fenichel G, Jankovic, J. *Neurology in Clinical Practice.* 4th ed. Philadelphia: Butterworth Heinemann; 2004.

Faridi K, Suchowersky O. Gilles de la Tourette's syndrome. *Can J Neurol Sci.* 2003 Mar;30 (Suppl):S64–S71.

Kenney C, Kuo SH, Jimenez-Shahed J. Tourette's syndrome. *Am Fam Physician.* 2008 Mar 1; 77(5):657–658.

Muller-Vahl, KR. The treatment of Tourette's syndrome: Current opinions. *Expert Opin Pharmacother.* 2002 Jul;3(7):899–914.

Ropper A, Brown R. *Principles of Neurology.* 8th ed. New York: McGraw Hill; 2005.

CHIEF COMPLAINT: **Family members reporting personality changes and memory loss.**

HISTORY OF PRESENT ILLNESS

A 66-year-old, right-handed woman was brought into the emergency department by her family for altered mental status. According to the patient's daughter, during the month prior to admission, the patient had had increasing memory loss and changes in her behavior. She would have intermittent outbursts of anger. She would not allow her family and friends into her apartment. Her speech became slurred, her answers would not make any sense, and often she would make statements out of context of the conversation being held. Patient was found disheveled in her apartment; her house was filthy and full of clutter. She was found to have nausea, vomiting, diarrhea, and it appeared that she was not eating properly. She was taken to the local emergency department where a noncontrast head CT was performed. The family brought the copy of the abnormal CT results.

PAST MEDICAL HISTORY

HTN, hypothyroidism, hypoparathyroidism, COPD, iron deficiency anemia, depression.

PAST SURGICAL HISTORY

Appendectomy, hiatal hernia repair.

MEDICATIONS

Cozaar 50 mg daily, Synthroid 25 mg daily, baby aspirin 81 mg daily, Nexium 40 mg daily, Rocaltrol 0.25 mg tab, three tabs daily, Oscal four tabs three times per day, Diltiazem 180 mg daily, Ferrous Sulfate 325 mg TID, Micardis 40 mg daily, Lexapro 5 mg BID, Advair and Atrovent inhaler, Spiriva.

ALLERGIES

NKDA.

REVIEW OF SYSTEMS

Denied fever, chills, night sweats, chest pain, and shortness of breath, palpitations, weight loss, and changes in urinary frequency or urgency.

PERSONAL HISTORY

Patient had smoked one pack a day for more than 40 years. She quit smoking about 6 years ago. Family denied any use of alcohol or recreational drugs. Prior to the month before admission, the patient had lived a fairly normal life and was gainfully employed. She was independent, lived alone, and managed all of her bills and household chores.

FAMILY HISTORY

Noncontributory.

PHYSICAL EXAMINATION

The patient was disheveled, agitated, and uncooperative with the examination. There were no signs of trauma, and she was afebrile. She had dry buccal mucosa and increased skin turgor.

NEUROLOGICAL EXAMINATION

Mental status: Examination was very limited. The patient was only oriented to person and not to place, time. She had no insight. Patient had poor attention and concentration. Her mood was slightly dysthymic. She had masked facies, dysarthria, and she was slow to respond to questions. She was unable to consolidate information.

CNs II–XII: Cranial nerves intact.

Motor: No drift, no tremors, normal bulk, and mild rigidity.

Sensory: Grossly normal and withdrew to pin prick equally, detailed examination deferred.

Reflexes: 2+ and symmetrical.

Plantars: Flexors.

Gait: Wide base.

Romberg: Negative.

Cerebellar: Negative.

STOP AND THINK QUESTIONS

➢ What are the signs and symptoms of extrapyramidal symptoms involvement?

➢ Would you classify this as a hyperkinetic or hypokinetic disorder?

DIAGNOSTIC TEST RESULTS

Laboratory results revealed an elevated white count, normocytic anemia, an increase in BUN and creatinine, and serum calcium greater than 11 mg/dL. Repeat serum calcium was 17.5 mg/dL.

Noncontrast head CT showed multiple calcifications in the bilateral basal ganglia, thalamus, and subcortical white matter, suggestive of Fahr's disease (Figure 22.1).

DIAGNOSIS: Fahr's syndrome.

HOSPITAL COURSE

The patient was medically managed for her dehydration and hypercalcemia. She was treated with intravenous fluids and furosemide 40 mg daily with resultant decrease of her serum calcium (8.9 mg/dL). She was started on keppra 500 mg bid for seizure prophylaxis, given the extent of her calcifications. Her mental status improved, and she became oriented to time, place, and person. She was more cooperative. Her attention and concentration improved, and she was able to consolidate information. However, some of her personality changes and mood swings persisted. There was not much improvement in her parkinsonism symptoms.

DISCUSSION

Bilateral basal ganglia calcification is a rare neurodegenerative disorder. It is characterized by abnormal calcium deposition and neuronal cell loss in the basal ganglia and cerebral cortex. There are two fundamental types:

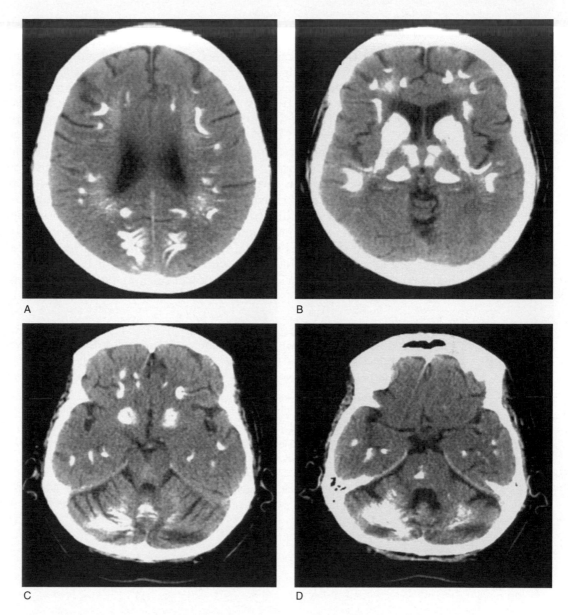

FIGURE 22.1 *Noncontrast head CT axial images showing multiple symmetric calcifications in the bilateral basal ganglia (A), thalamus (B), subcortical white matter (C), and cerebellum (D).*

1. Fahr's disease which refers to different causes of cerebral calcification (i.e., idiopathic striopallidodentate calcinosis, nonarteriosclerotic cerebral calcification, or idiopathic basal ganglia calcification).
2. Fahr's syndrome which is defined as symmetric and bilateral calcifications of the basal ganglia, associated with neuropsychiatric manifestations, preferentially occurring in patients with parathyroid disorders, particularly hypoparathyroidism.

Fahr's disease is often familial with autosomal dominant inheritance; however, a few cases have been reported to have an autosomal recessive pattern of inheritance with reports of occasional sporadic cases. The clinical course of Fahr's syndrome has a slowly progressive degenerative component. The deposition of calcium may lead to neuronal cell loss in the cerebral cortex, basal ganglia, and dentate nuclei. Patients can present with motor disorders (56% of cases) and exhibit signs and symptoms of Parkinsonism, dystonia, tics, and dysarthria. These motor disorders have been linked to the involvement of the frontostriatal motor system. Autopsy studies have revealed Wallerian degeneration of the corticospinal tracts. Seizure can occur in up to 22% of cases.

Neuropsychiatric manifestations such as psychosis, mood and personality changes, obsessive–compulsive behavior, and disorders in executive functioning occur in up to 40% of patients. These symptoms have been linked to corticosubcortical disconnection mediated by the basal ganglia with involvement of the frontostriatal and limbic circuits.

Clinical diagnosis is facilitated by the presence of early cognitive decline, neuropsychiatric symptoms, new onset motor disturbances, and the exclusion of other causes. Neuroimaging findings of bilateral, symmetric calcifications in the basal ganglia seen on CT are characteristic. There is no cure or treatment for Fahr's disease or syndrome. Supportive treatment is provided. Correction of calcium may improve the mental status as in our patient.

SUGGESTED READING

Cummings JL, Gosenfeld LF, Houlihan JP, McCaffrey T. Neuropsychiatric disturbances associated with idiopathic calcification of the basal ganglia. *Biol Psychiatry.* 1983;18:591–601.

Koller WC, Cochran JW, Klawans HL. Calcification of the basal ganglia: Computerized tomography and clinical correlation. *Neurology.* 1979;29:328–333.

Manyam BV. Bilateral strio-pallido-dentate calcinosis: A proposed classification of genetic and secondary causes. *Mov Disord.* 1990;5(Suppl 1):94S.

Manyam BV. What is and what is not "Fahr's disease." *Parkinsonism Relat Disord.* 2005;11:73–80.

Manyam BV, Walters AS, Narla KR. Bilateral striopallidodentate calcinosis: Clinical characteristics of patients seen in a registry. *Mov Disord.* 2001;16:258–264.

Manyam BV, Bhatt MH, Moore WD, Devleschoward AB, Anderson DR, Calne DB. Bilateral striopallidodentate calcinosis: cerebrospinal fluid, imaging, and electrophysiological studies. *Ann Neurol.* 1992;31:379–384.

Sudden Onset Tremors

Marjorie E. Bunch

CHIEF COMPLAINT: **Awakened with uncontrolled left arm shaking.**

HISTORY OF PRESENT ILLNESS

The patient is a 27-year-old, left-handed man who was suddenly awakened in the morning around 5 a.m. by the shaking of his left arm. He noted a violent movement in his shoulder, elbow, and wrist that he could not control. The shaking would come and go, lasting for less than 1 minute at a time. Each episode of shaking was preceded by a sensation of twitching in his upper arm which would then spread. While the shaking occurred in any position, with action or rest, it seemed to be triggered by sitting or lying down. He placed his right hand on his left arm to stop the movement, and then the shaking occurred intermittently in the right arm. When he stood up, he developed brief shaking in his right leg. The right leg and arm shaking resolved fairly quickly, but the left arm continued to shake intermittently, with decreasing frequency and amplitude throughout the morning and resolved completely by noon. He showed a brief video of the shaking that demonstrated coarse irregular tremor at the left wrist, also seen less prominently in the right wrist.

He felt soreness and tingling diffusely in his left arm, but there were no other sensory complaints. There was no complaint of weakness or involvement of the face or axial musculature. There was no pain in his neck or problems with balance.

PAST MEDICAL HISTORY

Frequent sinus headaches.

PAST SURGICAL HISTORY

No history of surgeries.

MEDICATIONS

Advil and Zyrtec-D as needed, typically at least 5 days per week.

ALLERGIES

NKDA.

PERSONAL HISTORY

Nonsmoker. Drinks 1 to 2 alcoholic beverages per night and more on the weekends. Denies recreational drug use. Lifts weights and exercises regularly.

FAMILY HISTORY

Father has diabetes mellitus. Maternal aunt died at age 10 and was diagnosed with cerebral palsy.

PHYSICAL EXAMINATION

Well developed, well nourished with a muscular build, and not distressed.
General examination was normal.

NEUROLOGICAL EXAMINATION

Mental status: Awake, alert, cooperative, oriented, with appropriate affect and fluent English.

CNs II–XII: Intact.

Motor: Extremely subtle left pronator drift and slight decreased frequency of finger popping with the left hand. Otherwise full strength, normal tone, and no atrophy, fasciculations, or tremor.

Sensory: Intact to pin prick, temperature, position, and vibration sense. Slightly diminished light touch diffusely over the left arm compared to the right.

Reflexes: 2+ and symmetric biceps, brachioradialis, triceps, patellar, and Achilles.

Plantars: Flexors.

Coordination: Finger-to-nose, rapid alternating movements, and heel-to-shin intact bilaterally.

Gait: Normal including heel and toe walking, tandem gait. Romberg negative.

STOP AND THINK QUESTIONS

➤ Is this neurological problem localizable? Where?

➤ What types of neurological problems are likely to wake someone up?

DIAGNOSTIC TEST RESULTS

Routine blood tests including thyroid studies were normal.

Three-day ambulatory EEG was normal.

MRI brain with and without contrast demonstrated a 1.6 × 0.8 × 0.8 cm heterogeneous lesion in the interpeduncular cistern extending to the right. The lesion had heterogeneous high signal on the T1WI and T2WI and exerted mild mass effect on the medial aspect of the right cerebral peduncle. Associated T2 and gradient echo low signal was suggestive of chronic hemorrhage (Figure 23.1).

CTA brain demonstrated a 1.9 × 1.9 mm outpouching of contrast extending posterolaterally from the P1 segment of the right posterior cerebral artery, consistent with aneurysm. Surrounding low density, approximately 1.6 × 0.9 cm, was suggestive of lipoma (Figure 23.2). Mild compression from mass effect upon the medial aspect of the right cerebral peduncle. The posterior cerebral arteries were otherwise unremarkable.

Cerebral angiogram demonstrated a P1 segment fusiform aneurysm with perforating branches extending posteriorly. No intervention was possible.

DIAGNOSIS: Right P1 aneurysm in a lipoma with associated hemorrhage causing mass effect on the cerebral peduncles bilaterally causing Holme's tremor, most prominent in the left arm.

DISCUSSION

The differential diagnosis of paroxysmal shaking includes frontal lobe simple partial seizures, which can wake someone up, be episodic, and recur. However, this would be unlikely in this case because the patient had shaking in each arm independently without change in mental status or other signs of cortical involvement.

Limb shaking transient ischemic attack would be unlikely to be so recurrent and transiently bilateral; also, the patient had no vascular risk factors as this is typically due to carotid occlusive disease. Psychogenic etiology is also a consideration with this presentation as the location of shaking seemed to vary dramatically, which is atypical for a focal neurological process.

164

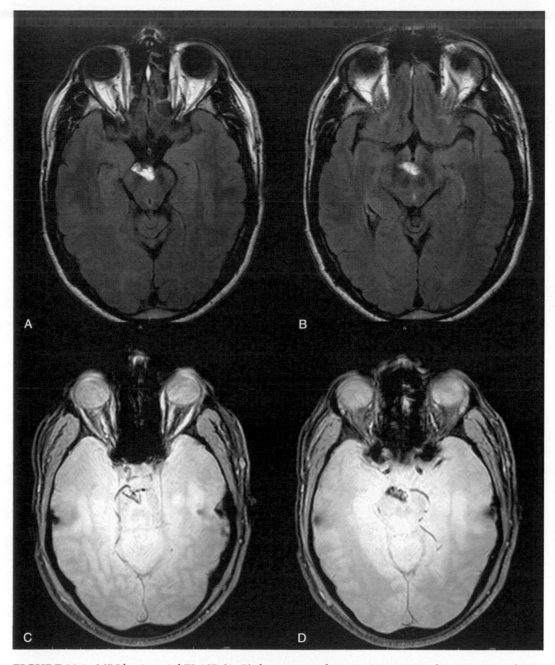

FIGURE 23.1 *MRI brain axial FLAIR (A, B) demonstrated a 1.6 × 0.8 × 0.8 cm heterogeneous lesion in the interpeduncular cistern extending to the right with mild mass effect on the medial aspect of the right cerebral peduncle. MRI gradient echo images (C, D) demonstrate low signal in the lesion suggestive of chronic hemorrhage.*

Many movement disorders involve shaking movements, such as hemiballismus, tics, myoclonus, and paroxysmal choreathetosis, but these do not fit the clinical description well. A tremor is rhythmic shaking and is typically categorized by type: rest, postural, or kinetic. This patient's shaking was unusual in that it was present both at rest and with

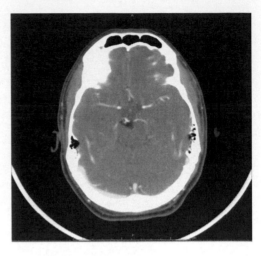

FIGURE 23.2 *CTA brain demonstrated a 1.9 × 1.9 mm outpouching of contrast extending postero-laterally from the P1 segment of the right posterior cerebral artery, consistent with aneurysm and surrounding 1.6 × 0.9 cm lipoma.*

movement. A tremor from medication or drug effect should not have improved so quickly nor been so lateralized. Most tremors disappear in sleep; however, there are some exceptions, such as palatal myoclonus. Given the coarse, irregular, high amplitude movement described in this case combined with the anatomic location of the lesion, this patient's tremor is most consistent with Holme's tremor.

Lipomas are benign findings, usually found in the midline of the brain. Aneurysms and lipomas are sometimes associated findings, but the nature of the relationship is unclear. One theory is that a congenital lipoma may cause aneurysmal defect in vasculature. Prognostic implications are also unclear; it is possible that the lipoma contained the hemorrhage and prevented further complications in this patient.

Holme's tremor, formerly referred to as "rubral tremor," is a characteristically 2- to 5-Hz tremor that can be of rest, postural, and intention type. Typically, it affects the proximal more than distal limb but can occasionally affect the neck and torso. It can be less rhythmic than other tremors and may or may not disappear in sleep. The movement can be high amplitude and very disabling. It usually takes weeks to months to develop after injury to the thalamus or midbrain, typically due to damage to cerebello-thalamic or nigrostriatal pathways. Hemorrhage is the most common etiology, but trauma and ischemia have also been documented causes.

TREATMENT

Traditionally, Holme's tremor has been treated with trials of levodopa, dopaminergic agonists, anticholinergics, or benzodiazepines, although poor response is typical. There are also some case reports of using levetiracetam with success. Stereotactic thalamotomy or deep brain stimulation can be used for refractory cases.

SUGGESTED READING

Deuschle G, Bain P, Brin M. Consensus statement of the Movement Disorder Society on Tremor. *Mov Disord.* 1998;13(S3):1–149.

Seung-Jae Lee et al. Monosymtpomatic rest tremor due to a midbrain ateriovenous malformation. *Mov Disord.* 2008;23(14):2094–2096.

Zhong J, Li S, Xu S, Wan L. Holmes' tremor caused by midbrain cavernoma. *Chin Med J.* 2007; 120(22):2059–2061.

CHIEF COMPLAINT: **Hands and feet have been tingling, and legs are weak.**

HISTORY OF PRESENT ILLNESS

A 28-year-old, right-handed male complained of tingling in his hands for the past 2 weeks that progressed to include his feet, along with shooting pains in arms and legs which he described as "like growing pains." Two days ago, he noticed weakness in his legs; he was unable to climb the stairs to his apartment. He also began choking on food and could not swallow solids anymore. He noted that 4 weeks ago, he had fever and chills followed by a couple of days of diarrhea. He described waves of nausea associated with profuse sweating and episodes of dizziness, lightheadedness, and nausea; these complaints would typically subside upon lying down.

He denied any history of travel. He denied history of diabetes or liver or kidney disease. He denied ever having experienced these symptoms in the past. He denied any bladder or bowel problems. He had no double vision, blurring of vision, or slurred speech.

PAST MEDICAL HISTORY
None.

PAST SURGICAL HISTORY
None.

ALLERGIES
NKDA.

PERSONAL HISTORY
Nonsmoker, no alcohol or illicit drug use.

FAMILY HISTORY
Maternal grandmother with CREST syndrome.

PHYSICAL EXAMINATION
Vital signs: 155/88, Heart rate, 101; respiratory rate, 18; O_2 sat 94% on room air.
General: No acute distress, breathing short/shallow breaths at time.
HEENT: Sclera non-icteric. No conjunctival injection. No lymphadenopathy. Trachea midline. Tympanic membranes looked healthy.
Pulmonary: Clear to auscultation bilaterally, taking poor volumes.
Cardiovascular: Normal S1/S2, no murmurs/rubs/gallops, sinus tachycardia 101/min.
Abdomen: Normal active bowel sounds. Nontender/nondistended.
Musculoskeletal: No atrophy, no joint pains, no redness, or swelling of joints.
Skin/extremities: No rash, no clubbing/cynanosis/edema, patent pulses.

NEUROLOGICAL EXAMINATION
Mental status: Awake and alert to time, place and person, good insight into recent events, normal affect. Speech fluent and followed three-step commands. Immediate memory 3/3.
CNs II–XII: Normal except for absent gag reflexes bilaterally.

Motor: 3+/5 weakness UE and LE except L gastrocnemius and soleus 4+/5, normal tone. No fasiculations or atrophy. No pronator drift.

Sensory: Intact to light touch, pin prick, vibration, proprioception, cortical sensations.

Reflexes: Trace triceps and brachioradialis bilaterally, absent reflexes in the lower extremities.

Plantars: Flexor.

Coordination: Finger-nose-finger and heel-to-shin intact.

Gait: Unstable due to weakness, unable to toe, heel or tandem walk; could not squat to 30% at hip without collapse.

Romberg sign: Absent.

Spinal tap was performed in the ED showing a protein level of 134, with no white blood cells.

He was soon unable to clear his secretions, especially upon vomiting, and required intubation for airway protection. On cardiac monitoring he was noted to have wide swings in heart rate and blood pressure.

STOP AND THINK QUESTIONS

➢ Why was the patient intubated?

➢ What are other possible etiologies for acute, diffuse weakness?

➢ What is the fastest way to obtain laboratory evidence to aid in the diagnosis?

➢ What is the best treatment for this neurological condition?

DIAGNOSTIC TEST RESULTS

1. Elevated CSF protein (90%) with no cells; this is referred as albuminocytological dissociation and can be delayed by 7 days after presentation.

2. Nerve conduction studies showing slowing of conduction (90%) and prolonged distal motor and F wave latencies, conduction block, decreased CMAP amplitudes, slowed motor conduction.

DIAGNOSIS: Guillian-Barré syndrome (GBS) or, more specifically, AIDP.

DISCUSSION

This disease was originally described by Guillian, Barré and Strohl as a triad of motor weakness, areflexia, and parasthesias with subtle sensory loss all in the context of a patient with high protein in the CSF (albuminocytological dissociation). AIDP is a disorder of peripheral nerves in which the myelin nerve sheathes are attacked by autoantibodies. This disease is the most common cause of acute paralysis in the Western world. There is often an antecedent illness or event, and the most common of these is respiratory illness most often CMV (15%) or Mycoplasma pneumoniae (10%), followed by a gastrointestinal illness (22%) most often Campylobacter jejuni (26%), and finally a prior surgery (5%). Other possible infections preceding AIDP include *Helicobacter pylori*, EBV, HSV or hepatitis. Vaccination against rabies, influenza, and *meningococcal meningitis* have been associated with GBS. HIV seroconversion can present as GBS.

The classical features are the onset of an aforementioned illness that is followed 1 to 4 weeks later by paresthesias and/or a symmetric, subacute motor weakness progressing over hours to days. The weakness is often described as an "ascending motor paralysis" which can be a deceptive description in that the weakness may involve the legs before the arms; however, the proximal muscles may be more profoundly affected than distal muscles. In 9% of cases, the weakness can be asymmetric. Often the cranial nerves are affected, usually later in the disease process. More than half of those with affected cranial nerves will have a bilateral facial paralysis (polyneuritis cranialis) which can even herald the onset of this disease. Usually, extraocular muscles are spared, but can be involved in a rare GBS variant named after the celebrated neurologist Charles Miller Fisher. Miller-Fisher syndrome is a clinical triad of *areflexia, ataxia* (due to a mismatch in proprioceptive and joint position sensory inputs from damaged nerves), and *opthalmoplegia*. Facial diplegia can be seen in this variant causing a seemingly flat affect due to decreased facial movements.

EMG/NCV can aid in diagnosis, as this study often reveals the widespread multifocal demyelination of the peripheral nervous system involving anywhere from the nerves up to the roots and anywhere in between. EMG/NCV demonstrating reduced conduction velocities is highly suggestive of GBS.

MRI with gadolinium may show enhancement of spinal roots. Sural nerve biopsy can show segmental demyelination, focal inflammation, and Wallerian degeneration.

DIFFERENTIAL DIAGNOSIS

Some other disease processes that can mimic the acute paralysis with loss of reflexes are exposures such as organophosphate/pesticide poisoning (marked GI symptoms including vomiting), heavy metal toxicity (arsenic, lead, thallium), botulinum toxicity (most often in the United States due to uncooked potatoes), ciguatoxin poisoning (large reef fish), and tick paralysis (multiple species, e.g., wood tick, dog tick, and others).

If reflexes are preserved, then metabolic derangements should be considered; severe hyper- or hypokalemia, hypophosphatemia, hypermagnesemia can also cause diffuse weakness, with preserved reflexes. If CSF shows pleocytosis (>50 cells) along with elevated protein, then acute Lyme, HIV, CMV, or West Nile virus meningoradiculopathies ought to be considered. If none of the above criteria are met, realize that acute CNS pathology such as brain stem/spinal cord compromise can initially present as a flaccid are flexic paralysis or so-called "spinal shock," and that an MRI of the central axis may be warranted. Myasthenia gravis should be considered if cranial nerves are primarily affected. In children

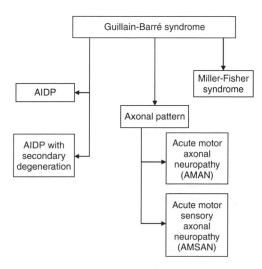

FIGURE 24.1 *Different forms of GBS.*

in areas of poor vaccine compliance, such as in the Eastern world, diphtheria and polio are among the more common causes of acute paralysis.

There are several different subtypes of GBS (Figure 24.1), which involve variations of the peripheral nervous system either affecting only motor or sensory nerves and sometimes axonal rather than myelin components, and even the autonomic nerves rather than somatic.

The following criteria are required for the diagnosis of GBS:

1. Progressive, bilateral weakness of all extremities
2. Loss of muscle stretch reflexes (formerly known as DTR)

The following are supportive features of diagnosis:

1. Absence of fever
2. Symmetry
3. Mild sensory involvement
4. Cranial nerve involvement
5. Autonomic involvement (65%)
6. Subacute course over days to 4 weeks
7. Recovery in 2 to 4 weeks after progression halts

TREATMENT

Thanks to the advent of PPV, the mortality rate of this illness has dropped from a staggering 33% to 5%. There are better critical care services available to prevent aspiration pneumonia, frank respiratory failure, and cardiogenic shock due to autonomic/hemodynamic instability. FVC and NIF should be checked every 4 hours for respiratory muscle compromise, along with pulse oximetry with the possibility of lung collapse due to poor ventilation. Indicators for concern of imminent respiratory compromise are as follows: rapid course with onset to admission in 7 days or less, bulbar compromise especially bilateral facial nerve palsies, and autonomic instability. The "20–30-40 rule" should be followed: VC < 20 ml/kg, NIF < 30 cm of H_2O, maximum expiratory pressure < 40 cm of H_2O, and when any of these respiratory measures have been breeched, monitoring in an ICU setting is appropriate. If the VC falls below 15 ml/kg (18 ml/kg in patients with severe buccal weakness) or PaO_2 falls below 70 mm Hg, then elective intubation should be performed for airway protection. If the patient is unable to lift his head off the bed, an acute course is evident. If VC falls to less than 60% of predicted, then emergent intubation and mechanical ventilation must be considered. Cardiac monitoring for autonomic instability is essential throughout the initial acute hospitalization. Cardiac conduction abnormalities from arrhythmia to heart block are not uncommon, and wide fluctuations in blood pressure are the rule. Pressor agents and antihypertensives should be avoided if possible. NSAIDs (provided renal function is not compromised due to low flow states or immune complex deposition which can be seen in this syndrome) and opiates (close attention to airway/respiratory function) are generally safe and efficacious for the painful parasthesias that mark this disease. With long immobilization, subcutaneous heparin and spontaneous compression stockings are essential to prevent deep venous thrombosis.

IVIG and PLEX have been shown to shorten recovery time if started within 2 to 4 weeks of onset of symptoms in GBS patients with marked weakness; these treatments have been shown to be roughly equivalent. The AAN guidelines recommend IVIG for *nonambulant* patients within 2 and possibly even 4 weeks after the onset of neuropathic symptoms. The

AAN guidelines recommend PLEX for the *nonambulant* patient within 4 weeks of presentation of neuropathic symptoms. Finally, the AAN guidelines recommend "consideration" of PLEX for the *ambulant* patient within 2 weeks of presentation of neuropathic symptoms. For patients who may not be able to tolerate intravascular volume shifts due to hemodynamic instability (e.g., elderly patients or patients with sepsis or active bleeds or heart disease), IVIG may be the better choice. IVIG given as a course of five treatments of 0.4 g/kg/d is preferred over PLEX (five 50 ml/kg exchanges given over a 1- to 2-week period) for interfacility ease of use and 24-hour access. In most academic centers, IVIG has become the first line treatment of choice, unless the patient has contraindications for IVIG, that is, a history of hyperviscosity syndromes, congestive heart failure, renal failure, or congenital IgA deficiency.

Recovery is usually rapid with improvement in the second month of illness; however, 18% of patients may not improve fully even after 2 years. DTRs are often the last to recover. Older age (>60 years), intubation/mechanical ventilation, rapid progression (<7 days), CMAP 20% of normal or less and axonal forms (not just demyelination) have all been found to portend a poor prognosis for recovery.

SUGGESTED READING

Bosch, EP. Guillain-Barré syndrome: An update of acute immune-mediated polyradiculoneuropathies. *Neurologist.* 1998;4:211–226.

Bradley, WG. *Neurology in Clinical Practice.* Philadelphia, PA: Elsevier; 2004:2336–2345.

Hughes RAC, Wijdicks EFM, Barohn R, et al. Practice parameter: Immunotherapy for Guillain–Barré syndrome: Report of the Quality Standards Subcommittee of the American Academy of Neurology. *Neurology.* 2003;61:736–740.

CHIEF COMPLAINT: There is something wrong with right arm and right leg.

HISTORY OF PRESENT ILLNESS

A 44-year-old, right-handed Caucasian man presented with right arm and leg weakness. The patient works as a carpenter. On the day prior to coming to the emergency room, he had noticed that his right side felt "stiff" and he had trouble holding his tools at work. His right arm also felt like it kept "going to sleep." The next morning, on waking up, he noticed that his entire right arm including his hand was weak, and when he tried to get out of bed, he had trouble walking. He noticed weakness on the right side of his torso as well. After a hot shower, he felt his symptoms were worse. He reported frequent urination for few months, but denied any incontinence of bowel or bladder.

Three years prior, the patient awakened one morning with a "crooked face." The right side of his face was paralyzed and felt numb for about 2 weeks, then gradually improved back to normal. He intermittently experienced double vision while his face was "crooked." At that time, his physician diagnosed him with "Bell's palsy."

PAST MEDICAL HISTORY

Bell's palsy.

PAST SURGICAL HISTORY

None.

ALLERGIES

NKDA.

PERSONAL HISTORY

Denied illicit drug use. He is a social alcohol drinker and smokes 1 pack of cigarettes per day. He is single and works as a carpenter. He is heterosexual and denied unprotected sex.

FAMILY HISTORY

No history of autoimmune or neurologic disorder, there is history of hypertension.

PHYSICAL EXAMINATION

Vital signs: Blood pressure, 130/70 mm Hg; heart rate, 75 bpm; respiratory rate, 12/min; temperature, 98.7°F.
General: No apparent distress.
HEENT: Atraumatic, normocephalic.
Neck: Supple, normal carotid pulses.
Pulmonary: Lungs clear to auscultation bilaterally.
CVS: Regular rate, no murmurs.
Abdomen: Nondistended, nontender, normal bowel sounds, but patient notably had trouble sitting up in bed, and his navel would pull to the left side as he was sitting up.
Musculoskeletal: No joint pain or swelling.
Skin: No rashes or abnormal pigmentation.

NEUROLOGICAL EXAMINATION

Mental status: Alert, awake, oriented to person, place, and time. Higher mental function including level of knowledge, language (comprehension, expression, naming, repetition, reading and writing), judgment, abstraction, memory, calculation, and praxis were all normal, memory 3/3.

CNs II–XII: Visual acuity 20/20 bilaterally. Visual fields full, fundoscopic exam normal, pupils were 4 mm bilaterally and equally reactive to light and accommodation, extraocular movements were intact, normal facial sensation, no facial weakness, normal hearing, palate normal, SCM/shoulder shrug normal, tongue normal.

Motor: Right pronator drift, normal bulk in all four extremities without atrophy. Slightly increased tone in the right leg. Strength 5/5 on the left side, 4/5 in the right leg.

Sensory: Light touch and two-point discrimination were decreased in the right hand, trunk, and leg. When tested on the trunk, there appeared to be a distinct sensory level at the T6 level dermatome on the right, but not on the left. Pain and temperature sensation were diminished on the left leg and left side of the trunk to approximately 3 inches above the level of the umbilicus. Proprioception was diminished at the hallux and ankle in the left foot compared to the right foot, but normal in the left arm.

Reflexes: Biceps, brachioradialis, triceps, patellar 2+ on the left, but 3+ on the right. Patellar reflex on the right elicited a crossed adductor reflex. Two beats of clonus were present in the left ankle, but sustained clonus for 10 beats was present on the right. Hoffman's and Babinski reflex were present on the right side but absent on the left.

Gait: Gait was wide based; he had a foot drag on the right.

Romberg: Positive with patient falling to the right side repeatedly.

When the patient was asked to flex his neck forward and touch his chin to his chest, he reported experiencing a "shock" sensation up and down his spine, radiating into his right leg. Romberg positive with patient falling to the right side repeatedly.

STOP AND THINK QUESTIONS

➢ Where will you localize the lesion?

➢ What is the name of the syndrome of hemiparesis with crossed sensory signs described in this patient's current examination?

➢ What clinical characteristics of a Bell's palsy should prompt imaging?

➢ What is the name of the sign that describes a sensation of electric shocks on neck flexion?

➢ What sign is it when there is a worsening of symptoms with increased temperature?

➢ What is the differential of recurrent brain and spinal cord lesions?

➢ What tests would help you properly diagnose, prognosticate and treat the patient?

DIAGNOSTIC TEST RESULTS

MRI brain with and without contrast (Figure 25.1) showed T2 hyperintense lesions in the brain stem (A) and in the supratentorial white matter (B, C), with open ring gadolinium enhancement (D) and T1 hypointensities referred as "black holes" (E).

MRI cervical spine revealed an enhancing lesion in the spinal cord at the level of C4 to C5 and nonenhancing lesions at the cevicomedullary junction and upper C2 (Figure 25.2).

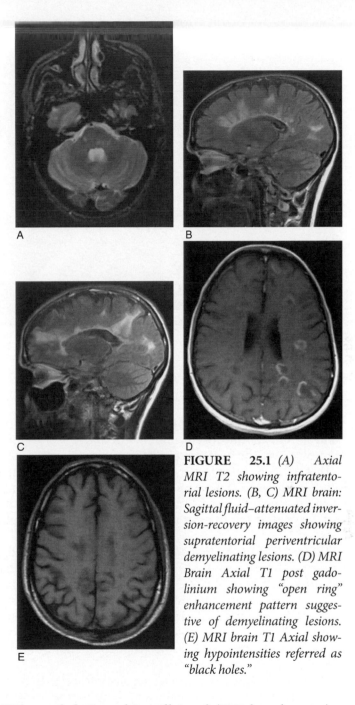

FIGURE 25.1 *(A) Axial MRI T2 showing infratentorial lesions. (B, C) MRI brain: Sagittal fluid–attenuated inversion-recovery images showing supratentorial periventricular demyelinating lesions. (D) MRI Brain Axial T1 post gadolinium showing "open ring" enhancement pattern suggestive of demyelinating lesions. (E) MRI brain T1 Axial showing hypointensities referred as "black holes."*

Spinal tap: CSF revealed nine white cells/mm³ (90% lymphocytes), protein 31 mg/dl, glucose 52 mg/ml, and five oligoclonal bands in the CSF that were not present in the serum. Cultures of CSF were negative.

Blood tests: HIV, Lyme, syphilis, HTLV, thyroid-stimulating hormone, angiotensin-converting enzyme, antithyroid, antinuclear, and anticardiolipin antibody testing were all negative. Fasting serum glucose and hemoglobin A1C were normal.

Chest X-ray was normal without hilar adenopathy.

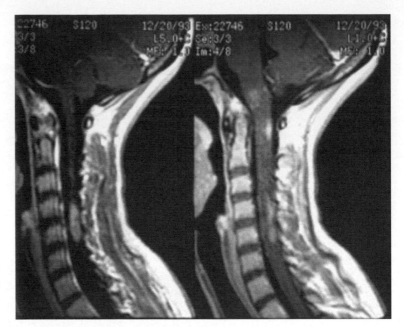

FIGURE 25.2 *MRI cervical spine, sagittal images showing demyelinating lesions in the cervical spine.*

DIAGNOSIS: **Relapsing–remitting multiple sclerosis (RRMS).**

DISCUSSION

The patient was treated with IV methylprednisolone 500 mg every 12 hours for 3 days with rapid significant improvement in motor and sensory symptoms. His symptoms continued to resolve over the next 4 weeks while undergoing regular physical therapy.

This patient's initial episode of facial paralysis accompanied by facial sensory loss and diplopia on vertical gaze was clearly not Bell's palsy and likely attributable to his right-sided pontine lesion seen on imaging. Facial paralysis that is accompanied by other cranial nerve abnormalities or is bilateral or recurrent should be investigated for underlying causes.

This patient presented with a partial Brown-Sequard syndrome due to an asymmetrical spinal cord lesion. MS lesions are frequently small and located postero-laterally in the cord. They tend to cause partial rather than complete transverse myelitis. Transverse myelitis with lesions that involve the entire cross section of the spinal cord and are longitudinally extensive causing severe bilateral motor, sensory, and autonomic (usually bladder) dysfunction is more commonly found in association with neuromyelitis optica (Devic's syndrome), as an isolated phenomenon, or with other autoimmune disorders rather than MS.

Lhermitte's sign (paresthesias on neck flexion) is thought to be due to cervical meningeal irritation. With neck flexion, there is stretching of the cord. Uhthoff's phenomenon is provocation of neurologic deficits with elevated body temperature and is thought to occur as a result of poor conduction across demyelinated or partially remyelinated axons. Recurrence of prior symptoms (pseudoexacerbations) can also occur in the setting of fever, infection, or other stressors.

This patient has RRMS. He has had two clinical events involving two distinct areas of the CNS, and these events were separated in time. He meets the revised McDonald's criteria for a diagnosis of MS. Along with requiring dissemination of the disease in space and time, the criteria also emphasize that MS is a diagnosis of exclusion, and an alternate cause must be ruled out before a diagnosis of MS is made. The revised criteria incorporate MRI findings to provide evidence of dissemination in space and time. Differential diagnosis of MS is vast and includes other demyelinating diseases like neuromyelitis optica and ADEM, infections such as syphilis, HIV, Lyme and HTLV, systemic autoimmune diseases such as Sarcoidosis, Systemic Lupus Erythematosis, Behcet's syndrome and Sjogren's disease, and primary or secondary CNS lymphomas and other malignancies and leukodystrophies. Chronic ischemic injury forms microvascular disease and CNS vasculitis can cause lesions mimicking MS (Table 25.1).

MS is the most common nontraumatic cause of neurologic disability in young adults, occurring in approximately 1 in 3,500 people. The highest prevalence is in North America and Western Europe. The female-to-male ratio is about 3:1. The general population risk of MS is 0.5% in women and 0.3% in men. Siblings of patients with MS have an increased risk ~3% and monzygotic twins about 30%. A family history of MS or other autoimmune disease (asthma, psoriasis, type I diabetes, etc.) is common. Peak age of diagnosis is the second to fourth decade of life, but it can also occur in children and older individuals.

There are several types of MS defined by the clinical course. The most common form of MS is the RRMS form characterized by relapses or episodes of neurologic dysfunction in between periods of relative clinical stability. About 85% to 90% of patients are diagnosed with this form. When patients with RRMS are followed over time, the relapses become less frequent, the recovery from relapses becomes incomplete, and they transition to a progressive stage called secondary progressive stage. A smaller number of patients, about 10% to 15% have a slowly progressive clinical course from the beginning, and this type of MS is called primary progressive MS. Distinguishing the different types of MS has therapeutic implications because currently available treatments have shown to be of benefit in the relapsing forms but have shown little benefit in the progressive forms. The clinical course of MS spans a wide spectrum with some patients having minimal deficits many years after the diagnosis, while others have a more aggressive course with rapid accumulation of disability.

TREATMENT

Treatment of MS involves treatment of acute relapses and the long-term disease modifying therapy.

Relapses are usually treated with high-dose steroids. A commonly used regimen is IV methylprednisolone 1000 mg daily for 3 to 5 days. Sometimes, higher doses of steroids may be required. ACTH, or oral prednisone may be used if IV steroids cannot be given due to

TABLE 25.1 *Differential Diagnosis of Multiple Sclerosis*

Other CNS Demyelinating Diseases	Vascular Disorders	Autoimmune Diseases	Infectious Diseases	Genetic Disorders	Neoplasms	Metabolic Disorders
ADEM, NMO, isolated ON, isolated TM	CNS vasculitis, CADASIL	SLE, Sjogren's syndrome, Behcet's disease, antiphospholipid syndromes, sarcoidosis	HTLV-associated myelopathy, Lyme disease, syphilis, HIV	Leber's hereditary optic neuropathy, hereditary spastic paraparesis, hereditary ataxias	CNS lymphomas, other malignancies	Leukodystrophies, vitamin B_{12} metabolism disorders

TABLE 25.2 *First-Line MS Treatments*

	IFN β 1b Betaseron®	IFN β 1a Avonex®	IFN β 1a Rebif®	Glatiramer Acetate Copaxone®
Injection	SC	IM	SC	SC
Frequency	Every other day	Q Weekly	3/week	Every day
Dose	8 MIU (250 µg)	30 µg	44 µg	20 mg
Side effects	Injection site pain, erythema, induration, flu-like symptoms, myalgias, depression, elevated liver enzymes, thyroid abnormalities, suppression of WBC count, lipodystrophy, need to monitor CBC with diff, LFT every 3 months then at least every 6 months, need to check TFT periodically, potential risk of developing neutralizing antibodies			Injection site pain, erythema, induration, transient hyperventilation, tachycardia, lipodystrophy

lack of IV access, insurance reasons, and so on. Severe relapses that are refractory to steroids are treated with plasma exchange. Another treatment that has been used for relapses is a course of IVIG.

Currently, there are six FDA-approved treatments for MS. Clinical trials have shown them to be effective in relapsing MS. Treatments are more effective earlier during the inflammatory stage rather than the later neurodegenerative phase of the disease. Four of these agents are used as first-line agents; they are the three interferons, and glatiramer acetate (refer to Table 25.2).

In patients who have very aggressive disease from the onset or those whose disease is not controlled on first-line agents, then second-line agents are employed. They are natalizumab (Tysabri®) or chemotherapeutic agents including mitoxantrone or cyclophosphamide. Some of the newer agents that are being used for MS currently include alemtuzumab, rituximab, fingolimod (Gilenya), and cladribine among others. In two phase III clinical trials, oral agent fingolimod reduced the rate of relapses in RRMS by over half compared both to placebo and to the active comparator interferon beta-1a.

Natalizumab is a humanized monoclonal antibody against α4β1 and α4β7 integrins. It prevents transendothelial migration of activated leukocytes into the CNS. It is administered as an IV infusion every 4 weeks. Side effects/adverse events include infusion associated reactions including chills, headache, and allergic reactions. There is the potential risk of opportunistic infections including PML.

Some of the common symptoms reported by MS patients include fatigue, spasticity, gait impairment, visual symptoms, pain, bowel/bladder issues, sexual dysfunction, cognitive impairment, and mood alteration including depression and anxiety. These have to be evaluated and treated by a multidisciplinary team including physical and occupational therapists.

SUGGESTED READING

Miller DH, Weinshenker BG, Fillippi, et al. Differential diagnosis of suspected multiple sclerosis: A consensus approach. *Multiple Sclerosis*. 2008;14:1157–1174.

Noseworthy JH, Lucchinetti C, Rodriguez M, Weinshenker BG. Multiple sclerosis. *NEJM*. 2000;343:938–952.

Polman CH, Reingold SC, Edan G, et al. Diagnostic criteria for multiple sclerosis: 2005 revisions to the "McDonald criteria." *Neurology*. 2005;58:840–846.

CHIEF COMPLAINT: **I am walking like I am drunk.**

HISTORY OF PRESENT ILLNESS

A 67-year-old, right-handed man awoke the night prior to admission with sudden onset headache, nausea and vomiting, dizziness, and severe imbalance. He arrived at the hospital 24 hours after the onset of symptoms, complaining of an occipital headache and gait instability. He had been to another emergency room prior and had been diagnosed with "gastroenteritis." He said that he never had headaches like this before and was otherwise in excellent physical condition, teaching martial arts. Now, he said, he could barely stand without falling over, and is walking as if he was drunk.

PAST MEDICAL HISTORY AND PAST SURGICAL HISTORY

The patient thought he might have been diagnosed with hypertension several years ago, but is not sure and almost never saw doctors.

MEDICATIONS

None.

ALLERGIES

None.

PERSONAL HISTORY

The patient had smoked one pack of cigarettes per day for the past 40 years.

FAMILY HISTORY

His mother died from breast cancer when the patient was a child, and the patient's father was still alive and well at age 90.

PHYSICAL EXAMINATION

Vitals: Blood pressure, 170/94; heart rate, 85; respiratory rate, 13; temperature, 98.5°F.
GPE: Unremarkable, though the patient appeared uncomfortable.

NEUROLOGICAL EXAMINATION

Mental status: Normal.
CNs I–XII: The patient had vertical and horizontal nystagmus. Rest of the cranial nerve examination was otherwise normal.
Motor: Normal bulk in all four extremities without atrophy. Strength was 5/5 throughout, and his tone was normal. No fasciculations or abnormal movements were seen.
Sensory: His sensory examination was intact to light touch, pin prick, joint position sense, and temperature.
Reflexes: 2+ throughout and symmetric.
Plantars: Flexors.
Coordination: He had dysmetria on the finger-nose-finger test, the heel-to-shin maneuver and while performing rapid alternating movements.

Gait: The patient's gait was very wide based, and he was unable to make more than a few steps without falling. He did not preferentially fall to either the left or the right. He could not even attempt to tandem and even had trouble sitting up straight in bed (truncal ataxia).

STOP AND THINK QUESTIONS

➢ The patient has classic signs and symptoms of cerebellar pathology. What is the difference between appendicular and truncal ataxia?

➢ Why are large, acute lesions in the midline cerebellum potentially fatal?

➢ What is the vascular supply to the cerebellum?

DIAGNOSIS: Acute bilateral infarction of the PICA with obstructive hydrocephalus and tonsillar herniation.

HOSPITAL COURSE

NCHCT revealed symmetric, bilateral hypodense lesions of the cerebellum in the territory of the medial branches of the PICA (Figure 26.1). There was edema of the cerebellum with moderate compression of the fourth ventricle and almost complete obliteration of the prepontine and cerebellopontine angle cisterns. The remainder of the ventricular system was enlarged, and there was evidence of transependymal flow of CSF, consistent with early, obstructive hydrocephalus. Additionally, soft tissue was seen in the foramen magnum posterior to the medulla, indicating tonsillar herniation.

Routine blood studies were normal.

12-lead EKG showed a normal sinus rhythm with occasional premature ventricular contractions, as well as left ventricular hypertrophy and left atrial enlargement.

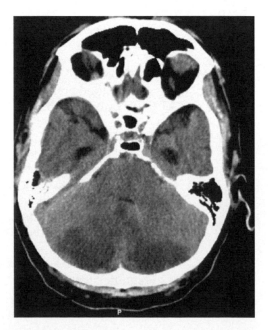

FIGURE 26.1 *Admission noncontrast CT of the head demonstrating hypodensities in bilateral cerebellar hemispheres, near-total effacement of the fourth ventricle, and dilated temporal horns consistent with acute hydrocephalus.*

The patient was admitted to an ICU, and he underwent frequent clinical examination and serial NCHCT studies. He was placed on dipyridamole, and aspirin was held in anticipation of possible CSF diversion, and because patient reported a prior adverse reaction.

Two days after admission, the patient was noted to have increased somnolence. A NCHCT revealed further enlargement of the lateral ventricles and near-complete effacement of the fourth ventricle. A right frontal ventriculostomy was placed, without any immediate improvement in the patient's level of alertness. Initial ICP was recorded at 20 cm H_2O. The ventriculostomy was left open to drainage at 10 cm above the external auditory meatus, and ICP subsequently remained less than 12 cm H_2O. Two days after placement of the ventriculostomy, the patient became progressively more alert, with resolution of his headache. He was found to have decreased nystagmus, but persistent gait ataxia. The fourth ventricle became more visible on NCHCT. CSF diversion was rapidly tapered, and the ventricular drain was removed eight days after admission. He was transferred out of intensive care and later to acute inpatient rehabilitation. At discharge, the patient was no longer complaining of headache, and his gait was significantly improved.

MRI of the brain obtained on hospital day five revealed an extensive area of restricted diffusion in the posterior, inferior portions of both cerebellar hemispheres, consistent with acute infarction (Figure 26.2).

MRA brain failed to visualize either of the PICA arteries, but showed normal AICA bilaterally.

Carotid Doppler revealed minimal (less than 50%) stenosis of both internal carotid arteries and anterograde flow in both vertebral arteries.

The patient was unable to tolerate a tranesophageal echocardiogram; however, a transthoracic echocardiogram failed to visualize cardiac or valvular thrombi. Additionally, continuous telemetry showed the patient to be in sinus rhythm throughout his ICU course.

DISCUSSION

Bilateral infarctions in the PICA territory are exceedingly rare. The first case was reported by Tada et al. in 1994 (1). Including this report, 20 cases of acute, bilateral infarcts in the PICA territory have been published (1–7). Clinically, gait ataxia is a universal symptom.

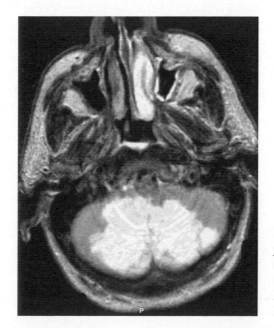

FIGURE 26.2 *MRI of the brain obtained on hospital day five. This T2WI demonstrates extensive edema bilaterally within the PICA territories of the cerebellum, consistent with recent infarction. DWI demonstrated restricted diffusion in the same location.*

Other symptoms commonly observed include dizziness, headache with nausea and vomiting, and horizontal nystagmus. Of note, this constellation of symptoms is identical to those often observed in cases of unilateral PICA infarction. Full recovery is the rule for patients with infarctions in the medial PICA territory. Whether the infarction is unilateral or bilateral, gait impairment is typically the last symptom to recover, as was the case with our patient (8). "Fatal gastroenteritis" refers to cerebellar pathology misdiagnosed as a gastrointestinal illness that eventually can lead to fatal complications for the patient.

Of all the major intracerebral vessels, the PICA is the most variable (9). At least one PICA is absent on up to 20% of cerebral angiograms of the posterior circulation. Several hypotheses have been advanced to explain cases of bilateral PICA territory infarction (4). These include the presence of a single artery supplying both territories, as well as a dominant PICA that supplies the medial territories bilaterally. Both mechanisms are consistent with the findings in this case. Gaida-Hommernick et al. demonstrated a single, unpaired PICA artery in a patient with a bilateral PICA territory infarction using cerebral angiography (5). Although this study was not performed in our patient, the absence of either PICA artery on the MRA suggests occlusion of a single PICA artery that supplied the medial cerebellar hemispheres bilaterally.

It has also been suggested that bilateral PICA territory infarction may occur in the context of normal vascular anatomy and unilateral PICA occlusion, with subsequent vasogenic edema leading to compression of the contralateral PICA (4). This seems unlikely in our case, as all the imaging data suggest a uniform progression of the entire area of the infarct from a single ischemic event. MRA examination has ruled out other possible mechanisms, including a single dominant AICA supplying both PICA territories, and both PICAs arising off a single occluded vertebral artery or an occluded basilar artery. In addition, a normal sinus rhythm on continuous cardiac telemetry, the absence of thrombi on echocardiogram, and the absence of infarction in other vascular territories argue strongly against simultaneous embolic infarction of both PICAs (4).

The risk of tonsillar herniation with brain stem compression and respiratory arrest is well appreciated in large, unilateral PICA infarctions (10–12). In addition to a case described by Sorenson et al., this is only the second documented case where a bilateral PICA territory infarction and the subsequent effacement of the ventricular system necessitated CSF diversion (3). This case emphasizes that although such infarctions are rare, and outcomes are usually favorable, clinicians need to be aware of potentially fatal complications. Our patient developed both obstructive hydrocephalus and tonsillar herniation. Because the clinical impact of these complications is easily mitigated by ventricular drainage, we believe observation in a monitored setting with frequent clinical assessment and serial imaging is essential. Additionally, the radiographic appearance of the infarction is symmetrical and does not conform to normal cerebral anatomy. Because of this, the pathology on the initial NCHCT in the emergency department, when the entire extent of the infarction might not yet be visible, can be easily overlooked or misinterpreted.

ACKNOWLEDGMENTS

We would like to thank Dr. Saran Jonas for his invaluable assistance.

REFERENCES

1. Tada Y, Mizutani T, Nishimura T, Tamura M, Mori N. Acute bilateral cerebellar infarction in the territory of the medial branches of posterior interior cerebellar arteries. *Stroke.* 1994;25:686–688.
2. Brusa L, Iannilli M, Bruno G, Gualdi GF, Schiaffini C, Lenzi GL. Bilateral simultaneous cerebellar infarction in the medial branches of the posterior interior cerebellar artery territories. *Ital J Neurol Sci.* 1996;17:433–466.

3. Sorenson EJ, Wijdicks EFM, Thielen KR, Cheng TM. Acute bilateral infarcts of the posterior inferior cerebellar artery. *J Neuroimaging*. 1997;7:250–251.

4. Kang DW, Lee SH, Bae HI, Han MH, Yoon BW, Roh JK. Acute bilateral cerebellar infarcts in the territory of posterior inferior cerebellar artery. *Neurology*. 2000;55:582–584.

5. Gaida-Hommernick B, Smekal UV, Kirsch M, Schminke U, Machetanz J, Kessler C. Bilateral cerebellar infarctions caused by a stenosis of congenitally unpaired posterior inferior cerebellar artery. *J Neuroimaging*. 2001;11:435–437.

6. Gurer G, Sahin G, Cekirge S, Tan E, Saribas O. Acute bilateral cerebral infarction in the territory of medial branches of posterior inferior cerebellar arteries. *Clin Neurol Neurosurg*. 2001;103:194–196.

7. Umashankar G, Gupta V, Harik SI. Acute bilateral inferior cerebellar infarction in a patient with neurosyphilis. *Arch Neurol*. 2004;61(6):953–6.

8. Amarenco P, Roullet E, Hommel M, Chaine P, Marteau R. Infarction in the territory of the medial branch of the posterior inferior cerebellar artery. *J Neurol, Neurosurg Psychiatry*. 1990;53(9):731–735.

9. Lazorthes G. La vascularisation arterielle du cervelet. In: Lazorthes G, ed. *Vascularisation et Circulation Cerebrales*. Paris, France: Masson; 1961;65–75.

10. Sypert GW, ALvord EC, Jr. Cerebellar infarction. A clinicopathological study. *Arch Neurol*. 1975;32(6):357–363.

11. Macdonell RA, Kalnins RM, Donnan GA. Cerebellar infarction: Natural history, prognosis, and pathology. *Stroke*. 1987;18(5):849–855.

12. Khan M, Polyzoidis KS, Adegbite AB, McQueen JD. Massive cerebellar infarction: "Conservative" management. *Stroke*. 1983;14(5):745–751.

Sudden Onset Confusion

Vincci Ngan

CHIEF COMPLAINT: **Confusion.**

HISTORY OF PRESENT ILLNESS

A 23-year-old, right-handed male presented to the emergency room with speech difficulties and confusion for 2 days. His family reported that he had not been answering questions appropriately. He had intermittent sharp frontal headaches associated with nausea and neck stiffness for the past 2 weeks, and he had low-grade fevers and chills for 1 week. Except for a trip to Montreal, Canada, 4 weeks prior to presentation, he had no travel history or sick contacts. The patient did not complain of weakness, tingling, numbness, double vision, or blurry vision. He had no cough, urinary symptoms, diarrhea, arthralgias, or other common neurological symptoms.

PAST MEDICAL HISTORY

None.

PAST SURGICAL HISTORY

Excision of a precancerous mole on his back 10 years ago.

MEDICATIONS

None.

ALLERGIES

None.

PERSONAL HISTORY

No use of tobacco, drugs, or alcohol. He is married and works in the IT department of a financial company.

FAMILY HISTORY

His father had hypertension and diabetes. His mother had no medical problems. There was no known neurological disease in his extended family.

PHYSICAL EXAMINATION

Vital signs: Temperature, 99.8°F; blood pressure, 121/83 mm Hg; pulse, 79; respiratory rate, 13.
General: Ill-appearing gentleman appearing his stated age.
HEENT: There was no nuchal rigidity.
Heart: Regular rate and rhythm, no murmurs.
Lungs: Clear to auscultation bilaterally.
Abdomen: Soft, nondistended, nontender.
Extremities: 2+ distal pulses.

NEUROLOGICAL EXAMINATION

Mental status: The patient was alert, oriented, and somewhat inattentive. His spontaneous speech was reduced, and he made some paraphasic errors. His comprehension, reading, writing, naming, and repetition were grossly intact.

CNs II–XII: Pupils were equal and reactive. Visual fields were full to confrontation. Fundoscopic examination revealed no papilledema. Extraocular movements were full. There was no facial asymmetry. Hearing was intact to finger rub bilaterally. His palate elevated symmetrically. There was no weakness in head turn or shoulder shrug. His tongue protruded midline.

Motor: There was no pronator drift. His strength was full to confrontation throughout.

Sensory: His sensation was intact to light touch, pin prick, and vibration.

Reflexes: He had normal reflexes throughout. Plantar response was flexors bilaterally.

Coordination: There was no dysmetria on finger-nose-finger or heel-knee-shin testing. There was no dysdiadochokinesia.

Gait: Normal.

STOP AND THINK QUESTIONS

➤ What are your worries in a patient with fever, headaches, neurological deficits, and changed mental status?

➤ Will you obtain neuroimaging first?

➤ Is spinal tap indicated in this case?

➤ How will you approach the case and what treatment would you initiate?

DIAGNOSIS: Herpes simplex virus (HSV) encephalitis.

HOSPITAL COURSE

The patient was admitted to the neurology service for further workup. His initial head CT showed multiple hyperdense lesions in the left inferior frontal and medial temporal lobes with associated edema concerning for hemorrhagic metastases, especially given his history of a precancerous skin lesion (Figure 27.1). His initial laboratory data were remarkable for sodium level of 127.

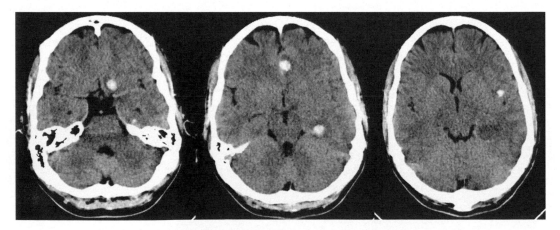

FIGURE 27.1 *Initial head CT without contrast.*

An MRI of the brain (Figure 27.2) was obtained the following morning and demonstrated large areas of abnormal signal intensity in the left medial and posterior temporal lobe, with areas of hemorrhage and irregular gadolinium enhancement, as well as multiple punctate areas of hemorrhage with edema in the left inferior frontal, left frontal parasagittal, left subinsular, left thalamic, and right posterior temporal lobes. Given the above

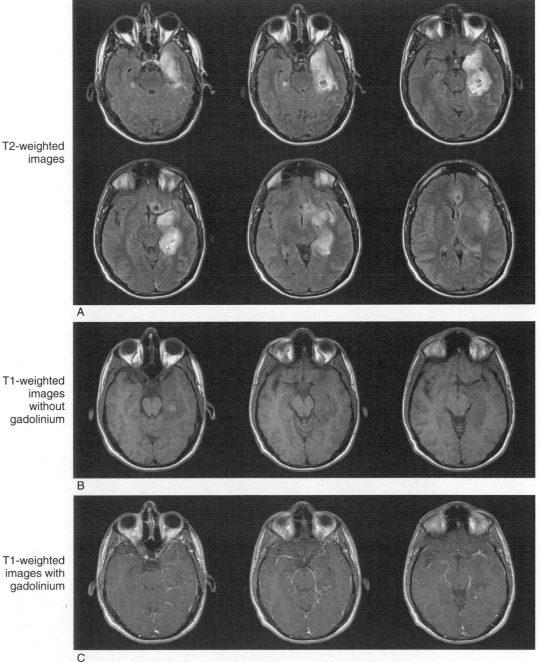

T2-weighted images

A

T1-weighted images without gadolinium

B

T1-weighted images with gadolinium

C

FIGURE 27.2 *MRI brain with and without gadolinium.*

findings, a neoplastic process was thought to be less likely, and infectious and inflammatory causes were entertained.

The patient became febrile to 104.1° F within 12 hours of admission, but his examination remained unchanged. Blood and urine cultures were obtained, which revealed no microorganisms. An echocardiogram did not demonstrate valve vegetations.

CSF showed 888 red cells, 244 nucleated cells with a lymphocytic predominance, normal glucose, high protein value of 146, and opening pressure of 40. Broad-spectrum antibiotics and Acyclovir were initiated for treatment of infectious encephalitis.

Over the next several days, the patient's mental status worsened, and continued to have fevers to 104° F. On hospital day 5, a repeat CT scan showed progression of the edema in the left temporal region, new areas of hypodensity in the left internal capsule, left frontal insular cortex, and right medial temporal lobes, as well as 6 mm left-to-right midline shift (Figure 27.3). Foscarnet was subsequently added due to his clinical deterioration.

Bacterial and fungal CSF cultures were negative, and HSV-1 DNA in the CSF was eventually isolated by PCR. In addition, the patient was found to have negative IgM and IgG HSV antibodies in his serum, suggesting that he had suffered primary CNS HSV-1 encephalitis.

Patient was continued on a 28-day course of Acyclovir and 14-day course of Foscarnet. He was ultimately stable for transfer to acute rehabilitation on hospital day 16. The patient's aphasia had improved: he made infrequent paraphasic errors, and his fluency was near normal.

DISCUSSION

HSV encephalitis is the most common form of fatal sporadic encephalitis in the United States, accounting for 10% to 20% of all cases of viral encephalitides. HSV-1 strains account for the majority of herpes encephalitis in adults; neonatal encephalitis is caused by either HSV-1 or HSV-2 strains. Initial infection with the herpes virus usually occurs in the oronasopharynx via contact with infected secretion. The virus then invades along the cranial nerves and lies dormant in the trigeminal ganglion. HSV-1 reactivation within the CNS can at times cause acute hemorrhagic, necrotizing encephalitis.

Fever and headache are the most common presenting symptoms of herpes encephalitis. Focal neurological findings, such as confusion, personality change, seizures, motor deficits,

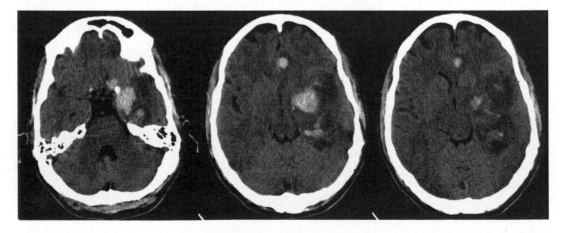

FIGURE 27.3 *Repeat head CT without contrast on hospital day 5.*

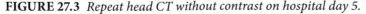

and aphasia commonly accompany systemic symptoms. Early recognition and initiation of antiviral treatment are essential in reducing morbidity and mortality.

CSF examination will often reveal an increased opening pressure, a lymphocytic pleocytosis of 10 to 1000 WBC/µL, xanthochromia or increased RBC count, as well as a moderately elevated protein count. Before the advent of PCR analysis, brain biopsy was considered the gold standard for the diagnosis of HSV encephalitis. Currently, HSV DNA detection in CSF by PCR testing has a sensitivity and specificity of >95%. CSF HSV PCR remains positive for at least 2 weeks and sometimes up to 4 weeks. CSF cultures are positive in only about 4% of adults and are therefore not routinely recommended.

Neuroimaging is often used to aid in the diagnosis. CT brain can be normal early in the illness, but hypoattenuation can be appreciated in the mesial temporal lobes and insular cortices 3 days after symptoms onset. MRI will show abnormalities 24 to 48 hours earlier than CT and will typically reveal asymmetric bilateral T2/FLAIR hyperintensities of the limbic system, the medial temporal and inferior frontal cortices, with diffusion restriction. Deep cortical structures are usually spared. Gyriform enhancement can be seen 1 week after the initial symptoms. Hemorrhagic lesions are a late feature of HSV encephalitis. Electroencephalogram in the majority of HSV cases will show intermittent slowing and occasionally periodic lateralized epileptiform dishcarges in the affected region.

The treatment of HSV encephalitis is early administration of antiviral therapy. Acyclovir has been shown to decrease the mortality and morbidity of the disease. All suspected cases of HSV encephalitis should receive Acyclovir 10 mg/kg IV every 8 hours for 14 to 21 days. There have been no prospective studies to evaluate the efficacy of corticosteroids in improving the outcome of HSV encephalitis.

The prognosis for untreated HSV encephalitis is extremely poor, with mortality approaching as high as 70%. Even with appropriate treatment, mortality rates can be about 20% to 30%. Survivors may suffer significant neurological deficits, such as cognitive impairment and behavioral abnormalities.

As stated, herpes encephalitis is the most common form of fatal sporadic encephalitis in the United States, with HSV-1 being the most common causative agent in adult cases. The clinical syndrome is characterized by headache, fever, seizures, focal neurological deficits, and impaired consciousness. Lumbar puncture with PCR analysis for HSV DNA, along with neuroimaging to assess for limbic system pathology, is recommended. If the diagnosis is clinically suspected, treatment with Acyclovir should be initiated without delay.

SUGGESTED READING

Boivin G. Diagnosis of herpesvirus infections of the central nervous system. *Herpes*. 2004;11(Suppl 2): 48A–56A.

Caliendo AM. PCR testing for the diagnosis of herpes simplex virus encephalitis. In: Hirsch MS, ed. *UpToDate*. Waltham, MA: UpToDate; 2011.

Kimberlin DW. Management of HSV encephalitis in adults and neonates: Diagnosis, prognosis and treatment. *Herpes*. 2007;14(1):11–16.

Klein RS. Herpes simplex type 1 encephalitis. In: Hirsch MS, ed. *UpToDate*. Waltham, MA: UpToDate; 2011.

CHIEF COMPLAINT: **I'm falling a lot, and my eyes are bad.**

HISTORY OF PRESENT ILLNESS

A 59-year-old, right-handed male complained of a progressive inability to move his eyes in all directions, difficulty swallowing, and increasing stiffness in his body making him unstable and causing him to fall often. The problems started with a sensitivity to light, requiring him to wear sunglasses even when indoors. At around the same time, he began coughing up liquids during meals. This soon progressed to difficulty swallowing solid foods. One year from onset of the sensitivity to light and swallowing difficulty, the patient began to stumble and fall, experiencing multiple falls thereafter. His son describes him tilting back and forth and occasionally collapsing like a "block of cement." Eventually, he experienced difficulty initiating his stride; he was thought to have PD by his neurologist, but a trial of Sinemet failed to help his symptoms. Over the next few months, his voice weakened, and around the same time, he developed the inability to look upwards, always having to tilt his head back to see objects above head level. He denies word finding difficulties or memory problems, but family has noticed that he does not engage or take interest in conversations. Every so often, he exhibits sporadic crying spells, but with no associated feelings of sadness. Once, he became really agitated and could have hurt his wife.

PAST MEDICAL HISTORY

Hypertension, hypercholesterolemia.

PAST SURGICAL HISTORY

None.

MEDICATIONS

Risperdal, Lexapro, Sinemet, Diovan, Zocor.

ALLERGIES

NKDA.

PERSONAL HISTORY

Heavy drinker for many years as a young adult, but quit 10 years ago. Denies smoking or drugs.

FAMILY HISTORY

Denies history of movement disorder or stroke.

PHYSICAL EXAMINATION

Blood pressure, 120/78 mm Hg; pulse, 66/min; respiratory rate, 14/min; afebrile.
No orthostatic hypotension.
General: Frequent tearing from eyes and wide stare. Hypophonic.

NEUROLOGICAL EXAMINATION

Mental status: Alert and consolidates, slight apathy. Does not initiate conversation, but answers appropriately to all questions. Hypophonic, fluent, comprehends and repeats appropriately. No apraxia, but when asked to clap three times, he keeps clapping multiple times.

CNs II–XII: Loss of voluntary eye movements in all directions of gaze. Oculocephalic reflexes intact, while vertical gaze "locked" in place. Eyes fixated in midline and conjugate, tears coming down at times. Pupils react equally to light, OS 20/25, intact visual fields, "startled" look, no flattening of nasolabial folds, no facial asymmetry, uvula and tongue midline, symmetric gag reflexes.

Motor: Strength 5/5 throughout distribution without pronator drift, atrophy or fasciculations. Mild cogwheeling R > L with mild rigidity in arms. No rigidity apparent in lower legs. Patient can perform heel tap bilaterally but cannot perform full raised leg tap due to inability to elevate legs. Bradykinetic on fine finger movements and heel tap.

Sensory: Intact to light touch and pain throughout.

Reflexes: 2+ symmetrical throughout but absent ankle jerks both sides.

Plantars: Toes down bilaterally.

Romberg: Positive, after 30 seconds patient falls back.

Coordination: FNF intact.

Gait: Trouble with initiating stride at times and small shuffling steps.

STOP AND THINK QUESTIONS

➢ What is the most likely diagnosis?

➢ What anatomical brain areas are involved in this disease?

➢ What is the prognosis for this disease?

DIAGNOSTIC TEST RESULTS

Routine laboratory results unremarkable, serum cholesterol 248 mg/dl; LDL 172 mg/dl. MRI brain without gadolinium: Sagittal T1 midline section of the brain illustrating midbrain atrophy and the classic "penguin sign" (Figure 28.1).

DIAGNOSIS: Progressive supranuclear palsy (PSP).

DISCUSSION

The differential diagnosis in this case is of the atypical Parkinson syndromes such as MSA and corticobasilar degeneration. Another consideration is normal pressure hydrocepahlus. However, very few diseases cause progressive loss of vertical eye movements and supranuclear palsy with rigidity, tilting/falls backward, and swallowing difficulties. In the first stages of PSP, it may be difficult to distinguish it from other atypical Parkinson syndromes, because all can cause rigidity, bradykinesia, trouble initiating gait, and swallowing difficulties. Among disorders involving the extrapyramidal pathways, PSP is distinct in that it causes *loss of vertical gaze, marked decreased blink rate* (3–5 times only in 1 minute), *severe truncal rigidity* that is out of proportion to appendicular rigidity (opposite of PD), *astonished facial expression*, and has *paucity of rest tremor*. Early falls and gait disturbances are not seen in typical PD cases (1).

PSP affects most patients by midlife (late 50s–early 60s) and causes dramatic deterioration thereafter over a 5- to 10-year period. It accounts for 5% to 6% of patients with

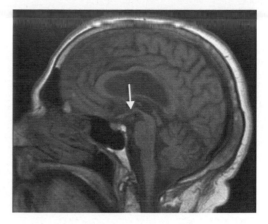

FIGURE 28.1 *MRI brain Sagittal T1 midline section of the brain illustrating midbrain atrophy and the classic "penguin sign," the white arrow pointing to the beak of the penguin.*

features of PD, and men are affected slightly more than women (1). The diagnosis is made from the history and examination and can be supported by imaging studies. Initial symptoms may be misleading as patients may complain of occasional unexplained falls, blurry vision, or photophobia (due to decreased eye blink), or the family may note that the patient is developing apathy or word-finding difficulties. Other symptoms that may present early are a weak voice and a pseudobulbar affect (crying or laughing that is dissociated from feelings). Usually within 1 year, patients develop frank postural instability and bradykinesia and later swallowing difficulties. Commonly, there is little or no tremor. Eye movements become slow, and then there is loss of vertical eye movements before horizontal eye movements. Initially, the downward gaze is affected. Examination also reveals slow saccades and eyelid opening apraxia and later swallowing difficulties. On examination, patients have prominent axial rigidity, with or without dystonia, most commonly retrotorticollis of the neck, and cogwheel rigidity. The face reveals facial hypomimia, a decreased blink rate (0–4/minutes vs. normal of 15), a fixed stare with loss of vertical gaze, and slowing of lateral saccades. In advanced stages, the eyes tend to follow the head as it moves. Over time, patients develop the classical "toppling like a tree" instability, ideomotor apraxias, and later corticospinal signs such as spasticity, hyperreflexia, extensor plantar responses, and muscle weakness. Sleep disorders such as insomnia, hypersomnia, periodic limb movements, and REM sleep disorders are common in patients with PSP (1).

There is no laboratory test for PSP. Recently, it has been suggested that MRI can help distinguish PSP from other degenerative disorders. While normal midbrain area is 115 mm^2, a midbrain area of <70 mm^2 was found to be 100% sensitive and 91% specific for PSP. Another useful feature is the ratio of midbrain tegmentum to pons area < 0.15, which excludes PD or MSA-P as the diagnosis 100% of the time. Together these spatial ratios create a hallmark imaging sign, "the penguin silhouette." Atrophy of the tectum and frontal regions is commonly seen on imaging (2).

The prognosis of PSP is grave and median survival is of 6 to 7 years. Early falls and bulbar symptoms herald a worse prognosis and more rapid deterioration. An average delay of 3 to 5 years has been seen as falls may not be recognized, or midbrain and pons abnormalities may not be appreciated early in the disease (1).

TABLE 28.1 *Supportive Symptomatic Therapy for PSP Patients*

Postural instability	Gait training, avoid and buffer falls, grab bars for the hallways and using stairs, walking aids or wheelchair, referral to physical therapists.
Dysphagia	Nutrition consult, video fluoroscopic studies to assess risk of aspiration, sit upright during meals and maintain head in a safe swallowing position, slow rate of feeding with small bites, avoid highly textured foods, encourage use of safe swallowing cups, monitor for weight loss, percutaneous endoscopic gastrostomy insertion (as needed)
Management of secretion problems	Glycopyrrolate, acetylcysteine, portable suction machine, avoid medications that dry up secretions

TREATMENT

Treatment is mostly supportive. Table 28.1 lists common interventions that can help improve the quality of life. Personality and mood changes, such as apathy, emotional incontinence, and inappropriate behavior, can be helped with medications. Nuedexta (dextromethorphan and quinidine sulfate) is a dual action glutamate inhibitor that can help symptoms of pseudobulbar affect.

REFERENCES

1. Lubarsky M, Juncos JL. Progressive supranuclear palsy: A current review. *The Neurologist*. March 2008;14(2):79–88.
2. Oba H, Yagishita A, Terada H, et al. New and reliable MRI diagnosis for progressive supranuclear palsy. *Neurology*. 2005;64:2050–2055.

Medically Refractory Seizures

Maria Stefanidou, Anuradha Singh, and Sarah Milla

CHIEF COMPLAINT: I want to get surgery done for my seizures.

HISTORY OF PRESENT ILLNESS

A 38-year-old, right-handed/ambidextrous female was referred to our Epilepsy Monitoring Unit for presurgical evaluation. She reported that her first seizure was at the age of 2, which was thought to be a febrile seizure. She did not have subsequent seizures until the age of 25. Since then, she has been experiencing multiple seizures and different seizure types. The frequency of seizures may vary from 5 to 20 seizures per day. Most of these sound like complex partial seizures that can last couple of minutes. She described episodes of déjà vu sensations followed by staring, difficulty understanding, and producing speech with or without brief periods of confusion and disorientation and purposeless hand movements. There are other times when she would start speaking gibberish or speak a perfect foreign language during her seizures without any recollection of events. Occasionally, she had suffered from secondarily generalized tonic-clonic seizures. She had four tonic-clonic seizures in her lifetime. She had multiple minor physical injuries. She was tried on multiple older and newer antiepileptic agents (AEDs) without any relief. She noticed increased frequency of her seizures around her menses.

She denied any history of head trauma with loss of consciousness, meningitis, or encephalitis. She was told that her MRI brain was abnormal. She endorsed feelings of depression but refused to consult a psychiatrist.

PAST MEDICAL HISTORY

Partial seizures, depression, asthma as a child, endometriosis.

PAST SURGICAL HISTORY

Hysterectomy (patient opted for hysterectomy for better control of seizures; however, hysterectomy did not bring her seizures frequency down).

MEDICATIONS

Tegretol XR 400 to 600 mg bid (opted to be only on single AED and lower dose because of tolerance issues).

PAST ANTIEPILEPTIC DRUGS

Lyrica, Diamox, Topamax, Lamictal, Depakote, Vimpat, Dilantin, Phenobarbital, Trileptal, Zonegran, Felbatol, Neurontin, Diazepam, Keppra.

PERSONAL HISTORY

Architect, unemployed because of frequent seizures; no smoking or drugs, occasional drinking.

FAMILY HISTORY

Negative for seizures; mother has bipolar disorder.

PHYSICAL EXAMINATION

Unremarkable.

NEUROLOGICAL EXAMINATION

Higher mental functions: Alert and oriented to time, place, and person; affect strange, pressured speech, dysthymic, good attention and concentration, judgment was normal; her immediate recall was 3/3 and recall of three objects after 5 minutes was 3/3. Comprehension, expression (fluency), repetition, reading, and writing were normal.

CNs II–XII: OU 20/20, Pupils equal and reactive, fundi normal, visual fields full by confrontation method, muscles of mastication, and facial muscles symmetric; face symmetric, hearing normal by whispering, uvula moved symmetrically, tongue midline, no tongue atrophy, no tongue fasciculations, sternocleidomastoids, and trapezii muscles showed normal strength.

Motor: Normal tone, no atrophy, strength proximally and distally in both upper and lower extremities was normal and is 5/5.

Sensory: Intact to light touch, pin prick, temperature, vibration and position sense. Cortical sensations were intact.

Reflexes: Biceps, triceps, brachioradialis, patellar, and ankle jerks were 2+ and symmetrical; there was no ankle clonus or Hoffman's.

Plantars: Flexors bilaterally.

Romberg: Negative.

Cerebellar: Finger-nose-finger in upper extremities and knee-shin-heel did not show any dysmetria.

Gait: Normal.

STOP AND THINK QUESTIONS

➢ Does this patient have focal or generalized epilepsy?

➢ What is catamenial epilepsy?

➢ What are the risk factors for seizures?

➢ What is a vagal nerve stimulator (VNS)?

DIAGNOSTIC TEST RESULTS

MRI brain: Abnormal area of bilateral gray matter heterotopias near the atria of the lateral ventricles (see Figure 29.1).

VEEG: Normal well-organized 9 to 9.5 Hz posterior dominant rhythm. Normal sleep architecture. Right hemispheric gamma activity in bursts lasting from 5 to 7 seconds was seen in both wakefulness and sleep. During seizures, patient had difficulty speaking. She spoke gibberish; there were push buttons for experiencing visual auras and déjà vu sensations.

Twelve complex partial seizures were captured. Five were with left hemispheric onsets, five had right hemispheric onsets, and two were nonlateralizable. *Ictal onsets* suggested independent extra temporal bilateral posterior quadrant onsets (see Figure 29.2A and 29.2B).

WADA (intracarotid amobarbital procedure) test results were indicative of left hemispheric language dominance. The left hemisphere memory performance following the right ICA injection was 11/12 (91.6%). The right hemisphere memory performance following the left ICA injection was 1/12 (8.3%). The difference of 10 points in memory scores between the hemispheres suggests right hemispheric memory dysfunction.

Neuropsychological Testing VCI: SS=107 POI: SS=138 PSI: SS=103

AMI: SS=101 VMI: SS=107 WMI: SS=102

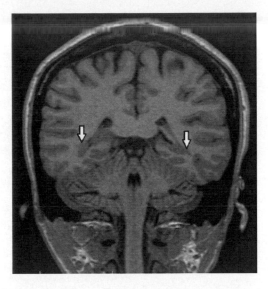

FIGURE 29.1 *(A) MRI brain coronal T1 images showing bilateral gray matter heterotopias near the atria of the lateral ventricles (indicated by arrows).*

Additional neuropsychological testing results: Most aspects of general intellectual functioning fell in the average range, with a significant strength in perceptual organization. Attention, memory, language skills, visuospatial skills, motor skills, and executive functions were intact.

Interictal cerebral SPECT showed diminished perfusion in the right occipital lobe, suggesting a right occipital lobe seizure focus.

Ictal cerebral SPECT demonstrated greater radiotracer in the right temporoparietal lobe. Occipital lobe uptake was asymmetric, greater on the right inferiorly and on the left superiorly.

Cerebral PET: Normal PET/CT of brain.

MEG/MSI: This is an abnormal MEG/MSI study demonstrating evidence for bilateral temporal and temporo-occipital cortical hyperexcitability. Although the left temporal discharges more frequently fit the statistical model, the overall frequency of discharges was only modestly more left hemispheric.

SSEP: This MSI study demonstrated normal localization of SSEP from the bilateral upper extremities to the contralateral postcentral gyri. No evidence of cortical reorganization or displacement was seen within either hemisphere. VEP: This MEG/MSI study demonstrated normal localization of VEP to the mesial occipital lobe without evidence of cortical reorganization or displacement. This abnormal MEG/MSI study is consistent with a diagnosis of a multifocal localization-related (partial) epilepsy with a bitemporal focus. Normal localizations for somatosensory and visual cortices were seen, which were distant from the identified epileptiform foci.

Multidisciplinary surgical conference: A bilateral strip survey study including depth electrodes in the regions of heterotopic gray matter was considered as an option to lateralize a single or predominant epileptic focus considering her high seizure burden rate. Patient refused the survey study and possible resection of seizure focus when she was told that the resection of the heterotopia could potentially cause a visual field defect. VNS was offered as a second alternative epilepsy surgery. Initially, the frequency of the seizures decreased to three to four per day around the time of her menses. In 2009, the frequency increased again to almost daily events. Patient could not tolerate higher settings of VNS.

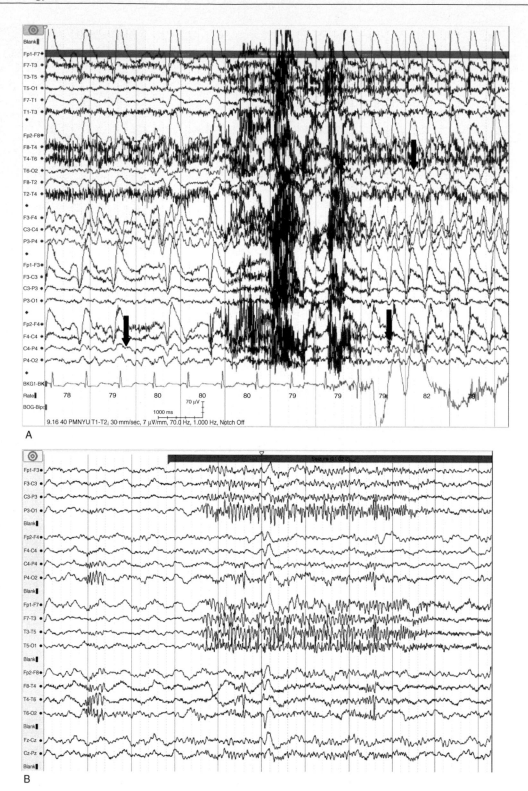

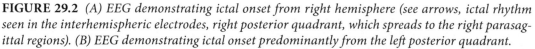

FIGURE 29.2 *(A) EEG demonstrating ictal onset from right hemisphere (see arrows, ictal rhythm seen in the interhemispheric electrodes, right posterior quadrant, which spreads to the right parasagittal regions). (B) EEG demonstrating ictal onset predominantly from the left posterior quadrant.*

DIAGNOSIS: Malformations of cortical development (MCD).

DISCUSSION

Our patient definitely meets the criteria of medically refractory seizures as she has tried both narrow and broad spectrum first- and second-generation antiepileptics. She failed several antiepileptics partly because of tolerance issues. The presence of aura makes you think of partial epilepsy, and multiple seizure types raise suspicion of multiple seizure foci. The presence of bilateral periventricular gray matter heterotopia and independent ictal onsets do not support a good surgical outcome but palliative surgical resection of predominant seizure focus can still be offered. Medication side effects, poorly controlled seizures, low self-esteem, anxiety, depression, inability to drive, limited job options despite a college degree and lack of sustained relationships are some of the quality-of-life issues that our patient has been dealing with since early adulthood. The patient tried drastic measures such as hysterectomy on her own because of definite worsening of seizures around her menses and in the ovulatory phase. The menstrual cycle-related seizure disorder is referred to as catamenial epilepsy. Herzog et al. (1997) have described three different patterns seen with catamenial epilepsy. In women with epilepsy, seizures can be influenced by variations in sex hormone secretion during the menstrual cycle. This type of epilepsy has generally been defined as an increase in seizure frequency beginning immediately before or during menses. However, three distinct patterns of catamenial epilepsy have been described: perimenstrual, periovulatory, and luteal. Different therapeutic approaches can be employed to treat catamenial epilepsy, including acetazolamide (carbonic anhydrase inhibitor), cyclical use of benzodiazepines (clobazam, lorazepam) or conventional AEDs, and hormonal therapy or ganaxolone (GABA-A receptor modulator). However, evidence for the effectiveness of these treatment approaches comes from small, unblinded series or anecdotal reports.

Patient opted for VNS. VNS received approval from Food and Drug Administration in 1997. It is approved for adjunctive therapy in medically resistant cases in patients older than 12 years of age. VNS system consists of an implanted pacemaker-like generator and nerve stimulation electrodes, which deliver intermittent stimulation to the left vagus nerve. Left vagus stimulator is stimulated at regular intervals based on preprogrammed settings. The right vagus nerve is not implanted because it has rich cardiac innervations. The *nucleus of the tractus soliatrius in the medulla receives dense innervations by the synapsing vagal afferents and projects its efferents widely to various subcortical and brain stem regions.* The exact mechanisms of action of VNS are really not clear but in animal models, VNS has been seen to desynchronize the EEG.

VNS therapy is delivered via a small pacemaker-like device that is implanted just under the skin during a short outpatient procedure that does not involve the brain. The device is implanted in the left chest area, and thin, flexible wires connect the device to the left vagus nerve in the neck. Once activated by the physician, the device sends precisely timed and measured mild pulses to the left vagus nerve. Using a dose adjustment system, physicians can adjust the timing and amount of stimulation the patient receives. It is usually performed on an outpatient basis under regional or general anesthesia. The pulse generator is powered by a single battery, with a battery life of 3 to 8 years, depending on the parameter settings. When battery replacement is necessary, usually only the pulse generator is changed, and the bipolar leads are left in place. Normal mode stimulation parameters refer to the stimulation throughout the day (24 h/d) and seven days a week. On-demand stimulation is triggered by a magnet stimulation and is referred as magnet-mode stimulation (refer to Table 29.1).

MCD comprise a broad spectrum of disorders that may be the underlying cause in up to 40% of treatment-resistant epilepsy in children (1,2). They may also be associated with

TABLE 29.1 *VNS Parameters for Normal Mode and On-Demand Stimulation*

Parameter	Range	Typical
Output current (mA)	0–3.5	1–2
Signal frequency (Hz)	1–30	20–30
Pulse width (μs)	130–1000	250–500
Signal on-time (s)	7–60	30
Signal off-time (min)	0.2–180	5
Magnet output current (mA)	0–3.5	Normal model output current plus 0.25 mA
Magnet pulse width (μs)	130–100	Same as normal mode pulse width
Magnet on-time (s)	7–60	30–60

developmental delay and motor dysfunction. Identification of these malformations is now possible due to advent of high-resolution MRI, though there are still subtle MCD that elude visualization. These disorders are so far understood as the result of disruption of one or more of the major steps of cortical development, namely:

1. Cell proliferation/maturation/apoptosis in the germinal matrix (stem cells located in the subependymal layer of the wall of the ventricles).

2. Neuronal migration.

3. Cortical organization (formation of lamina and synaptic connections) (3).

This disruption may be genetically determined or acquired and in some poorly characterized conditions it is felt to be heterogeneous in nature. The most utilized classification of these disorders was proposed by Barkovich in 2005 and is based on the primary stage of development when disruption is believed to have led to the anomaly (Table 29.2) (4). This is an area, though, of continuous evolution as more knowledge becomes available on the genetic signature, pathological findings, imaging characteristics, and clinical behavior/ prognosis of these conditions.

It is beyond the scope of this chapter to describe MCDs in great detail, but we will attempt to provide basic knowledge of commonly encountered MCDs such as FCD, HME, heterotopia, lissencephaly, polymicrogyria, schizencephaly, DNET, and ganglioglioma. Figures 29.3 to 29.11 depict various forms of MCDs for review of our readers.

FCD

The most commonly encountered MCD in the presurgical evaluation of refractory partial epilepsy and the most common cause of epilepsy in children is FCD (3). This comprises a broad spectrum of lesions characterized mainly by cortical dyslamination, cytoarchitectural lesions, and abnormalities of the underlying white matter. Their main clinical manifestation is seizures that can start at any age (usually childhood) and tend to be resistant to medications in up to 40% of cases (5).

So far, the most widely accepted classification differentiated these dysplasias in two groups, but in this review, we will use the very recent ILAE proposed classification that breaks them down into three categories taking into account electroclinical, imaging, neuropathological findings, as well as postsurgical outcome (6) (see Table 29.3).

FCD TYPE I

FCD type I is characterized by abnormal cortical layering either compromising radial migration and maturation of neurons (type IA) or the six-layered tangential composition

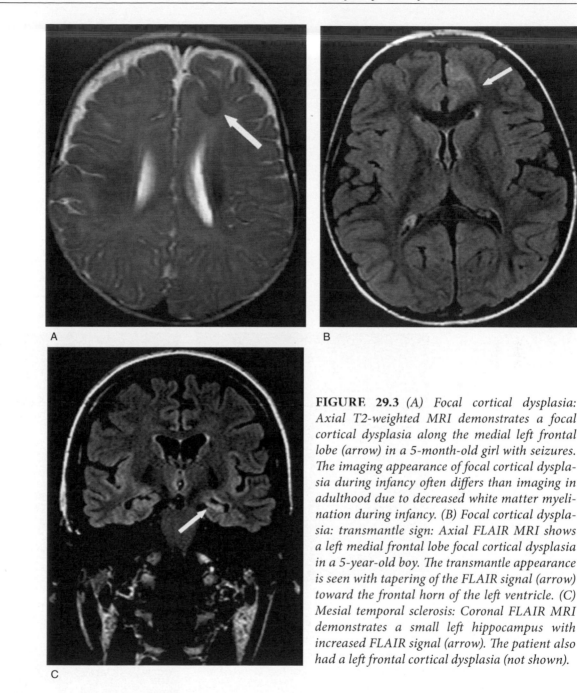

FIGURE 29.3 *(A) Focal cortical dysplasia: Axial T2-weighted MRI demonstrates a focal cortical dysplasia along the medial left frontal lobe (arrow) in a 5-month-old girl with seizures. The imaging appearance of focal cortical dysplasia during infancy often differs than imaging in adulthood due to decreased white matter myelination during infancy. (B) Focal cortical dysplasia: transmantle sign: Axial FLAIR MRI shows a left medial frontal lobe focal cortical dysplasia in a 5-year-old boy. The transmantle appearance is seen with tapering of the FLAIR signal (arrow) toward the frontal horn of the left ventricle. (C) Mesial temporal sclerosis: Coronal FLAIR MRI demonstrates a small left hippocampus with increased FLAIR signal (arrow). The patient also had a left frontal cortical dysplasia (not shown).*

of the neocortex (type IB). When there is a combination of both processes it is classified as type IC. Immature small diameter neurons and hypertrophic pyramidal neurons outside layer 5, as well as normal neurons with disoriented dendrites may also be encountered. In a fully myelinated brain, these dysplasias may be characterized by blurring of the gray-white matter junction with typically normal cortical thickness and moderately

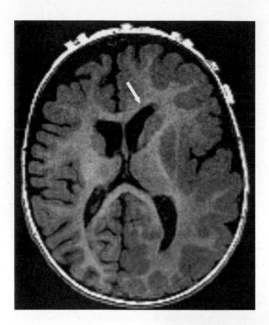

FIGURE 29.4 *Hemimegalencephaly—Thin section axial T1-weighted MRI shows the left hemisphere larger than the right, with thicker cortex as well as a straightened frontal horn on the ipsilateral side (arrow), often seen in hemimegalencephaly.*

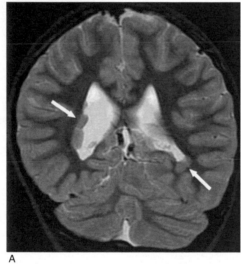

A

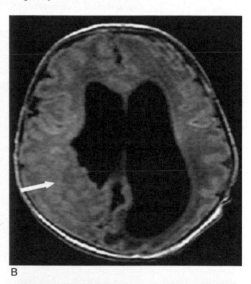

B

FIGURE 29.5 *(A) Heterotopia: Periventricular nodular heterotopia: Coronal T2-weighted MRI shows bilateral foci of periventricular nodular heterotopia along the ventricular surface. These foci (arrows) followed gray matter signal on all sequences, distinguishing them from other pathology, such as subependymal nodules in tuberous sclerosis. (B) Heterotopia: Subcortical heterotopia: Axial T1-weighted MRI in a newborn with seizures demonstrates an extensive area of subcortical heterotopia (arrow) in the right parietal lobe. (C) Heterotopia: Band heterotopia: Coronal T2-weighted MRI shows shallow gyri with a thick layer of gray matter (black arrow) separated from the thin cortex by a thin layer of myelinated white matter (hypointense thin layer between the cortex and band heterotopia, indicated with a white arrow).*

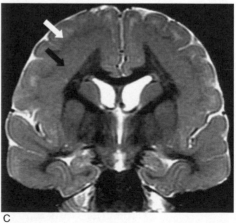

C

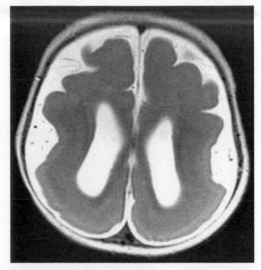

FIGURE 29.6 *Lissencephaly: Axial coronal T2-weighted MRI shows overall paucity of gyri with a thickened and flattened appearance. Pattern is more posteriorly affected, suggestion LIS 1 mutation.*

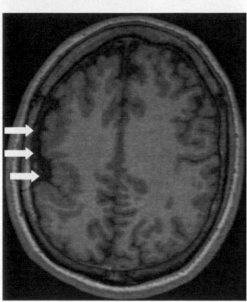

FIGURE 29.7 *Polymicrogyria: Thin section T1-weighted MRI shows right sided polymicrogyria (arrows) extending superiorly from the sylvian fissure into the frontal and parietal lobes. Note absence of named gyri in the affected region, such as the pre and post central gyri.*

increased white matter signal abnormality on T2 and FLAIR images and decreased signal intensity on T1-weighted imaging. It is most usually encountered in the temporal lobe (6).

FCD TYPE II

FCD type II is characterized by higher seizure frequency compared to the type I lesions. On pathology there is disrupted cortical lamination (cannot differentiate individual cortical layers except layer I) and specific cytologic abnormalities that include dysmorphic neurons (enlarged cell body and nucleus, malorientation, abnormally distributed Nissl substance, cytoplasmic accumulation of neurofilament proteins) either without balloon cells (type IIA) or with balloon cells (type IIB). Balloon cells are the hallmark of type IIB

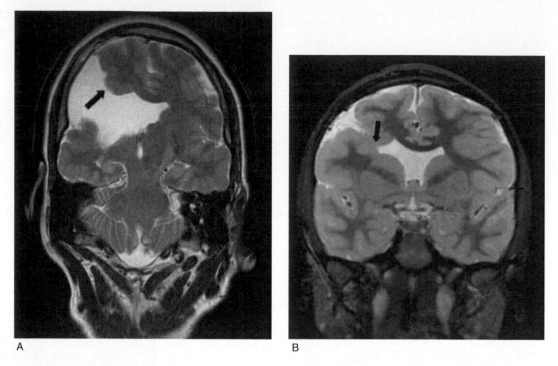

FIGURE 29.8 *(A) Schizencephaly: Open-lip—Coronal T2-weighted image demonstrates absence of the septum with a large gray-matter lined cleft in the right frontal lobe with no approximation of the gray-matter lined sides ("lips") of the cleft; (B) Schizencephaly: Closed-lip—Coronal T2-weighted image demonstrates close apposition of the gray matter lined clefts causing an "outpouching" of the right lateral ventricle at the region of the closed-lip schizencephaly.*

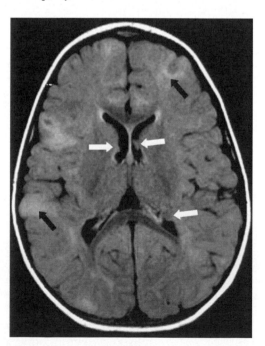

FIGURE 29.9 *Tuberous sclerosis: Axial FLAIR image demonstrates FLAIR high-signal hamartomas, also known as "tubers" (black arrows). Small nodules along the ventricular surface (white arrows) do not follow T1 gray matter on all sequences (distinguishing them from gray matter heterotopia), have evidence of calcification (not shown) and are classic subependymal nodules of tuberous sclerosis.*

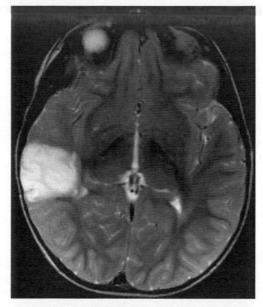

FIGURE 29.10 *Dysembryoplastic Neuroepithelial tumors (DNET): Axial T2-weighted MRI shows a focal T2 hyperintense lesion in the right temporal lobe cortical and subcortical regions. Associated cortical dysplasia was detected adjacent to the DNET neoplastic tissue.*

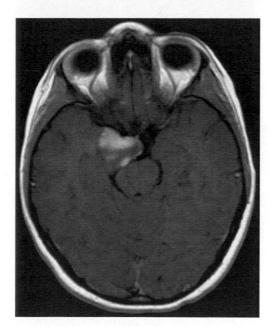

FIGURE 29.11 *Ganglioglioma: Postcontrast T1-weighted MRI demonstrates foci of enhancement within this well circumscribed right mesial temporal lobe mass.*

and they are characterized by a large cell body and opalescent glassy eosinophilic cytoplasm, which lacks Nissl substance (6).

Type IIA lesions are not always easily identified on MRI. Type IIB dysplasias are characterized by marked blurring of the gray-white matter junction on T1W and T2FLAIR images, due to hypo- or dysmyelination of the subcortical white matter that may also mimic cortical thickening. There is increased white matter signal changes on T2W and FLAIR images that frequently tapers toward the ventricles ("transmantle" sign) reflecting

TABLE 29.2 *Classification of Cortical Malformations of Brain*

I. ***Malformations due to abnormal neuronal and glial proliferation or apoptosis***
   A. Decreased proliferation/increased apoptosis or increased proliferation/decreased apoptosis-abnormalities of brain size.
      1. Microcephaly with normal to thin cortex
      2. Microlissencephaly (extreme microcephaly with thick cortex)
      3. Microcephaly with extensive polymicrogyria
      4. Macrocephalies
   B. Abnormal proliferation (abnormal cell types)
      1. Non-neoplastic
         a. Cortical hamartomas of tuberous sclerosis
         b. Cortical dysplasia with balloon cells
         c. HME
      2. Neoplastic (associated with disordered cortex)
         a. DNET (dysembryoplastic neuroepithelial tumor)
         b. Ganglioglioma
         c. Gangliocytoma
II. ***Malformations due to abnormal neuronal migration***
   A. Lissencephaly/subcortical band heterotopias spectrum
   B. Cobblestone complex/congenital muscular dystrophy syndromes
   C. Heterotopia
      1. Subependymal (periventricular)
      2. Subcortical (other than band heterotopia)
      3. Marginal glioneuronal
III. ***Malformations due to abnormal cortical organization (including late neuronal migration)***
   A. Polymicrogyria and schizencephaly
      1. Bilateral polymicrogyria syndromes
      2. Schizencephaly (polymicrogyria with clefts)
      3. Polymicrogyria or schizencephaly as part of multiple congenital anomaly/mental retardation syndromes
   B. Cortical dysplasia without balloon cells
   C. Microdysgenesis
IV. ***Malformations of cortical development, not otherwise classified***
   A. Malformations secondary to inborn errors of metabolism
      1. Mitochondrial and pyruvate metabolic disorders
      2. Peroxisomal disorders
   B. Other unclassified malformations
      1. Sublobar dysplasia
      2. Others

the involvement of radial glial-neuronal bands. Type II lesions are more commonly encountered in extratemporal regions and in particular in the frontal lobe (6).

According to the above classification association of type II FCD with hippocampal sclerosis/tumors or cavernomas are considered as "dual pathology."

FCD TYPE III

FCD type III refers to cortical lamination abnormalities associated with a principal lesion, usually located in the same area/lobe. The principal lesion and the FCD are felt to be etiologically linked and do not fall under the category of "dual pathology." Four variants are identified:

Type IIIA is associated with HS.

Type IIIB is associated with tumors (ganglioglioma, dysembryoplastic neuroepithelial tumor or other epilepsy related neoplesms).

Type IIIC is associated with vascular malformations (cavernomas, AVMs, telangectasias, meningoangiomatosis).

Type IIID is associated with any other principal lesion acquired early in life (prenatal or perinatal ischemic injury, traumatic brain injury, inflammatory or infectious process) (6).

This classification, as noted by the authors will require further testing, but identifies a third category of FCD that is essentially an FCD type I plus a principal lesion and has been found to have similar prognosis to that seen when the principal lesion is found in isolation and removed surgically. In these cases, seizure freedom may reach 70% to 80% post-operatively (6).

Experimental evidence points to intrinsic epileptogenicity of these lesions. Continuous epileptiform discharges are frequently seen in patients with FCD and in two thirds of the cases there are regional EEG findings on scalp recording related to the anatomical location of the malformation (5).

High resolution multiplanar MRI is considered the gold standard for the evaluation of these patients. Another imaging modality utilized to identify FCDs is the 18F FDG-PET scan that has a sensitivity of 75% to 100% in localizing the lesions. It is particularly useful in identifying subtle FCD (MRI sensitivity 13% compared to 86% sensitivity with FDG-PET) (3). Since it is a functional study of the brain it also helps delineate better the epileptogenic zone (region of the brain responsible for generating the seizures) when it spreads beyond the region of structural abnormality identified on the MRI. In the interictal phase, areas of metabolic hypoactivity correlate with epileptogenic tissue that appears hyperactive if the study is performed in the ictal state. Co-registration of the two modalities may be very helpful in determining the exact area to be resected when surgical intervention is contemplated. Other modalities used are MEG that identifies inter and intra ictal dipole sources that correlate with epileptogenic tissue, as well as DTI that quantifies and gives a detailed anatomical map of the microstructure of the brain.

Detailed invasive pre-surgical evaluation is mandatory in FCD since it may evolve eloquent cortex and the lesion visualized on MRI may be only the 'tip of the iceberg" with higher epileptogenicity identified in neighboring MRI-undetectable dysplastic regions that comprise the epileptogenic zone (5). Seizure freedom rates vary considerably following resection of FCDs and evidence from cohorts that have predominantly MRI positive FCDs have demonstrated seizure freedom ranging between 54% and 72%.In a series of MRI negative patients, when pathology indicated a FCD, seizure freedom rates were between 50% to 56% (7).

The three-tired ILAE classification system of FCD distinguishes isolated forms (FCD Types I and II) from those associated with another principal lesion (FCD Type III) as indicated in Table 29.3.

HME

HME is the unilateral hamartomatous excessive growth of all or part of one cerebral hemisphere secondary to defects that may occur at one or more of the three embryogenic stages mentioned above (8). The posterior regions of the hemisphere (parietal, occipital, posterior aspect of the temporal lobe) appear more involved. It is a very rare condition, but may account for up to 30% to 50% of cases among children who underwent hemispherectomy for the treatment of refractory epilepsy (9).

Histologic analysis shows involvement of both neuronal and glial cells with anomalous giant neurons variably scattered in the different cortical layers, as well as within the white matter (8).

TABLE 29.3 *Different Types of Focal Cortical Dysplasia*

FCD Type I (isolated)	Focal cortical dysplasia with abnormal radial cortical lamination (FCD Type Ia)	Focal cortical dysplasia with abnormal tangential cortical lamination (FCD Type Ib)	Focal cortical dysplasia with abnormal radial and tangential cortical lamination (FCD Type Ic)	
FCD Type II (isolated)	Focal cortical dysplasia with dysmorphic neurons (FCD Type IIa)		Focal cortical dysplasia with dysmorphic neurons and balloon cells (FCD Type IIb)	
FCD Type III (associated with principal lesion)	Cortical lamination abnormalities in the temporal lobe associated with hippocampal sclerosis (FCD Type IIIa)	Cortical lamination abnormalities adjacent to a glial or glioneuronal tumor (FCD Type IIIb)	Cortical lamination abnormalities adjacent to vascular malformation (FCD Type IIIc)	Cortical lamination abnormalities adjacent to any other lesion acquired during early life, e.g., trauma, ischemic injury, encephalitis (FCD Type IIId)

FCD Type III (not otherwise specified, NOS): if clinically/radiologically suspected pricipal lesion is not available for microscopic inspection. Please note that the rare association between FCD Types IIa and IIb with hippocampal sclerosis, tumors, or vascular malformations should not be classified as FCD Type III variant.

On clinical examination, infants have macrocephaly at birth that is usually asymmetric and in some cases hypertrophy of the ipsilateral body (hemigigantism) or just one body segment (usually the face). The classic neurological triad of HME is refractory epilepsy (90% of cases), mild to severe developmental delay and slowly progressive contralateral hemiparesis/hemianopia (9).

Three variants are identified. In the isolated form, there are no other associated abnormalities, and the prognosis depends on the severity of the epilepsy and the neurological deficits. In the systemic form, there is partial or total hemigigantism and concurrent neurocutaneous syndromes (neurofibromatosis, tuberous sclerosis, epidermal nevus syndrome, Ito's hypomelanosis, and Klippel-Trenauney syndrome). In the total HME form, there is additional involvement of the ipsilateral cerebellum and brain stem (9).

Seizures are the predominant feature and evolve in semiology over time. Onset is usually within the first few days of life with partial motor seizures, asymmetric spasms, asymmetric, and lateralized myoclonic jerks that gradually evolve to constitute different epilepsy syndromes. They first tend to correspond to the Ohtahara syndrome with tonic, partial and myoclonic seizures, and burst suppression seen on EEG, followed by West syndrome with asymmetrical spasms and hemihypsarrhythmia on EEG and finally Lennox-Gastaut syndrome with tonic/atonic seizures and atypical absences. In the end, epilepsia partialis continua may be seen. Interictal discharges have also been identified in the healthy hemisphere (9).

On MRI, there is an enlarged hemisphere seen with increased white matter volume, cortical thickening with agyria, pachygyria, polymigrogyria, or lissencephaly and blurring of the gray–white matter junction. Often, a large, ipsilateral irregularly shaped ventricle is also seen. On MRI/spectroscopy, a decreased N-acetylaspartate/creatine ratio can be found in the dysplastic hemisphere (9).

Surgical treatment is usually an anatomic or functional hemispherectomy that is usually considered in the presence of hemiparesis (10). Seizure control may be expected in up to 60% of cases, a lower rate compared to that seen with hemispherectomy for different etiologies. It is thought that difficulties in the complete disconnection of the malformed hemisphere because of its severe anatomical distortion, as well as the possible involvement in a molecular basis of the "healthy" hemisphere account for this difference. The procedure may be complicated by perioperative bleeding, due to associated vascular anomalies, and postoperative hydrocephalus. Following hemispherectomy, motor and visual performance tends to remain stable, but cognitive performance tends to improve with increase in intelligence quotient and psychomotor development (9).

HETEROTOPIA

Heterotopia is generated by a defect in the migration of neurons originating in the periventricular region. Subsequently, ectopic neuronal tissue is seen within the white matter. Intrinsic epileptogenicity has been shown with intracranial recordings of these lesions. There are three types identified on MRI:

1. **PNH.** PNH consists of confluent nodules of gray matter along the lateral ventricles (1). It usually affects females during the second decade of life who present with epilepsy, that may or may not be resistant to treatment, and normal to borderline intelligence. Coagulopathy and cardiovascular abnormalities have also been observed (1). Classical bilateral PNH (BPNH) has been linked to inherited or sporadic filamin A gene mutations on chromosome X that cause prenatal lethality in almost all males and 50% recurrence risk in the female offspring of women with BPNH (11). It is the most common MCD associated with the presence of more than one class of epileptogenic substrate ("dual pathology"). When it is associated with hippocampal sclerosis, ictal onsets tend to appear simultaneously over both structures or be confined to the mesial temporal lobe. In patients with the latter finding selective amygdalohippocampectomy has been performed (5); however, other series have shown that best results are obtained when the majority of the PNH is also excised. This is rarely feasible as they can be extensive and their location is not always amenable to surgical intervention.

2. **Focal subcortical heterotopia.** This is associated with focal cortical thinning and decrease in the volume of the underlying white matter. Cognitive deficits are more commonly seen than in PNH. Ictal onsets tend to occur simultaneously within the heterotopia and the overlying dysplastic cortex and complete excision of both is associated with better prognosis (5). Extensive or bilateral presence of the abnormality limits the surgical options.

3. **Band heterotopia.** Layers of gray matter are found in subcortical white matter separated from the cortex by a thin layer of white matter. On MRI, these lesions are isointense to cortex in every sequence and do not enhance. The thickness of the band correlates with the severity of the seizures.

LISSENCEPHALY

Lissencephaly is another disorder in which neuronal migration is defective. It is a rare condition, and affected children have early developmental delay with eventual severe mental retardation. The brain surface is smooth and gyration may vary between agyria (complete lack of gyri) and pachygyria that is characterized by thickening of the cortex and shallow sulci. The cortical architecture is disorganized, and there is blurring of the white–gray matter junction. SBH is considered the mild end of this spectrum of disorders and the thicker the heterotopic band, the higher the possibility of it being associated with a pachy-gyric cortical surface and worse clinical prognosis (11).

Seizures that tend to be refractory occur in over 90% of cases with onset prior to 6 months of age in up to 75%. Seizure phenotype varies and may include infantile spasms, focal motor and generalized tonic seizures, complex partial seizures, atonic and myoclonic seizures, and atypical absences. EEG findings vary, but diffuse high amplitude fast rhythms are considered to be highly specific for this malformation (11).

In 85 % of cases, a genetic defect has been identified. Lissencephaly with posteriorly predominant gyral abnormality is caused by mutations of the LIS1 gene on chromosome 17. Anteriorly predominant lissencephaly in hemizygous males and SBH in heterozygous females are caused by mutations of the XLIS (DCX) gene on chromosome X. Mutations in the tubulin alpha 1A gene, a third gene that also participates in the intrinsic motility of neural progenitor cells, have also been identified (2). Miller-Dieker syndrome is caused by large deletions of LIS1 and contiguous genes (1). Children, in addition to the lissencephaly, have distinct facial features with prominent forehead, bitemporal hollowing, short nose with upturned nares, protuberant upper lip, and small jaw (2). A syndrome of autosomal recessive lissencephaly with cerebellar hypoplasia has also been described with mutation identified in the reelin gene (11) and phenotype with seizures, developmental delay, hypotonia, and ataxia.

Surgery is usually ineffective, but sometimes callosotomy is considered.

POLYMICROGYRIA

Polymicrogyria is one of the most common MCD characterized by many small microgyria separated by shallow sulci, a slightly thickened cortex, neuronal heterotopias, and often enlarged ventricles (12). The disturbance is believed to occur during either the late phase of neuronal migration or early in the phase of cortical organization. Histologically, it is a diverse condition with derangement of the normal six-layered lamination of the cortex and sulcation, as well as fusion of the molecular layer across sulci (13). Polymicrogyria has been described as a consequence of congenital infections (particularly cytomegalovirus infection), localized or diffuse in utero ischemia (usually in the distribution of the middle cerebral artery), and genetic mutations (associated with 22q11.2 deletions) (11, 13). It may be focal, multifocal, diffuse, unilateral (40%), bilateral symmetric, or bilateral asymmetric. Age at presentation and clinical severity depend on the extent of cortical involvement with bilateral involvement or involvement of more than half of a single hemisphere being poor prognostic factors (13). The most common localization (60%–70%) is bilateral perisylvian polymicrogyria, and patients may manifest pseudobulbar palsy, learning difficulties, spastic quadriparesis, and epilepsy. The cortex surrounding the Sylvian fissure is involved in up to 80% of the cases with the frontal, parietal, temporal, and occipital lobes being involved with decreasing incidence (13).

Epilepsy in patients with polymicrogyria may be partial or generalized, but the intrinsic epileptogenicity of the malformation has not been verified with intracranial recordings (12). CT head may show areas of calcification. On MRI, findings show excessive gyration, cortical thickening, and irregularity of the gray–white matter junction. Polymicrogyria may be seen on the lips of schizencephaly.

In cases of unilateral polymicrogyria associated with contralateral hemiplegia, hemispherectomy or multilobar resections may be considered, and the use of MEG and EEG/f-MRI bold response has been used to define a more restricted epileptogenic region that can be resected (5). Focal resections are rare in the literature and tend to have poor prognosis.

SCHIZENCEPHALY

Schizencephaly is one of the rarest MCD. It is characterized by the presence of a transcortical cleft with open or fused lips, extending from the ventricles to the pia with subsequent communication between the ventricles and the subarachnoid space, lined with dysplastic gray matter and often polymicrogyria along its edges. Bilateral involvement is associated with a more severe clinical picture with microcephaly and severe developmental delay, where small unilateral closed lip clefts may be incidental findings in normal individuals. They are most commonly seen in the perisylvian region (11).

Vascular, infectious, and genetic causes are thought to be playing a role. De novo mutations in the EMX2 gene on chromosome 10 have been described, but a pattern of inheritance has not yet been elucidated (11).

Seizures are seen in 81% of patients and usually present before 3 years of age. The majority of the patients have partial seizures with no distinctive EEG pattern identified (11). The epileptogenic area tends to involve larger areas than those visualized on MRI.

As in polymicrogyria, limited surgical experience indicates that these structural abnormalities may point to, rather than contain, the critical part of the epileptogenic zone.

DNET

DNET are benign neoplastic cortical malformations due to abnormal neuronal and glial proliferation. These are cortically based but subcortical extension may be seen in 30% of cases giving these tumors a triangular appearance. These appear hyperintense on T2WI, which may enhance in one third of the cases. These tumors are well-defined lobulated tumors, which at times may erode the overlying calvarial bone. The most common location is temporal (60%) followed by frontal lobes (30%). These are solid tumors but cystic and microcystic components may occur. These tend to occur near the areas of cortical dysplasia (14).

GANGLIOGLIOMAS

Gangliogliomas fall under neoplastic MCDs and tend to occur in older children and young adults. Removal of ganglioglioma causes amelioration of seizures. These are well-defined tumors that frequently show cystic changes and may calcify. The most common location of gangliogliomas is the temporal lobe, followed by the parietal, frontal, and occipital lobes. These tumors may or may not show enhancement on gadolinium administration.

REFERENCES

1. Guerrini R. Genetic malformations of the cerebral cortex and epilepsy. *Epilepsia.* 2005;46(Suppl 1):32–37.
2. Pang T, Atefy R, Sheen V. Malformations of cortical development. *The Neurologist.* 2008;14(3):181–189.
3. Colombo N, Salamon N, Raybaud C, Ozkara C, Barkovich J. Imaging of malformations of cortical development. *Epileptic Disord.* 2009;11(3):194–205.
4. Barkovich AJ, Kuzniecky RI, Jackson GD, Guerrini R, Dobyns WB. A developmental and genetic classification for malformations of cortical development. *Neurology.* 2005;65:1873–1887.
5. Luders H and Schuele US. Epilepsy surgery in patients with malformations of cortical development. *Curr Opin Neurol.* 2006;19:169–174.
6. Blumcke I, Thom M, Aronica E, et al. The clinicopathologic spectrum of focal cortical dysplasias: A consensus classification proposed by an ad hoc task force of the ILAE diagnostic methods commission. *Epilepsia.* 2011;52(1):158–174.
7. Chern JJ, Patel AJ, Jea A, Curry DJ, Comair YG. Surgical outcome for focal cortical dysplasia: An analysis of recent surgical series. *J Neurosurg Pediatrics.* 2010;6:452–458.

8. Andrade CS, Da Costa Leite C. Malformations of cortical development. Current concepts and advanced neuroimaging review. *Arq Neuropsiquiatr.* 2011;69(1):130–138.

9. Di Rocco, Battaglia D, Pietrini D, Piastra M, Massimi L. Hemimegalencephaly: Clinical implications and surgical treatment. *Childs Nerv Syst.* 2006;22:852–866.

10. Sisodiya SM. Surgery for malformations of cortical development causing epilepsy. *Brain.* 2000;123:1075–1091.

11. Guerrini R, Carrozzo R. Epileptogenic brain malformations: Clinical presentation, malformative patterns and indications for genetic testing. *Seizure.* 2001;10:532–547.

12. Burneo JG, Bebin M, Kuzniecky RI, Knowlton RC. Electroclinical and magnetoencephalographic studies in epilepsy patients with polymicrogyria. *Epilepsy Res.* 2004;62:125–133.

13. Barkovich AJ. Current concepts of polymicrogyria. *Neuroradiology.* 2010;52:479–487.

14. Sisodiya SM. Malformations of cortical development: Burdens and insights from important causes of human epilepsy. *Lancet Neurol.* 2004;3:29–38.

Left Arm Numbness and Slurred Speech

Jai S. Perumal

CHIEF COMPLAINT: **Speech is not clear and left arm goes numb.**

HISTORY OF PRESENT ILLNESS

A 20-year-old, right-handed, African American woman referred to the neurology clinic for left arm numbness and slurring of speech. The patient woke up in the morning one day, 3 weeks prior to clinic visit with pins and needles in her entire left arm. She thought she had "slept wrong" on the left side and waited for it to resolve. The next day, she found that her speech was slurred. She denied weakness of arms or legs. She denied any hearing, swallowing, or visual problems. She did not experience any headaches, any head trauma, falls, or balance problems. There was no infection or vaccination preceding the episode. She has never experienced such symptoms in the past. She has no significant past medical history. She denied any joint pains, skin problems, history of travel.

PAST MEDICAL HISTORY

As above.

PAST SURGICAL HISTORY

None.

MEDICATIONS

None.

ALLERGIES

NKDA.

PERSONAL HISTORY

Denied smoking, alcohol, or illicit drug use.

FAMILY HISTORY

No history of autoimmune or neurologic disorder.

PHYSICAL EXAMINATION

Vital signs: Blood pressure, 110/70 mm Hg; heart rate, 88/min; respiratory rate, 11/min; temperature 98.2°F.
General: NAD.
HEENT: Atraumatic, normocephalic.
Neck: Supple, normal carotid pulses.
Pulmonary: Lungs clear to auscultation bilaterally.
CVS: Regular rate and rhythm, no murmurs.
Abdomen: Nondistended, nontender, normal bowel sounds.
Musculoskeletal: No joint pain or swelling.
Skin: No rashes or abnormal pigmentation.

NEUROLOGIC EXAMINATION

Mental status: Alert, awake, oriented to person, place, and time; higher mental function including level of knowledge, language (comprehension, expression, naming, repetition, reading, and writing), judgment, abstraction, memory, calculation, higher executive, and praxis were all normal.

CNs II–XII: Visual acuity 20/20 bilaterally. Visual fields full, fundoscopic examination normal, pupils were equally reactive to light and accommodation, extraocular movements were intact, normal facial sensation, no facial weakness, normal hearing, palate normal, sternocleidomastoid/shoulder shrug normal, tongue midline, and no atrophy.

Motor: Strength 5/5 bilaterally, normal bulk and tone.

Sensory: Normal to light touch, pin prick, vibration, and joint position.

Romberg test was negative.

Reflexes: Biceps, brachioradialis, triceps, patellar, and ankle were 2+.

Plantars were downgoing bilaterally.

STOP AND THINK QUESTIONS

➢ What is your diagnosis?

➢ What are Dawson's fingers?

➢ Are lesions in the corpus callosum specific for MS?

➢ Does a normal exam exclude a diagnosis of MS?

➢ How will you distinguish between ADEM and the initial episode of MS?

➢ What is the influence of ethnicity in MS?

➢ Will you start long-term disease modifying therapy?

DIAGNOSTIC RESULTS

MRI brain showed several T2 hyperintense lesions in the periventricular, subcortical, and deep white matter (Figure 30.1A). On sagittal, FLAIR images there were several lesions in the corpus callosum (Dawson's fingers, Figure 30.1B).

MRI cervical spine revealed lesions at C2 and C5.

Blood tests: Anti nuclear AB, Anti SSA. Anti SSB, TFT, LFT, RF, ESR, Lyme, HIV were normal.

CT thorax was normal.

DIAGNOSIS: **Clinically isolated syndrome (CIS) with high risks of conversion to clinically definite multiple sclerosis (MS).**

HOSPITAL COURSE

She was admitted to the hospital and had quite an extensive work up including MRI brain and spine and blood tests and was told she might have MS. She was treated with IV solumedrol 1 g/d for 5 days with complete resolution of her symptoms. On discharge from the hospital, she was advised to follow up in the neurology clinic. After discussing the diagnosis and benefits versus risk of treatment options, the patient started treatment with glatiramer acetate.

DISCUSSION

This patient has a CIS with high risk of conversion to CDMS. CIS can be thought of as the earliest presentation of relapsing remitting MS. In a study with the longest follow-up

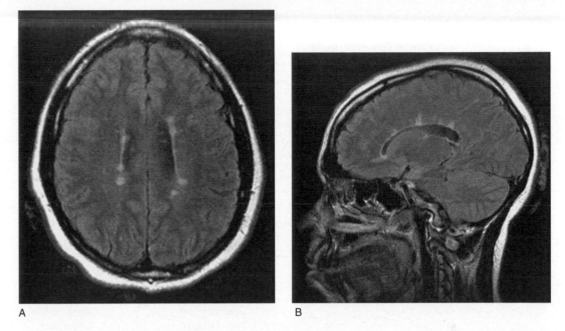

FIGURE 30.1 *(A) MRI Brain FLAIR axial shows several T2 hyperintense lesions in the periventricular, subcortical, and deep white matter. (B) Sagittal FLAIR images showing several lesions in the corpus callosum, Dawson's fingers.*

patients with CIS, 82% of patients with initial abnormal MRI went on to have CDMS, and importantly, 21% of CIS patients with normal initial MRI developed CDMS as well when followed for 20 years (1). The diagnostic criteria of multiple sclerosis are listed in Table 30.1. Thus, it is important to initiate treatment in those with initial abnormal MRI and follow those with initial normal MRIs closely both clinically and with periodic MRIs. CDMS is when patients have two clinical attacks separated in time and space (refer to Table 30.2).

Dawson's fingers are MS lesions that are perventricular, rather ovoid, and oriented perpendicular to the long axis of the lateral ventricles. They are due to inflammatory lesions around the veins. They were initially described in brain specimen by James Dawson who was a pathologist. Nowadays, Dawson's fingers are described on MRI scans. Often nonspecific white matter changes can be mistaken for MS. Lesions in the corpus callosum are more specific for MS. Another inflammatory disorder that causes extensive lesions in the corpus callosum is Susac's disease (triad of encephalopathy, hearing loss, and microangiopathy of retina).

TABLE 30.1 *Diagnostic MR Imaging Criteria Suggestive of Multiple Sclerosis*

Paty's Criteria	Fazekas' Criteria	Barkhof's Criteria
Four lesions or three lesions, one of which is periventricular	Three lesions, including two of the following characteristics: Infratentorial location Periventricular location Lesion > 6 mm	Gadolinium-enhanced lesion or the presence of ≥9 T2 lesions one infratentorial lesion one juxtacortical lesion three periventricular lesions

TABLE 30.2 *MRI Criteria to Demonstrate Dissemination of Lesions in Time*

Original McDonald Criteria	2005 Revisions
1. Positive CSF and	1. One year of disease progression
2. Dissemination in space by MRI evidence of	2. Plus two of the following:
≥9 T2 lesions	
≥2 cord lesions	Positive brain MRI
4–8 brain lesions and 1 cord lesion	Positive spinal cord lesions
4–8 brain lesions with +VEP	Positive CSF for OCB or IgG index or both
<4 brain lesion, 1 cord lesion and +VEP	
3. Dissemination in time by MRI *or* Continued progression for 1 year	

TABLE 30.3 *Differences Between CIS and ADEM*

	CIS/MS	ADEM
Clinical		
Patient population	More common in adults	Rare in adults
Preceding infection or vaccination	Not commonly found	Often present
Disease course	Relapsing	Most cases monophasic
Alteration of consciousness, aphasia, seizures, vomiting	Not common	Often seen
MRI		
Gray matter lesions-cortical and basal ganglia	Not often	Often seen
Corpus Callosum lesions	Frequent	Less Frequent
CSF		
Cell count	Rare above 50/ml	Higher counts can be seen
Protein	Rare above 100 mg/dl	Higher levels can be seen
OCB	Present in 90%, elevation is persistent	20%–50% reported in studies in adults, Often transiently elevated.

Patients with relapsing–remitting disease, especially early in the disease course can have a normal neurologic examination in between the episodes and so a normal examination does not exclude a diagnosis of MS. At the time of initial presentation, it can sometimes be difficult to distinguish between polysymptomatic CIS due to MS and acute disseminated encephalomyelitis. Though there is no absolute clinical presentation or investigation that helps differentiate the two, a list of factors that might help is shown in Table 30.3 (2, 3). Altered level of consciousness, seizures, and aphasia as a part of the initial clinical presentation, gray matter involvement on MRI brain, and lack of oligoclonal bands in CSF might be more suggestive of ADEM rather than CIS due to MS.

The incidence of MS in African Americans is less than that of Caucasians, but studies have demonstrated that they may have a more aggressive disease with faster accumulation of disability. Studies have also shown that African Americans might show less response to standard MS treatments than Caucasians (4).

Several clinical trials evaluating the efficacy of current disease modifying therapies in CIS patients have shown that treatments prolong the time to second event and thus conversion of CIS to CDMS reduced the number of patients converting to CDMS and showed beneficial effects on MRI parameters of the disease (5). All the first-line MS treatments including the three interferons, interferon β 1a IM (Avonex®), interferon β 1a SC (Rebif®), interferon β 1b SC (Betaseron®), and glatiramer acetate (Copaxone®) have demonstrated efficacy in CIS patients, and hence it is recommended that these patients start long-term disease modifying therapy.

REFERENCES

1. Finisku LK, Brex PA, Altman DR, et al. Disability and T2 MRI lesions: A 20-year follow up of patients with relapse onset multiple sclerosis. *Brain* 2008;131:608–817.
2. de Seze J, Debouverie M, Zephir H, et al. Acute fulminant demyelinating disease. *Arch Neurol.* 2007;64(10):1426–1432.
3. Schwartz S, Mohr A, Knauth M, et al. Acute disseminated encephalomyelitis—A follow up study of 40 adult patients. *Neurology.* 2001;56:1313–1318.
4. Cree BAC, Khan O, Bourdette D, et al. Clinical characteristics of African American vs Caucasian Americans with multiple sclerosis. *Neurology.* 2004;63:2039–2045.
5. Jacobs LD, Beck RW, Simon JH, et al. and the CHAMPS Study Group. Intramuscular interferon beta 1a therapy initiated during a first demyelinating event in multiple sclerosis. *NEJM.* 2000;343:898–904.

Dementia and Personality Changes

Sarina S. Shah and Adrian T. Chan

CHIEF COMPLAINT: **Fall from a two-story window.**

HISTORY OF PRESENT ILLNESS:

A 68-year-old, right-handed male presented to the emergency room following a fall from a large second-story window in his apartment that he was attempting to open. He was found awake on the sidewalk by a passerby "writhing in pain." He was unable to clarify if there was a loss of consciousness or not. He was noted to be restless, combative, and confused in the ER, for which he was given Ativan and Haldol and had to be restrained. The patient appeared to have an adverse reaction to the medications with increased rigidity and posturing. His confusion subsequently increased, and an adequate history was not attainable from him.

Immediate psychiatric evaluation excluded the possibility of suicide attempt. The patient's family was contacted. The family members seemed puzzled by the changes in his personality over the past year. They reported increasing intermittent periods of confusion, recent episodes of urinary incontinence, and difficulty sleeping. Patient did not seek any medical attention for these symptoms. During the hospital stay, patient seemed to experience visual hallucinations as he reported seeing "lions." He reported weakness and pain throughout his body in addition to a slight visual impairment that was not specific to one eye.

PAST MEDICAL HISTORY

Hypertension, diabetes mellitus.

PAST SURGICAL HISTORY

Appendectomy.

MEDICATIONS

Hydrochlorothiazide, Enalapril, Metoprolol, Metformin, Lantus.

ALLERGIES

No known food or drug allergies.

PERSONAL HISTORY

The patient lived alone in an apartment. He was unemployed. He denied use of tobacco, alcohol, and illicit drugs.

FAMILY HISTORY

No relevant family history.

REVIEW OF SYSTEMS

Significant for pain in his right forearm with associated swelling, redness, and warmth.

PHYSICAL EXAMINATION

Vital signs: Blood pressure, 145/90; pulse, 88/regular; no evidence of orthostatic hypotension; respiratory rate, 16/min; temperature, 98.0°F.

No meningeal signs, no tongue biting.

NEUROLOGICAL EXAMINATION

Higher mental functions: The patient was noted to be oriented to name, state, city, and year but not to specific location or time. He had decreased attention to commands. He was impulsive and confused at times. His responses to questions were incomplete and seemed unreliable. He did not attempt to do serial sevens; he could not spell the word "world" backwards. He could not draw a clock. He scored 20/30 on the MMSE. He could not copy Rey complex figure. His digit span and immediate memory was poor. He had no apraxia.

CNs II–XII: were unremarkable. Visual acuity of 20/30 OD and 20/25 OS, normal conjugate eye movements, and gross visual threat stimuli did not reveal any visual field cuts. Rest of the cranial nerve examination was unremarkable.

Motor: Tone was increased in all four extremities (lower more than upper). Strength was 4/5 in all extremities.

Sensory: Deferred because of poor attention.

Reflexes: 1+ bilaterally.

Plantars: Flexors bilaterally.

Gait: Unsteady and narrow based with a stooped posture. He could clear the foot off the ground but was bradykinetic.

Pull test did reveal postural instability. He was noted to have a pill-rolling resting tremor of his right hand. There was no cogwheel rigidity.

STOP AND THINK QUESTIONS

➤ Did he have a seizure precipitating a fall from the window?

➤ Is he suffering from complex partial seizures explaining his intermittent episodes of confusion?

➤ Is he in delirium or does he have dementia?

➤ Do visual hallucinations make you think of any particular neurological condition(s) in a patient with slow but progressive mental status change?

➤ How would you proceed with the work up?

DIAGNOSTIC TEST RESULTS

Complete blood count, chemistry, and hepatic panel were normal. Urine for toxicology was negative.

Head CT revealed a minimal subarachnoid hemorrhage in the anterior aspect of the left Sylvian fissure not requiring surgical intervention.

EEG revealed mild diffuse cerebral dysfunction; there were no periodic sharps/spikes.

POSSIBLE DIAGNOSIS: Diffuse Lewy body (DLB) dementia, Parkinson's disease (PD), Alzheimer's disease (AD).

DISCUSSION

Given the history of sudden fall with symptoms of delirium or acute confusional state, one has to rule out toxic-metabolic states, drug-related side effects, or recreational drug intoxication, or infections as possible etiologies of delirium. Other neurological causes of acute confusional states, such as seizure and stroke, need to be excluded as well.

Careful history and collateral information from the family members point to a neuro-degenerative disorder in this case. This patient has suffered cognitive changes in the past year, indicating a possible dementia. The presence of both visual hallucinations and fluctuating cognition fulfills the criteria for DLB. Lack of history of early symptoms of Parkinsonism before the onset of dementia also supports the diagnosis of DLB rather than Parkinson's disease with dementia. Table 31.1 summarizes the differentiating features of PD, AD, and DLB. The significant parkinsonian symptoms that are brought out after being given neuroleptics are also supportive of an underlying parkinsonian disorder.

DLB is the second most common type of dementia (first is AD) (1). The Lewy Body Dementia Association estimates 1 to 2 million Americans have DLB (2). Diagnostic criteria for DLB are categorized as essential, core, suggestive, and supportive features (3). They are as follows.

- Essential features: dementia.
- Core features: (2 of 3 = probable DLB; 1 of 3 = possible DLB): fluctuations in attention and alertness, visual hallucinations (recurrent, well formed, detailed), spontaneous features of Parkinsonism.
- Suggestive features: (1 or more with at least 1 of the above core features = probable DLB; 1 or more = possible DLB): REM sleep behavior disorder (RBD), severe neuroleptic sensitivity, low dopamine receptor uptake in basal ganglia seen by SPECT/PET.
- Supportive features: falling, syncope, loss of consciousness, depression, hypoperfusion of occipital lobe on SPECT/PET, low uptake w/MIBG myocardial scintigraphy.

Early cognitive features include getting lost, misjudging distances, failing to see stop signs or other cars, and impaired job performance (4). The MMSE reveals impaired figure copying, clock drawing, serial sevens, and spelling "world" backwards (4). One should note that often, until they have advanced disease, patients with DLB can have relatively good MMSE scores when compared with patients suffering from AD. Early on in the course of DLB, orientation and memory are relatively preserved compared with AD, and attention span as well as visual spatial orientation tends to be affected earlier than AD. However, these deficits eventually occur in both diseases. Fluctuating cognition is a distinctive feature of DLB and may be useful in differentiating DLB from other Dementias, but one should note that fluctuating cognition can also occur in AD and FTD, and clinically it may be difficult to get a clear history of fluctuating cognition. At times, these symptoms are very similar to those of an epileptic syndrome, and often the latter has to be ruled out.

While parkinsonism is often a reliable indicator that a patient may have DLB, parkinsonian symptoms may be subtle and not noted by the family members. Bradykinesia and postural instability or shuffling gait is more readily seen, while tremor is often absent, or very subtle without the classic pill-rolling tremor.

The presence of prominent hallucinations and paranoid delusions is a more striking features of DLB, and it is useful clinically to distinguish DLB from AD. Though patients with AD can often have paranoid delusions, they tend to occur later on in the disease, and it is interesting to note that a number of these patients are also found to have coexisting DLB at autopsy. A more distinctive characteristic of patients with both Parkinson's disease and DLB is the early and significant loss of sense of smell, which occurs to a much lesser extent in AD patients (5).

RBD, a hallmark of DLB, occurs when there is no normal muscle atonia during vivid dreams (3). Patients act out the dream with vocalizations and violent behavior. Patients

TABLE 31.1 *Comparison of Three Possible Diagnoses (1–4)*

	Diffuse Lewy Body Dementia	Parkinson's Disease	Alzheimer's Disease
Age of onset	40–70 years	Around 70 years	>late 60s (<65 years is designated early onset)
Signs and symptoms	Early-onset dementia (attention, executive function, visuo-spatial), parkinsonism, delusions, visual hallucinations, fluctuations in mental status, myoclonus, REM sleep behavior disorder (early finding), syncope, orthostasis, severe neuroleptic sensitivity. Compared to PD: less severe tremor and more postural instability Compared to AD: more visuo-spatial deficit, less language and memory deficit compared to AD	Resting tremor (early, pill rolling), rigidity (possibly cogwheel), flexed posture, bradykinesia, masklike facies, hypophonia, micrographia, difficulty starting and stopping walking, hurried shuffling steps, blepharoclonus, Myerson sign (sustained blink response to tapping over bridge of nose), loss of smell, dementia (30%)	Cognitive impairment, memory loss (early symptom), normal consciousness, aphasia, anomia, acalculia, apraxia, social/psychiatric symptoms (late finding), mutism (terminal finding), incontinence (terminal finding)
Pathologic findings	Lewy bodies (α-synuclein) throughout cortex and subcortex	Lewy bodies in basal ganglia, loss of pigment in substantia nigra	General cortical atrophy (especially in medial temporal lobe), amyloid plaques and neurofibrillary tangles, loss of cholinergic neurons
Diagnosis	Clinical MRI: less hippocampal atrophy than AD; SPECT/PET: decreased occipital lobe blood flow, low dopamine receptor uptake in basal ganglia; Neuropsychological	Clinical	Clinical CT/MRI: cortical atrophy especially of medial temporal lobe and enlarged ventricles; PET: amyloid deposits
Treatment	Acetylcholinesterase inhibitors (rivastigmine, donepezil, galantamine), atypical antipsychotics (quetiapine, risperidone, clozapine)	Carbidopa/levodopa, amantadine, dopamine agonists (pramipexole, ropinirole), selegiline, entacapone, muscarinic ACh antagonists (benztropine, trihexyphenidyl). Surgical: thalamotomy, pallidotomy. Deep brain stimulation	Acetylcholinesterase inhibitors (rivastigmine, donepezil, tacrine, galantamine), glutamate antagonist (memantine)
Prognosis	Death 7 years following appearance of cognitive symptoms	Variable, may be >20 years until death	Death 5–10 years following appearance of symptoms

also experience daytime somnolence. Diagnosis is made by polysomnography, which shows increased EMG tone during REM sleep and movements during sleep.

The pathological hallmark of DLB is the presence of Lewy bodies (Figure 31.1) that extend into the limbic and cortical regions, as compared with PD, where Lewy bodies are mainly confined to the substantia nigra and not present in the cortical region. Lewy bodies are stained positive for ubiquitin and more specifically for Alpha-synuclein (Figure 31.2). The use of Alpha-synuclein antibody to highlight the Lewy bodies in pathology specimen has become the gold standard for diagnosis of DLB. AD type changes are often found in these patients that may or may not be significant enough to warrant a dual diagnose of AD (6). In fact, pure Diffuse Lewy Body disease without AD type change is rather uncommon. Diffuse Lewy Body disease is the terminology used for describing the pathological findings

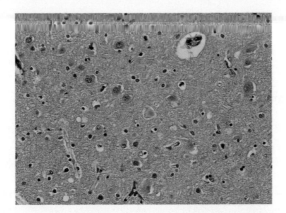

FIGURE 31.1 *Numerous eosinophilic Lewy bodies are seen in the frontal cortex of a patient with dementia with Lewy body.*

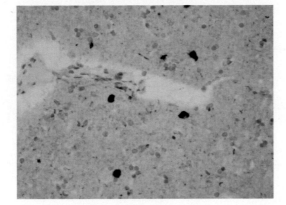

FIGURE 31.2 *Lewy bodies are highlighted by the alpha synuclein immunostain. Note that some alpha synuclein positive neurites are also highlighted.*

of Lewy bodies in the brain, whereas dementia with Lewy Body is the clinical term used to describe the clinical syndrome as defined by the consensus criteria. Therefore, for all patients presenting with symptoms of DLB, it is important to note that a coexistence of Alzheimer's disease is still a possibility.

Management of DLB is extremely difficult. These patients are relatively insensitive to dopaminergic therapy, and even though parkinsonism can be improved with L-dopa, the side effects of increased confusion and hallucinations often lead to the cessation of any dopaminergic medication. Despite this, very low doses of L-dopa can be tried and titrated up very slowly. Dopamine agonists and amantadine should be avoided as these will very often cause more confusion and hallucinations and are relatively ineffective antiparkinsonism medication.

Haldol and other typical neuroleptics should be avoided in treating hallucinations, as typical neuroleptics can cause a severe hypersensitivity reaction that causes severe rigidity and confusion, and these patients are at a higher risk of developing neuroleptic malignant syndrome (6). Other dopamine blocking agents such as anti-emetics should also be avoided. Newer generations of neuroleptics are safer but can possibly cause similar symptoms. The most commonly used neuroleptic is quetiapine which, though occasionally can cause drowsiness and confusion, is effective in controlling hallucinations and paranoia at low doses and rarely causes significant side effects.

Other medications such as benzodiazepine or anticholinergics should be avoided and should not be routinely used as tranquilizers, as they often cause confusion in patients with dementia. Finally, there are as yet no effective treatments for the progressive dementia in

DLB. Cholinesterase inhibitors may have subtle benefit in improving confusion and concentration but are in general not very effective (3,6).

REFERENCES

1. Hanson JC, Lippa CF. Lewy body dementia. *Int Rev Neurobiol.* 2009;84:215–228.
2. Tarawneh R, Galvin JE. Distinguishing Lewy body dementias from Alzheimer's disease. *Expert Rev Neurother.* 2007;7(11):1499–1516.
3. Bonanni L, Thomas A, Onofrj M. Diagnosis and management of dementia with Lewy bodies: Third report of the DLB Consortium. *Neurology.* 2006;66(9):1455.
4. Simon RP, Greenberg DA, Aminoff MJ. *Clinical Neurology.* 7th ed. Lange Medical Books/McGraw Hill Medical, New York, NY; 2009.
5. McShane RH et al. Anosmia in dementia is associated with Lewy bodies rather than Alzheimer's pathology. *J Neurol Neurosurg Psychiatry.* 2001;70:739–743.
6. McKeith IG. Dementia with Lewy bodies. *Br J Psych.* 2002;180:144–147.

CHIEF COMPLAINT: **I have the worst headache of my life.**

HISTORY OF PRESENT ILLNESS

A 58-year-old, right-handed female presented to the ER after experiencing sudden onset headache that morning while having a bowel movement. The headache was holocephalic but she described pain and stiffness particularly in her neck. The pain was 9/10 in severity, "intense" in nature, and was constant. There was no difference in her symptoms with positional changes. The headache was associated with nausea. She denied vomiting, light or sound sensitivity, fever, chills, and bowel or bladder problems, and seizure activity. There was no loss of consciousness. She denied a prior history of headaches and had never experienced similar symptoms. She stated that it was the worst headache of her life. She took ibuprofen to try to alleviate the pain but had only minimal relief.

PAST MEDICAL HISTORY

Graves disease s/p radioablation therapy 2005, now with hypothyroidism.

PAST SURGICAL HISTORY

Tonsillectomy as child, bilateral subdural hematoma evacuations at age 5 (details not known to the patient).

MEDICATIONS

Synthroid 125 mcg by mouth daily.

ALLERGIES

No known allergies.

PERSONAL HISTORY

Born in Mexico though raised in the United States, formerly smoked one to two packs of cigarettes daily but currently smokes one to two cigarettes daily, social alcohol use once weekly, denied illicit drug use.

FAMILY HISTORY

Noncontributory.

PHYSICAL EXAMINATION

Vital signs: Blood pressure, 148/91 mmHg; pulse, 60/min; respiratory rate, 16/min; O$_2$ saturation, 96%; temperature, 96.6°F.

The patient appeared uncomfortable, lying still on ER stretcher, no rashes, and normal cardiac/lung/abdominal/musculoskeletal examination.

Head and neck examination: No obvious facial symmetry, mild nuchal rigidity with pain on attempted flexion of neck.

NEUROLOGICAL EXAMINATION

Mental status: Alert, oriented to time, place and person, fluent speech without dysarthria, able to register and recall three objects, intact attention and concentration.

CNs II–XII: Visual acuity 20/20 bilaterally, pupils equal and reactive, extra ocular movements intact, no nystagmus, visual fields full, facial sensations intact, facial symmetry, tongue midline and no atrophy, palate elevation symmetric, equal shoulder shrug and head turn though some pain with movements of the neck.

Motor: No pronator drift, full 5/5 strength in both upper and lower extremities to confrontation, normal bulk and tone.

Sensory: Symmetric light touch, pin prick, temperature, position, and vibration sense in all four extremities.

Reflexes: 2+ symmetric upper and lower extremity reflexes, plantar flexors bilaterally, no clonus or Hoffman's sign.

Coordination: Normal finger-to-nose bilaterally, normal heel-knee-shin, rapid fine finger movements, normal rapid alternating movements.

Gait: Steady, normal stride and arm swing, able to tandem, walks on heels and toes, Romberg negative.

DIAGNOSTIC TEST RESULTS

Labs: Basic metabolic panel, CBC, hepatic panel, coagulation factors unremarkable.

Chest X-ray: No evidence of cardiopulmonary disease.

Head CT without contrast: Hyperdense signal is seen in the sulci/subarachnoid space, compatible with SAH (Figure 32.1A and 32.1B). No intraparenchymal or ventricular hemorrhage. No evidence of obstructive hydrocephalus. Figure 32.1C shows axial CT status post clipping of right middle cerebral aneurysm.

Three-vessel cerebral angiogram: On day one, patient underwent cerebral angiogram to potentially diagnose and treat the underlying cause of SAH. The vessels catheterized included the right internal carotid artery, the left internal carotid artery, and the left vertebral artery. On catheterization of the right internal carotid artery, the arterial phase images were notable for a large aneurysm arising from the right A1/A2 junction incorporating the origin of a large internal frontal branch of the right anterior cerebral artery. The right A1 was dominant. The aneurysm projected anteriorly and superiorly, with a secondary daughter aneurysm on the posterior aspect of the dome, likely representing the site of rupture. The aneurysm neck was wide. Arterial phase images also demonstrated a small aneurysm at the bifurcation of the right MCA measuring approximately 3 mm in diameter. No evidence of arterial venous shunting, vascular stenosis, or venoocclusive disorder. No abnormalities noted with catheterization of the left internal carotid artery or the left vertebral artery.

STOP AND THINK QUESTIONS

➢ What is the differential diagnosis in someone presenting with headache, neck rigidity, and nausea?

➢ What are the examination maneuvers one can perform to evaluate for meningeal irritation?

➢ What tests/studies will you pursue to reach a diagnosis?

➢ Based on the findings of the head CT and cerebral angiogram, what is the next step in management?

➢ What are the important steps in the medical management of this patient?

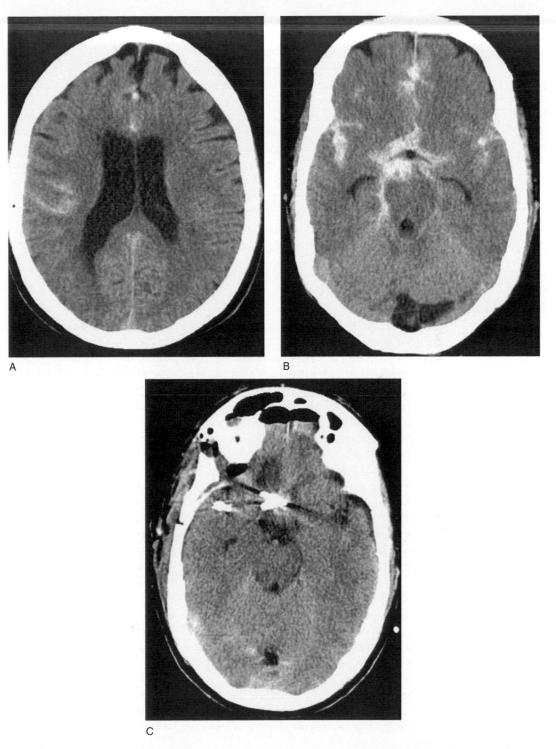

FIGURE 32.1 *(A,B) NCHCT axial images showing hyperdense signal showing subarachnoid hemorrhage seen in the sulci, cisterns, and subarachnoid space. (C) Status post clipping of right middle cerebral artery aneurysm.*

DIAGNOSIS: Subarachnoid hemorrhage (SAH) secondary to cerebral aneurysmal rupture.

HOSPITAL COURSE

Based on the above findings of spontaneous subarachnoid bleed on history and head CT, the patient was started on a Nicardipine drip for blood pressure control, Nimodipine to help prevent vasospasm, and Keppra for seizure prophylaxis. After the initial cerebral angiogram revealed multiple aneurysms including the likely site of rupture, neurosurgical clipping was pursued. The patient underwent a right pterional craniotomy; the right ACA A1/A2 segment aneurysm and the right MCA aneurysm were then surgically clipped. On day 6, patient had repeat cerebral angiogram showing mild vasospasm of the right A2 segment of the callosomarginal artery. Triple H therapy was initiated to treat vasospasm: hypertensive hypervolemic hemodilution. Intravenous medications and large volumes of intravenous fluids was used to elevate blood pressure, increase blood volume, and thin the blood, driving blood flow through and around affected vessels. The patient was ultimately stabilized, and transferred to acute inpatient rehabilitation for three weeks. A repeat head CT showed resolving SAH. The patient was discharged home from rehabilitation with appropriate follow-up appointments.

DISCUSSION

Hemorrhagic strokes account for 20% to 30% of strokes in developed countries and are a form of acute neurological injury resulting from bleeding into the head. Five percent to ten percent of hemorrhagic strokes are SAHs characterized by bleeding into the subarachnoid CSF containing sulci, fissures, and cisterns. The remaining 10% to 20% of hemorrhages is caused by intracerebral hemorrhages where the bleeding occurs directly into the brain parenchyma. Rapid identification of the type of acute stroke is essential as the intervention is fundamentally different based on whether the stroke is hemorrhagic or ischemic. SAH following aneurysmal rupture has a high fatality rate at 50% with between 10% and 15% of patients dying before they arrive at the hospital.

Etiology

The leading cause of nontraumatic SAH is aneurysmal rupture, accounting for 85% of SAH. Saccular aneurysms occur at branching points along cerebral vessels and at the bifurcation or origin of side branches. The majority of saccular aneurysms (80%–85%) are located in the anterior circulation at the origins of the posterior or anterior communicating arteries or at the MCA bifurcation. Posterior circulation aneurysms tend to occur at the basilar tip or posterior–inferior cerebellar artery origin. Fusiform aneurysms are less common than saccular aneurysms and account for 10% to 15% of SAH. These aneurysms consist of enlargement or dilatation of the entire circumference of the involved vessel.

Intracranial aneurysms are acquired cerebrovascular anomalies that develop throughout a patient's lifetime. These aneurysms have been detected at a frequency of 1% to 9% and approximately 6 to 10 million people in the United States have intracranial aneurysms. The annual risk of rupture for any aneurysm is 0.7%, though the risk can be more accurately predicted by the aneurysm size and location. Aneurysms greater than 6 mm in diameter have a much greater risk of rupture. In addition, aneurysms located in the posterior communicating arteries or posterior cerebral circulation are also at greater risk.

Approximately 10% to 15% of SAH is nonaneurysmal and does not have an identifiable cause such as those listed below. The more rare causes of SAH account for <5% of all cases. Inflammatory lesions and vasculitides causing SAH include primary CNS vasculitis, vasculitis involving medium and small vessels such as Polyarteritis nodosa, Churg-Strauss syndrome, and Wegner granulomatosis, and other pathologies including Behcet disease and mycotic aneurysms. There are noninflammatory lesions and vasculopathies that may cause SAH such as arterial dissection, arteriovenous malformations, cavernous angioma, amyloid angiopathy, cerebral venous thrombosis, and moyamoya. Finally, coagulopathies, neoplasms, and the use of drugs such as anticoagulants and sympathomimetics can precipitate the development of SAH.

Risk Factors

Risk factors for the development of SAH include hypertension, smoking, heavy alcohol use, and the use of drugs such as cocaine has also been implicated. Most aneurysmal SAHs are nongenetic in origin; however, there are some rare inherited conditions that have been associated with an increased risk of cerebral aneurysm and SAH. These include autosomal dominant polycystic kidney disease, glucocorticoid-remediable aldosteronism, and Ehler Danlos syndrome.

Clinical Manifestations

SAH is generally characterized by a thunderclap headache that is a sudden onset, severe, unprecedented headache. The following descriptions are typical in SAH: "my head was torn open," "my head was hit with a hammer," "my head exploded," "unbearable," "worst headache ever." The headache peaks within minutes and can last from 1 hour to 15 days and rarely 3 to 4 weeks. The majority of headaches is bilateral (70%) and in 66% of cases is generalized; 20% of the time the headaches are occipital, and 10% are parietal. Unilateral headaches occur 30% of the time and are typically frontal or frontoparietal.

While headache is the predominate clinical manifestations, patients may also experience meningeal irritation, less marked focal neurological signs, transient disturbances in consciousness, and periretinal hemorrhage. Blood in the subarachnoid space can produce meningeal irritation thus causing Kernig's sign, Brudzinski's sign, or nuchal rigidity. Sixty-four percent of patients exhibit these signs of meningeal irritation. In addition, 50% of patients may experience vomiting. Focal neurological signs occur based on the severity and location of the hemorrhage, increased intracranial pressure, and the occurrence of hydrocephalus, presence of a hematoma, and complications that can occur, such as vasospasm or cerebral infarction. Patients with a ruptured aneurysm of the MCA may exhibit swallowing disturbances, aphasia, hemianopsia, or motor deficits. Patients with anterior cerebral artery aneurysm rupture may exhibit increased deep tendon reflexes and paraparesis. Oculomotor palsy may occur in internal carotid-posterior communicating artery aneurysms.

Disturbances of consciousness have been observed in 50% of cases of SAH. These episodes of loss of consciousness can be short-lived, lasting a few minutes, or can last up to weeks. Respiration may be affected in SAH and can change in response to elevated intracranial pressure and subsequent compression of the brain stem. Body temperature may also become elevated to 38 to 39 °C. Systolic blood pressure is elevated in 75% to 90% of patients following aneurysm rupture and can rise to over 200 mmHg. EKG changes have also been described in patients without pre-existing heart disease. Some of these EKG changes include: atrial and ventricular dysrhythmias, changes in QRS complex, prolongation of the QT interval, ST elevation, T wave abnormalities, prominent U wave. These EKG changes are likely secondary to autonomic disturbances and in some cases may be caused by myocardial damage.

Clinical grading scores based on physical examination findings have been developed to assess eventual functional outcome following aneurysmal SAH. The two most commonly used scores are the Hunt and Hess and WFNS (Table 32.1). The most important predictive factors include level of consciousness on admission, the patient's age (inverse correlation), and the amount of blood on head CT (inverse correlation). WFNS scoring is based on the Glasgow coma scale points and associated neurological symptoms.

In addition to the clinical manifestations mentioned, 27% to 60% of patients experience warning signs and symptoms. These warning signs and symptoms may be caused by: compression of the aneurysm, minor bleeding at the aneurismal wall, vasospasm, or small leakage into the subarachnoid space. Some of these warning signs and symptoms include a generalized or localized headache which may be worse than usual but is less intense than that accompanying a major bleed. Patients may also describe visual disturbances, facial pain, ocular pain, nausea, and dizziness. These warning signs can precede symptomatic SAH by 10 to 110 days. Table 32.2 below correlates the location of headaches with the location of intracranial aneurysms.

Diagnostic Tests

Noncontrast head CT with or without lumbar puncture is the first line of imaging for the detection of acute intracranial hemorrhage. CT is commonly used both for its logistic and diagnostic advantages. It is widely available, with few if any contraindications, results are rapidly available, and patients can be safely monitored during the procedure. Noncontrast head CT is highly sensitive for acute and subacute SAH; it is 98% sensitive for SAH within 12 hours of symptom onset and 93% sensitive at 24 hours. Over time, the dilution and evolution of blood products lead to a decreased density of blood and thus a decrease in the sensitivity of CT for detecting SAH.

TABLE 32.1 *Clinical Grading Scores to Assess Functional Outcome Following SAH*

Grade	Hunt and Hess Score	WFNS Score
0	Unruptured aneurysm	Unruptured aneurysm
1	Asymptomatic or mild headache and slight nuchal rigidity	GCS 15 without hemiparesis
1a	Fixed neurological deficit without other signs of SAH	
2	Severe headache, stiff neck, no neurological deficit except cranial nerve palsy	GCS 14–13 without hemiparesis
3	Drowsy or confused, mild focal neurological deficit	GCS 14–13 with hemiparesis
4	Stuporous, moderate or severe hemiparesis	GCS 12–7 with or without hemiparesis
5	Coma, decerebrate posturing	GCS 6–3 with or without hemiparesis

GCS, Glasgow Coma Scale.

Table 32.2 *Correlation Between the Location of Headaches and Site of Cerebral Aneurysms*

Location of Headache	Anterior	Middle	Posterior	Vertebrobasilar	All Sites
Occipital (%)	24	20	19	39	21
Frontal (%)	14	15	19	3	15
Temporal (%)	3	9	13	6	8
Not localized (%)	35	28	29	30	32
None (%)	24	28	20	22	24
Total number of cases	381	253	292	36	962

Hemorrhage evolution is a dynamic process, hence the change in findings on imaging over time. Five stages have been described, and while the naming and molecular composition of each stage is agreed upon, there are discrepancies between the timing of each stage. In the hyperacute phase, blood contains oxyhemoglobin intracellularly. In the acute stage, blood loses its oxygen and becomes deoxyhemoglobin. In the early subacute phase, intracellular deoxyhemoglobin is converted to methemoglobin by oxidative denaturation. This stage is followed by the late subacute phase in which cell lysis leads to extracellular methemoglobin. Finally, in the chronic stage, methemolgobin is converted to hemosiderin and ferritin.

The pattern of SAH bleeding can be predictive of the location of an aneurysmal rupture (if the SAH was caused by aneursymal rupture). If blood is located in the interhemispheric fissure, it is often caused by a ruptured anterior cerebral artery aneurysm. In patients with intracerebral or SAH detected on CT, CTA is a less invasive alternative to catheter angiography for the detection of aneurysms. CTA has a 77% to 100% sensitivity for detecting aneurysms >3 mm in size. A negative CTA should be followed by catheter cerebral angiography as this method is more sensitive for detecting aneurysms <4 mm.

Using DSA or MRA, the specific underlying cause can also be further elucidated. MRA has a sensitivity of 85% to 100% for detecting aneurysms > 5 mm in size. MR can be used to detect hyperacute and subacute SAH. In the hyperacute phase, blood products in the subarachnoid space appear hyperintense on T1 and proton density-weighted imaging due to the increased protein content. On FLAIR sequences, blood-containing CSF appears hyperintense. CT, FLAIR, and proton density-weighted sequences are equally sensitive for the detection of SAH if done within 12 hours of symptom onset. MR is also useful for the accurate detection of chronic hemorrhage, small ischemic infarcts, and differentiating acute from chronic ischemia.

A negative noncontrast head CT can reliably exclude larger volume SAH; however, to rule out SAH with a negative CT, the Stroke Council of the American Heart Association strongly recommends a lumbar puncture. Classic findings on lumbar puncture include an elevated opening pressure and RBC count that does not diminish from CSF tube one to tube four. It is important to differentiate a traumatic tap, in which the RBC counts per collection tube declines in successive tubes, from nontraumatic bleeding. Decreasing RBC counts in serial tubes cannot be used to reliably distinguish between SAH and a traumatic tap and further tests should be done.

The CSF should be centrifuged and examined for xanthrochromia, which may require 12 hours to develop. Xanthrochromia, which is a yellow or pink tint to CSF fluid representing hemoglobin degradation products, is highly suggestive of SAH. The presence of xanthrochromia indicates that blood has been in the CSF for at least 2 hours and the tint can last up to 2 weeks. While xanthrochromia can be detected visually by comparing a tube of CSF with a tube of plain water against a white background in bright light, spectrophotometry can also be used. Spectrophotometry is highly sensitive (>95%) for detecting bilirubin if the lumbar puncture is preformed at least 12 hours after SAH.

TREATMENT

Patients with SAH should be stabilized; their ventilation, oxygenation, and circulation should be secured before attempting to prevent complications of SAH. Rebleeding is a complication with the highest risk of occurring within the first 24 hours after aneurysmal rupture. In order to prevent this complication, the aneurysm must be isolated from cerebral circulation. Temporary vessel occlusion using cerebroprotective techniques, such as hypothermia, induced hypertension, and mannitol, have been used to facilitate safe dissection near the aneurysm. Surgical clipping and endovascular coiling are both effective means of isolating the aneurysm. In the ISAT, 2100 patients with SAH amenable to either surgery or coiling were enrolled. The study showed that endovascular coiling was associated with a lower risk of death or dependency at 1 year compared with surgical clipping. While coiling requires angiographic surveillance, the net benefit in functional outcome remains in favor of endovascular coiling. Though this study demonstrates the advantages of endovascular coiling, individual patient characteristics including age, medical comorbidities, size location, and morphology of the aneurysm should be considered by a multidisciplinary team to determine the best management for the patient. Other proposed mechanisms for reducing the rate of aneurismal rebleeding include bed rest, blood pressure control, and the use of antifibrinolytic medications.

Hydrocephalus, an enlargement of the ventricular spaces, is another frequent complication in patients with SAH, occurring 9% to 67% of the time. Acute hydrocephalus develops within 3 days after SAH whereas chronic hydrocephalus develops later. Patients clinically presented with a decrease in the level of consciousness. On physical examination, patients may also exhibit a downward deviation of the eyes and small pupils. Hydrocephalus is confirmed by CT with radiologic criteria including expansion of the temporal horns, convexity of the third ventricular walls, rounding of the frontal horns, effacement of sulci, enlargement of ventricles out of proportion to sulcal dilatation. Treatment can involve external ventricular drainage, placement of a lumbar drain, or serial lumbar punctures.

Cerebral vasospasm is a narrowing of cerebral arteries and is an important complication of SAH. Symptomatic vasospasm occurs in 17% to 21% of patients following SAH. Cerebral vasospasms can clinically manifest with vague symptoms such as headache or confusion. Delayed cerebral infarction can also be attributable to vasospasm; this complication occurs in 20% of patients with SAH. Fisher et al. tried to correlate the index of vasospasm risk based on hemorrhage pattern on the initial head CT. Patients with diffuse thick subarachnoid clots are at a higher risk of vasospasm compared to other groups where no blood or only a thin layer of blood is detected.

Cerebral vasospasms are most commonly monitored by transcranial Doppler and conventional angiography. The primary treatment goal for patients experiencing vasospasm and subsequent cerebral infarction is to improve cerebral blood flow. Hypertensive hypervolemic hemodilution is the mainstay of treatment (refer to Table 32.3). However, despite the use of this treatment, there is a lack of well-controlled studies to support its efficacy. Endovascular therapies include transluminal balloon angioplasty and intraarterial infusion of vasodilators such as nicardipine. For prevention of vasospasm and delayed cerebral infarction, nimodipine, a calcium channel blocker, is recommended. Patients with aneurysmal SAH should be given 60 mg of nimodipine every 4 hours by enteral route from admission to 21 days after.

Table 32.3 *Management of Vasospasm in Patients With Cerebral Aneurysms*

Cerebroselective calcium channel blockers: Nimodipine (Nimotop) 30-60mg q4h
Aggressive Hypervolemic, Hypertensive, Hemodilution (HHH) therapy (maintaining systolic BP to 160-200mg with pressor agents; volume expansion: with colloids)
Early clipping of aneurysm reducing chances of rebleeding
Recognition of early signs of vasospasm (hyponatremia or increased velocities on the Transcranial Doppler studies)
Triliazad (lipid peroxidation inhibitor)
Thrombolytic and endovascular therapies in the future

Finally, hyponatremia occurs in 10% to 30% of patients with aneurysmal SAH and is likely caused by cerebral salt wasting. Treatment involves salt and fluid replacement and may also include use of fludrocortisone and concentrated saline (sodium chloride 3%).

SUGGESTED READING

Dupont SA, Wijdicks EF, Lanzino G, Rabinstein AA. Aneurysmal subarachnoid hemorrhage: An overview for the practicing neurologist. *Semin Neurol.* 2010;30(5):545–554. Epub 2011 Jan 4.

Fisher CM, Kistler JP, Davis JM. Relation of cerebral vasospasm to subarachnoid hemorrhage visualized by computerized tomographic scanning. *Neurosurgery.* 1980;6(1):1e9.

Molyneux AJ, Kerr RSC, Yu LM, et al. International Subarachnoid Aneurysm Trial (ISAT) Collaborative Group. International subarachnoid aneurysm trial (ISAT) of neurosurgical clipping versus endovascular coiling in 2143 patients with ruptured intracranial aneurysms: A randomized comparison of effects on survival, dependency, seizures, rebleeding, subgroups, and aneurysm occlusion. *Lancet* 2005;366(9488):809–881.

Okawara SH. Warning signs prior to rupture of an intracranial aneurysm. *J Neurosurg.* 1973;38:575–580.

Report of World Federation of Neurological Surgeons Committee on a Universal Subarachnoid Hemorrhage Grading Scale. *J Neurosurg.* 1988;68(6):985.

Shinohara Y. Hemorrhagic stroke syndromes: Clinical manifestations of intracerebral and subarachnoid hemorrhage. *Handb Clin Neurol* [0072–9752] Shinohara. 2009;93:577–594.

Smith SD, Eskey CJ. Hemorrhagic stroke. *Radiol Clin North Am.* 2011;49(1):27–45.

Wijdicks EF, Kallmes DF, Manno EM, Fulgham JR, Piepgras DG. Subarachnoid hemorrhage: Neurointensive care and aneurysm repair. *Mayo Clin Proc.* 2005;80(4):550.

Headache and Blurring of Vision

Anuradha Singh, Arielle Kurzweil, and Mohammad Fouladvand

CHIEF COMPLAINT: **I have a headache and I can't see right.**

HISTORY OF PRESENT ILLNESS

A 25-year-old, right-handed female was referred to the ER for insidious headache and visual disturbance. She had been experiencing a daily headache for the last several months, usually upon awakening in the morning. The headache was bilaterally in the front and back of the head, and was a dull, constant ache. The headache would dissipate after taking ibuprofen or would resolve on its own within a few hours. She also complained of blurry vision worse in her left eye despite wearing glasses. She had never experienced headaches prior to the onset 3 months ago. She denied other common neurological symptoms, weakness, tingling, numbness, double vision, speech, or swallowing difficulty. She denied any fever, nausea, vomiting, photophobia, photophobia, joint pains, or skin rash. She has been using birth control pills for a couple of years and has not noticed any association with its use. She has gained 30 pounds over the past few months. She denied any previous history of blood clots, TIA, stroke, or recurrent abortions.

PAST MEDICAL HISTORY

Polycystic ovarian syndrome, gastroesophageal reflux disease, anxiety.

PAST SURGICAL HISTORY

Cervical cone biopsy.

MEDICATIONS

Birth control pills, Prevacid, Spironolactone, Ativan 1 to 2 mg as needed for anxiety.

ALLERGIES

Sulfa medications (rash).

PERSONAL HISTORY

Lives alone, a writer, denied tobacco or illicit drug use, rare alcohol use.

FAMILY HISTORY

Her father has coronary artery disease and diabetes.

PHYSICAL EXAMINATION

Vitals: Blood pressure, 131/89 mmHg; pulse, 76/min; respiratory rate, 18/min; O_2 saturation, 96%; temperature, 98.4°F; height, 5'3"; weight, 286.3 lbs. Morbidly obese female appearing somewhat uncomfortable. No obvious facial symmetry, neck supple without meningismus.

NEUROLOGICAL EXAMINATION

Mental status: Alert, oriented to time, place and person, normal affect, fluent speech without dysarthria, able to register and recall three objects, intact attention, and concentration.

CNs II–XII: Visual acuity 20/25 bilaterally with corrective lenses, pupils 4 mm bilaterally and reactive, extraocular movements intact, no ptosis or proptosis, no nystagmus, visual fields full, fundoscopic examination shows bilateral disc elevation and bilateral swelling of the disc margins without disc atrophy, facial sensation intact, facial symmetry, tongue midline, palate elevation symmetric, equal shoulder shrug and head turn though some pain with range of motion movements of neck.

Motor: No pronator drift, full 5/5 strength in both upper and lower extremities to confrontation, normal bulk and tone.

Sensory: Symmetric light touch, pin prick, temperature, position and vibration sense in all four extremities.

Reflexes: 2+ symmetric upper and lower extremity reflexes, plantar flexors bilaterally, no clonus or Hoffman's sign.

Coordination: Normal finger-to-nose bilaterally, normal heel-knee-shin, rapid fine finger movements, normal rapid alternating movements.

Gait: Steady, normal stride and arm swing, able to tandem, walks on heels and toes, Romberg negative.

STOP AND THINK QUESTIONS

➤ What do the findings of the fundoscopic examination indicate?

➤ What is the differential diagnosis in a patient with early-morning headaches and visual changes?

➤ What would be the next steps in the workup of this patient?

DIAGNOSTIC TEST RESULTS

Serum labs: Basic metabolic panel, complete blood count, hepatic panel, coagulation factors unremarkable. Serum HCG negative.

CSF studies: Clear and colorless, opening pressure 33 mm Hg, glucose 47, protein 23, white blood count 3, red blood count 0, Gram stain negative.

Head CT without contrast: Normal.

MRI Brain with gadolinium: Normal.

MRA/MRV brain with gadolinium: Normal.

STOP AND THINK QUESTIONS

➤ What do the lumbar puncture results signify?

➤ What is the diagnosis?

➤ What is a common cranial nerve palsy that can be seen in patients with idiopathic intracranial hypertension (though is not seen in this patient)?

➤ What are the treatment options for this patient?

DIAGNOSIS: **Idiopathic intracranial hypertension (IIH).**

HOSPITAL COURSE

After the lumbar puncture revealed an elevated opening pressure but otherwise normal CSF studies, as well as normal brain imaging, the patient was diagnosed with idiopathic intracranial hypertension, also known as pseudotumor cerebri. The patient was counseled on weight loss and encouraged to pursue exercise and a healthier diet. In addition, she was initially treated with diamox, a carbonic anhydrase inhibitor. However, she did not tolerate this medication well due to gastrointestinal side effects. Ultimately, she underwent bilateral optic nerve fenestrations to preserve her vision. Should her symptoms return, CSF shunting can be considered in the future.

DISCUSSION

The intracranial pressure is exerted by the cranium on the brain tissue, CSF, and the brain's circulating blood volume. At rest and in supine state, it is normally 7 to 15 mm Hg. CSF is produced in choroid plexuses of lateral, third, and fourth ventricles. The rate of production is about 20 cc/h. It is absorbed into the arachnoid villi. Table 33.1 lists the causes of increased ICP.

Elevation in ICP can be graded from mild to severe or very severe.

Normal ICP	0–15 mm Hg
Mild elevation	16–20 mm Hg
Moderate elevation	21–30 mm Hg
Severe elevation	31–40 mm Hg
Very severe elevation	≥41 mm Hg

Pseudotumor cerebri is also referred as idiopathic intracranial hypertension, which is characterized by increased ICP and absence of space-occupying lesion on brain imaging. This is a diagnosis of exclusion. It is more common in females between the ages of 15 to 44 years. In general population, the prevalence is 0.9–1:100,000 people in general population.

The modified Dandy criteria to diagnose IIH are as follows:

- Awake and alert patient
- Signs and symptoms of increased ICP
- Normal neurological examination and localizing signs except VI cranial nerve palsy
- Normal CSF composition except for increased CSF pressure (> 20 mm Hg in non-obsese patients and >25 mm Hg in obese adults

TABLE 33.1 *Causes of Increased ICP*

Mechanism	Pathology
Generalized brain swelling	Pseudotumor cerebri, ischemia-anoxia states, hypercarbia, acute liver failure, Reye hepatocerebral syndrome, diffuse axonal injury, malignant hypertension
Focal mass effect	Ischemic infarct with cytotoxic edema, tumors with vasogenic edema, infections/abscess, intraparenchymal hemorrhage, epidural or subdural hematoma
Increase in venous pressure	Venous sinus thrombosis, obstruction of superior mediastinal and jugular veins, heart failure
Obstruction to CSF flow and or obstruction	Meningeal disease (infectious or inflammatory/granulomatous, hemorrhagic, or carcinomatous/lymphomatous; Arnold Chiari malformation

- Absence of deformity, displacement, and obstruction of ventricular system
- No other identifiable cause of ICP

Neuroimaging of the brain can possibly show:

- Empty sella
- Flattening of posterior sclera
- Enhancement of prelaminar optic nerves
- Intraocular protrusion of prelaminar optic nerve
- Distension of preoptic subarachnoid space
- Vertical tortuosity of orbital optic nerve

Clinical symptoms of IIH include headache, nausea, vomiting, and transient visual obscurations, blurred or double vision, vision loss, pulsatile tinnitus. Other symptoms include pain in the neck or the back of the eye. Rarely, torticollis, numbness hands and feet, radiating pains to limbs, facial pain and numbness, dizziness, and balance problems can be seen. Various medical illnesses are associated with IIH (refer to Table 33.2).

Spinal tap in IIH has diagnostic and therapeutic value. It checks the high pressure confirming the suspicion of IIH. Clear CSF excludes infectious, inflammatory, and carcinomatous etiologies. It provides therapeutic relief to the patient. CNS infections, malignancy, cerebral venous thrombosis, and pseudopapilledema (anomalous elevation of optic nerve head) should be ruled out. Papilledema is optic disc swelling seen in patients with elevated intracranial pressure. See Figure 33.1 for an example of patient with papilledema. There are four stages of papilledema.

1. Early stage: hyperemic disc with blurring of the disc margin, peripapillary retinal hemorrhages.
2. Advanced stage: Bilaterally swollen, hyperemic discs with flame-like retinal hemorrhages, cotton-wool spots, macular hemorrhage, and exudation.
3. Chronic stage: prominence of disc, cup disappear, and hard exudation.
4. Atrophic stage: pale papilla, gliosis, and narrowing of the retinal vessels.

Benign IIH is a misnomer because it is not so benign. It can cause irreversible visual loss by causing optic atrophy. Treatment includes withdrawal of incrementing agents, if any, and weight reduction by healthy diet, exercise, nutrition consult, or bariatric surgery. Acetazolamide (Diamox), a carbonic anhydrase inhibitor, can be started at 250 mg qid or 500 mg bid and can be increased to 1000 mg qid. Steroids may paradoxically be used in the treatment of IIH. Diuretics such as furosemide are also tried in the treatment of IIH.

TABLE 33.2 *Associations With IIH*

Sex	Females > Males
Obesity	BMI more than 29
Drugs	Tetracycline, hypervitaminosis A, steroids, oral contraceptives, NSAIDs, nalidixic acid, nitrofurantoin, minocycline, tamoxifen, lithium, phenytoin, sulphonamides, Penicillin, Carbidopa, levodopa, danazole, cyclosporine, Indomethacin, steroids therapy or withdrawal, growth hormone
Miscellaneous	Anemia, Chronic kidney disease, pregnancy, menarche, polycystic ovarian syndrome, Cryoglobulinemia
Endocrinopathy	Hypothyroidism, hypoparathyroidism, Addison's disease, Cushing's syndrome, Levothyroxine therapy

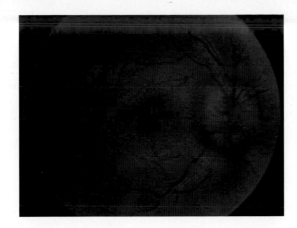

FIGURE 33.1 *Papilledema is characterized by blurring of the optic disc margins, increased congestion, and engorgement of veins.*

Enough fluid should be taken out to decrease the closing pressure to about 15 mm of Hg. Serial LPs are required in these patients.

Surgical measures include:

■ **ONSF**: It is a surgical procedure in which slits are made in the optic nerve sheath to reduce the pressure on the optic nerve. After entering the orbits via a surgical incision in the skin, the eyeball is pushed to one side. The ophthalmologist identifies the optic nerve, and slits are made in the optic nerve sheath to relieve the pressure. Typically, the beneficial effect of ONSF is limited to the ipsilateral optic nerve. In patients with bilateral visual loss, this procedure should be performed in the more affected eye.

■ **Ventriculoperitoneal shunt:** A communicating catheter is inserted that shunts CSF from the ventricles of the brain into the peritoneal cavity via a surgically implanted tube. Bur hole is placed and a catheter is inserted into the ventricle. A U-shaped incision is placed behind the ear, and second catheter is placed under the skin behind the ear and moved down the neck and chest, and into the peritoneal cavity. A valve (fluid pump) is placed underneath the skin behind the ear that is attached to both catheters. The valve opens up whenever excess fluid drains out of it into the peritoneum. Complications of shunt such as infections, shunt obstruction, or overdrainage require shunt revisions.

SUGGESTED READING

Bienfang, D. Overview and differential diagnosis of papilledema. Up-to-date. 8/2007.

Brodsky, MC, Vaphiades, M. Magnetic resonance imaging in pseudotumor cerebri. *Ophthalmology.* 1998;105:1686.

Chapman and Fishman. Idiopathic intracranial hypertension (pseudotumor cerebri) in children. Up-to-date. 8/2007.

Friedman DI. Pseudotumor cerebri. *Neurosurg Clin N. America.* 1999;10: 609–621.

Gordon, K. Pediatric pseudotumor cerebri: Descriptive epidemiology. *Can J Neurol Sci.* 1997;24:219.

Kupersmith MJ et al. Effects of weight loss on the course of idiopathic intracranial hypertension in women. *Neurology.* 1998;50:1094.

Pseudotumor cerebri. MedlinePlus.

Radhakrishnan K et al. Idiopathic intracranial hypertension. *Mayo Clinic Proceeding.* 1994;69:169.

Soler D et al. Diagnosis and management of benign intracranial hypertension. *Arch Dis Child.* 1998;78:89.

Wall M. Idiopathic intracranial hypertension. *Neurol Clin.* 1991;9:73.

Slurred Speech and Balance Problems

Shahzad Raza, Jerome J Graber, and Anuradha Singh

CHIEF COMPLAINT: **Speech is not clear and balance is not good.**

HISTORY OF PRESENT ILLNESS

A 51-year-old, right-handed male presented with progressive walking problems and slurring of speech. Speech problems started 6 months ago. Around the same time, he noticed mild headaches in his temples. He denied any nausea or vomiting with the headaches. He had never suffered from headaches during adolescence. He reported several falls in the past 2 to 3 months. The frequency of falls had increased in the past 3 months from 1 to 2 times per week to 4 to 6 times a day. He could no longer hold objects with his right hand for the past 2 months. He denied any loss of sensations. However, he complained of occasional mild fever in the evening for the past month. He denied any cough, chest pain, dizziness, memory changes, seizures or headaches, or visual disturbances.

PAST MEDICAL HISTORY

Diagnosed with hyperlipidemia 5 years ago.

PAST SURGICAL HISTORY

Appendectomy at the age of 20.

MEDICATIONS

Simvastatin 10 mg once daily.

ALLERGIES

NKDA.

PERSONAL HISTORY

Nonsmoker, social alcohol use, no illicit drugs.

FAMILY HISTORY

No family history of cancer.

PHYSICAL EXAMINATION

General: Middle-aged man in no apparent distress.
Vitals: Pulse, 82/min; temperature, 98.2°F; blood pressure, 140/87mm Hg; respiratory rate, 6/min; no postural hypotension.
HEENT: Normocephalic and atraumatic. No alopecia or dermatitis. Oropharynx clear. Neck supple. No palpable cervical or supraclavicular lymphadenopathy.
Pulmonary: Clear to auscultation bilaterally.
Cardiovascular: Regular rate and rhythm, S1 and S2 normal.
Abdomen: Soft, nontender, and nondistended.
Musculoskeletal: decreased strength lower extremities.
Skin: No clubbing, cyanosis, redness, rash, or edema.
Peripheral pulses: Normal.

NEUROLOGICAL EXAMINATION

Mental status: Awake, oriented to time, place and person but uncooperative. His memory of current and past events was intact. However, patient had apraxia, micrographia, and mild anomia. His comprehension was good. The affect was flat.

CNs II–XII: Unremarkable. Normal fundi without papilledema.

Motor: No signs of atrophy, normal tone in muscles. Patient had right pronator drift. Strength 4/5 in upper and lower extremities (poor effort) except right upper extremity distal strength was 3/5. Difficulty with gripping and holding pencil.

Sensory: Light touch, pain, temperature, vibration, proprioception, and cortical sensations normal.

Reflexes: Right hyperreflexia (3+) compared to the right (2+); no Hoffman's, no clonus.

Plantars: Flexors bilaterally.

Coordination: Mild bilateral dysmetria, left more than right.

Romberg's sign: Negative.

Gait: Could not tandem walk but otherwise normal.

STOP AND THINK QUESTIONS

➤ How will you work up this patient who has focal neurological deficits and a history of intermittent fevers at night?

➤ Which diagnoses are unlikely considering the progressive nature of his symptoms?

DIAGNOSTIC TEST RESULTS

MRI brain with or without gadolinium (Figure 34.1) demonstrates a large mass measuring 4 × 2 cm involving the deep periventricular white matter of the left frontal lobe, which extends via the body of the corpus callosum to the periventricular white matter of the right frontal lobe, anteriorly at the level of the genu of the corpus callosum and posteriorly to the splenium of the corpus callosum (A). There is also an abnormal patchy area of increased T2/FLAIR signal involving the left middle cerebellar peduncle (B). The lesion showed Gd-enhancement bilaterally as evident in the axial T1W (C). Sagittal T1W post gad images (D and E) show left-sided lesion showing Gd-enhancement and surrounding vasogenic edema.

Pathology (refer to Figure 34.2): H&E stains under magnifications 20× (A) and 40× (B) depict population of lymphocytes with basophilic nuclei and prominent nucleoli. Special immunostains using B-cell marker CD20 (C) and T-cell marker CD3 (D) reveal positivity to CD20 antigen and CD3 antigen respectively. The majority of tumor cells stain positive for CD20, a marker expressed on most B cells. Rituximab is a cytolytic monoclonal antibody against CD20 used in lymphoma. Note that CD3 immunostain highlights reactive, smaller T cells that are usually present in a B-cell lymphoma.

DIAGNOSIS: Primary CNS Lymphoma (HIV negative).

DISCUSSION

PCNSL used to be a rare form of extranodal, high-grade, non-Hodgkin's lymphomas that are confined to the brain or spinal cord at presentation. It accounts for approximately 1% of non-Hodgkin's lymphomas. Majority of these (~80%) are diffuse large B-cell lymphomas. T-cell PCNSL presents in a younger age group than B-cell PCNSL and is rare. Other rare CNS angiotropic lymphomas fill the lumina of small cerebral vessels and tend to cause vascular occlusion and hemorrhagic infarcts.

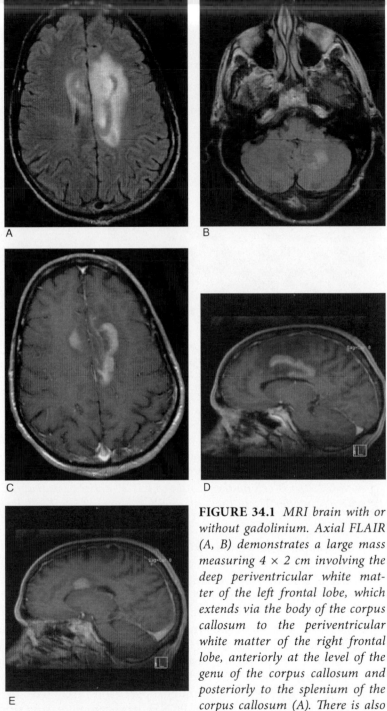

FIGURE 34.1 *MRI brain with or without gadolinium. Axial FLAIR (A, B) demonstrates a large mass measuring 4 × 2 cm involving the deep periventricular white matter of the left frontal lobe, which extends via the body of the corpus callosum to the periventricular white matter of the right frontal lobe, anteriorly at the level of the genu of the corpus callosum and posteriorly to the splenium of the corpus callosum (A). There is also an abnormal patchy area of increased T2/FLAIR signal involving the left middle cerebellar peduncle (B). The lesion showed Gd-enhancement bilaterally as evident in the axial T1W (C). Sagittal T1W post-gad images (D, E) show left-sided lesion showing Gd-enhancement and surrounding vasogenic edema.*

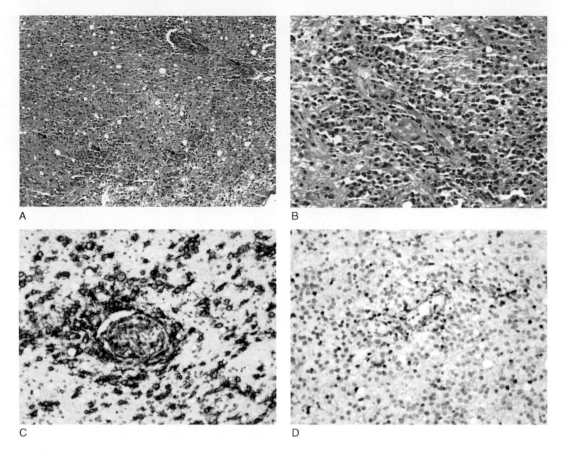

FIGURE 34.2 *Microscopic sections of primary CNS lymphoma. H&E 20x (A) and 40x (B) shows numerous round blue lymphoid cells invading the brain parenchyma in an angiocentric pattern clustering around blood vessels (see blcak arrows in A). Special immunostains (40x magnification) with CD20, a B-cell marker (C) shows CD 20 antigen positivity; CD3, a T-cell marker highlights reactive, smaller T cells that are usually also present in a B-cell lymphoma (D).*

In comparison, secondary CNS lymphomas metastasize to the CNS from a primary site outside the nervous system. Secondary immunodeficiency states such as HIV infection or use of immunosuppressants after organ transplantation or Hodgkin's disease are main conditions associated with PCNSL. Rare primary immunodeficiency states such as ataxia telangiectasia and severe combined immunodeficiency syndromes can be associated with PCNSL. EBV is implicated in the pathogenesis of all immunocompromised patients. It is caused by deficient control of EBV with immortalization of EBV-infected B cells. EBV DNA can be detected in the neoplastic tissue obtained by brain biopsy. Polymerase chain reaction can be performed on CSF to detect EBV DNA, though false positive CSF results can occur. PCNSL patients without immunosuppression rarely have evidence of EBV in the tumor cells or CSF. The incidence of PCNSL has been increasing since the 1980s, partially due to an increased prevalence of HIV and transplant survivors, but also in immunocompetent individuals for unknown reasons. A sharp decrease in the incidence of PCNSL in people with HIV has been noted since the introduction of more effective antiretroviral therapy in 1995. The peak incidence in immunocompetent patients is in the fifth to seventh decades of life with a 3:2 to 2:1 male/female ratio. In comparison, immunocompromised patients are frequently diagnosed in the third and fourth decades, and nearly all are males. The life-time risk of PCNSL in patients with solid organ transplant (kidney, heart) approaches 3%.

PCNSLs are most commonly occur in the supratentorial regions and favor periventricular regions of the brain, but can also occur in the cerebellum, brain stem, and spinal cord. Intraocular lymphoma is a type of PCNSL that occurs only in the eye, but has a high rate of eventual diffuse CNS relapse. CNS lymphomas tend to infiltrate extensively along the corpus callosum and other deep white matter tracts. They frequently traverse the ependyma to involve the ventricular surface or spread peripherally into the overlying leptomeninges. Meningeal involvement with invasion of the subarachnoid space is common in PCNSL. Histologic examination shows perivascular cuffing and sheets of lymphoid tumor cells infiltrating the brain tissue with expansion of the Virchow-Robin spaces.

The most typical presentation of PCNSL in an immunocompetent patient is progressive focal symptoms indicative of a mass lesion. Seizures or changed mental status may be some other presenting symptoms. Patients with AIDS are more likely to present with an encephalopathy. This correlates with the more often multifocal, diffuse enhancement pattern seen on MRI of the brain. A history of concurrent infections is quite common, and the median CD4+ count is 20/mm^3. The risk factors for PCNSL in immunocompetent patients are not very clear. Nature, intensity, and duration of immune suppression are factors in determining the risk of developing PCNSL. Differential diagnosis of a patient with suspected PCNSL depends on the patient's immune status and radiographic appearance of the lesions. More diffuse cognitive and MRI abnormalities suggest the possibility of some infectious encephalitides caused by toxoplasmosis, herpes zoster, cytomegalovirus, cryptococcal, or AIDS/dementia complex.

MRI of the brain shows a hypointense lesion or lesions on long TR-weighted images, which enhance densely and homogeneously after gadolinium administration. Multifocal lesions are present at the time of diagnosis in 25% to 50% of immunocompetent patients and in 60% to 80% of AIDS patients. Lesions are multifocal in 50% of patients with AIDS. Hemorrhage is not an uncommon presentation due to the angioinvasive nature of the tumor. MRI also gives information about leptomeningeal enhancement, hydrocephalus, and concurrent alternative diagnoses, such as other infections in patients with AIDS such as toxoplasmis or fungal infections. Thallium 201 SPECT scanning is appropriate in patients with AIDS to help distinguish between infectious processes and PCNSL.

CSF cytologic examination and an ophthalmologic evaluation that includes a slit-lamp examination should always be obtained, since definitive diagnosis can be made if tumor cells are found in the CSF or vitreous, sparing the need for more invasive brain biopsy. Even when the diagnosis is already established, these tests are necessary to establish the extent of disease as this can have prognostic and therapeutic implications. In some cases, specialized testing of CSF for monoclonal gene rearrangements in immunoglobulin chains or monoclonal populations of CD20-expressing B cells by FACS or flow cytometry may help elicit the diagnosis. A spinal MRI should be obtained in all patients to assess for the presence of leptomeningeal disease, since these patients may need placement of an Ommaya reservoir for intrathecal chemotherapy, though this is controversial. Chest and abdominal CT scans with contrast should be obtained because a minority of patients will be found to have an extraneural source for their cerebral lymphoma. Whole body PET scanning has a higher yield. Abdominal (especially retroperitoneal), breast, sinus, and testes are systemic lymphoma sites with a higher predilection for CNS metastases. Bone marrow biopsy is also indicated in all patients prior to treatment. Patients with evidence of both systemic and CNS lymphoma will require dual therapy for optimal treatment of both sites of disease, since CNS penetration of systemic lymphoma chemotherapy regimens is poor. Since the disease diffusely infiltrates brain tissue beyond what is visible on MRI, craniotomy and debulking of lesions have been proven to have no role in PCNSL and only introduce the risk of causing greater complications. Stereotactic brain biopsy may be necessary in those patients who have lesions located in areas of the brain that are difficult to access (e.g., brain stem). Steroids cause rapid lysis of lymphoma cells and may produce a nondiagnostic specimen, so they should be avoided prior to diagnostic procedures except in cases of life-threatening edema.

More than 80% of PCNSLs are densely cellular, aggressive non-Hodgkin's B-cell lymphoma. Macroscopically, these can be well demarcated despite their infiltrative nature. Infiltration to the meninges and subependymal layer may be evident. Immunocompetent patients usually have a small, noncleaved cell or immunoblastic subtype. Microscopic examination shows perivascular sheets of lymphoma cells separated by areas of necrosis. Perivascular distribution of lymphocytes may be evident in other encephalitides but vascular invasion shown by lymphomas can help distinguish it from other pathological processes. Polymorphous cells are seen most commonly, some of which resemble centroblasts and centrocytes. Cells have prominent nuclei with single or multiple nucleoli, many apoptotic bodies. EBV virus can be revealed by immunohistochemistry or in-situ hybridization. Small-cell PCNSLs are more infiltrative but produce less necrosis compared to large-cell PCNSLs. B-cell lymphomas can be differentiated from T-cell lymphomas by using antibodies to the following antigens:

- CD20 and CD79a (B-cell marker)
- CD3 and CD45Ro (T-cell marker)

TREATMENT

The goal of treatment is eradication of both contrast-enhancing mass lesions and microscopic infiltration of brain, spine, leptomeninges, and vitreous. Successful therapy in immunocompetent patients leads to a median survival duration as long as 44 months. Treatment must be designed to maximize efficacy and minimize toxicity to cerebral white matter.

SURGERY

The role of surgery is to establish a tissue diagnosis, and this is best obtained by stereotactic biopsy which is the most appropriate method for diagnosis of PCNSL Because of the multifocal nature of this tumor, extensive resections have been proved to produce no survival benefit and increase the risk of postoperative deficits. When PCNSL is suspected and biopsy is considered necessary, surgeons and pathologists should be alerted to diagnostic consideration of PCNSL so that steroids can be avoided and surgical planning for stereotactic biopsy with intraoperative pathologic consultation can be obtained.

RADIATION

Historically, whole-brain irradiation with corticosteroids had remained the standard treatment for primary CNS lymphoma. Radiation frequently produces response, but there is high rate of disease relapse within 6 to 12 months after radiation when used as monotherapy. Focal radiation is not indicated for PCNSL due to the multicentric and infiltrating nature of the disease. With higher long-term responses obtained with the combination of radiation and high-dose methotrexate chemotherapy, there has been a greater appreciation of the incidence of radiation-induced leukoencephalopathy, which occurs in up to 90% of patients over the age of 60. Radiation leukoencephalopathy occurs due to damage to blood vessels, oligodendrocytes, and CNS stem cells after ionizing radiation, and manifests months to years after radiation as progressive memory loss, dementia, gate imbalance, and urinary incontinence, sometimes mimicking normal pressure hydrocephalus with diffuse T2/FLAIR white matter changes on MRI. Given that long-term survival is possible and even expected in individuals under 60 with good performance status, trials have been exploring the possibility of using lower dose radiation or even eliminating it altogether by using combination chemotherapy regimens.

CHEMOTHERAPY

Methotrexate-based chemotherapy regimens have been the most successful treatment strategies to date. Methotrexate is a folate analogue that interferes with DNA synthesis and repair. For treatment of PCNSL, patients receive high-dose systemic methotrexate at doses greater than 3 mg/m² to penetrate the blood brain barrier. Close monitoring and adjustment of intravenous fluids and leucovorin rescue necessitate inpatient administration of this drug, which can produce serious toxicity, including renal failure, infections, thrombosis, and bone marrow suppression. Therefore, patients should be referred to centers familiar with treating PCNSL whenever possible, especially if clinical trials are available. Other chemotherapies include lomustine, procarbazine, cytarabine, vincristine, and rituximab, a monoclonal antibody against CD20, a surface antigen expressed on most B-cell lymphomas. A phase II randomized study showed that the addition of high-dose cytarabine for 2 months in patients who responded to methotrexate was more effective than methotrexate alone in maintaining long-term freedom from relapse.

Historically, survival times from the onset of symptoms to death with no treatment or surgical resection alone ranged from 0.9 to 4.6 months. The median survival for whole brain radiotherapy alone varies from 12 to 18 months, and only 3 to 4% of patients survive for 5 years.

Combination chemotherapy and radiation therapy more than doubled survival time but such success was achieved at the price of a greater than 50% incidence of dementia in those who survived more than 18 months on these regimens.

Median survival times for treatment programs that include high-dose methotrexate-based chemotherapy range from 33 to 42 months. Age less than 60 and good KPS are favorable prognostic indicators. Prophylactic use of antiepileptic drugs should be avoided and their use should be confined to perioperative use and the minority of PCNSL patients who experience seizures.

In immunosuppressed patients, restoration of immune function when possible can produce responses by itself or in combination with chemotherapy. In patients with HIV, antiretroviral therapy should be initiated immediately. Reducing immunosuppression in transplant patients is a more complex decision, but in some cases, loss of the donor organ (i.e., resuming dialysis should a donated kidney be rejected) should be weighed against the risk of death from PCNSL if chemotherapy is ineffective.

SUGGESTED READING

Abrey LE, DeAngelis LM, Yahalom J. Long-term survival in primary CNS lymphoma. *J Clin Oncol.* 1998;16:859–863.

Buhring U, Herrlinger U, Krings T. MRI features of primary central nervous system lymphomas at presentation. *Neurology.* 2001;57:393–396.

Graber J, Omuro A. Pharmacotherapy in primary CNS lymphoma: Progress beyond methotrexate? *CNS Drugs.* 2011;25:447–457.

Subacute Onset of Balance Problems

Anuradha Singh and Shahzad Raza

CHIEF COMPLAINT: **I do not know why I am falling so often.**

HISTORY OF PRESENT ILLNESS

A 62-year-old, right-handed female presented with unsteadiness and difficulty maintaining her balance for the last 4 months. Her symptoms had a gradual onset. Her husband had witnessed few falls. She tends to fall on her left side. She does not lose consciousness during the falls. In the past month, she has been falling 3 to 4 times a day. She denied any preceding symptoms before the fall. She did not complain about confusion or disorientation after the falls. She did not give any history of dizziness, vertigo, headache, or seizures. She denied any history of fever, bowel and bladder dysfunction, or visual and hearing problems. She had similar complaints 5 years ago and saw a neurologist. Her work-up revealed a brain tumor.

PAST MEDICAL HISTORY

Uterine fibroids, osteoporosis and benign "brain tumor."

PAST SURGICAL HISTORY

Craniotomy in 2003, myomectomy in 1990, tonsillectomy in 1977.

MEDICATIONS

Keppra 500 mg for seizure prophylaxis.

ALLERGIES

Betadine.

PERSONAL HISTORY

Nonsmoker, social alcohol use, no drugs.

FAMILY HISTORY

No family history of cancer.

PHYSICAL EXAMINATION

General physical examination: A very pleasant Caucasian female, well developed, well nourished in no apparent distress.
Vitals: Pulse, 76; temperature, 97°F; respiratory rate, 14; blood pressure, 130/78 mm Hg. No postural hypotension.
HEENT: Normocephaic and atraumatic. No alopecia or dermatitis. Oropharynx clear. Neck is supple. No palpable cervical or supraclavicular lymohadenopathy.
Pulmonary: Clear to auscultation bilaterally.
Cardiovascular: Regular rate and rhythm, S1 and S2 normal.
Abdomen: Soft, nontender, and nondistended. Gentilia normal.
Musculoskeletal: Normal bulk, no joint tenderness.
Skin: No clubbing, cyanosis, redness, rash, or edema.
Peripheral pulses: Normal.

NEUROLOGICAL EXAMINATION

Mental status: Alert, awake, oriented to time, place, and person. Affect was normal. She had good knowledge of current events. Her judgment, abstract thinking, calculation, and praxis were normal. She could recall only two items out of three.

CNs II–XII: Was significant for visual field defect in the left inferolateral quadrant.

Motor: No sign of atrophy, normal tone. Strength 5/5, No pronator drift.

Sensory: Patchy altered light touch and pin prick on the left side, arm more than leg.

Reflex: Biceps (2+) brachio (2+), triceps (2+), patellar (2+), Achilles (2+).

Plantars: Flexors.

No Hoffman's or ankle clonus.

Coordination: Coordination was normal.

Gait: Could not tandem.

Romberg: Negative.

STOP AND THINK QUESTIONS

➢ Why is this patient falling so often?

➢ Would you worry about brain tumor recurrence?

➢ What are the benign brain tumors of the CNS that can have recurrence?

➢ What is the significance of inferior quadrantonopia and decreased sensations on the left side of the body?

DIAGNOSTIC TEST RESULTS

MRI brain (Figure 35.1) showed a 6.6 cm extra axial homogenously enhancing mass on T1c, arising from the right posterior falx, which exerts significant mass effect upon the right parietal, temporal, and occipital lobes, associated with parenchymal T2/FLAIR signal abnormality and moderate right-to-left midline shift and midbrain compression.

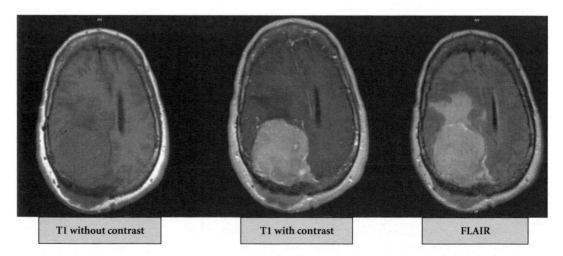

| T1 without contrast | T1 with contrast | FLAIR |

FIGURE 35.1 *Preoperative MRI brain. Axial images showing 6.6 cm extra axial enhancing mass arising from the right posterior falx with significant mass effect upon the right parietal, temporal, and occipital lobes. The mass is associated with sucal effacement, vasogenic edema, and moderate right-to-left midline shift.*

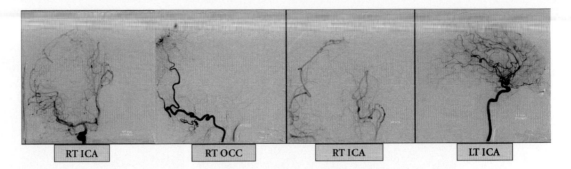

RT ICA RT OCC RT ICA LT ICA

FIGURE 35.2 *Preoperative cerebral artery angiogram. Large right parietal occipital parasagittal meningioma with significant mass effect and displacement of multiple branches of the anterior cerebral arteries and the right posterior cerebral artery, and deep venous structures. There is occlusion of the leptomeningeal branches of right anterior cerebral, right middle cerebral, right occipital arteries.*

Carotid angiogram (Figure 35.2) showed large right parietal occipital mass with significant mass effect and displacement of multiple branches of the anterior cerebral arteries and the right posterior cerebral artery, and deep venous structures. There is an occlusion of leptomeningeal branches of right anterior cerebral, right middle cerebral, and right occipital arteries. Venous phase images disclosed a leftward shift of the internal cerebral vein and a complete occlusion of the superior sagittal sinus throughout its parietal and occipital segments. The straight sinus is displaced leftward and partially compressed. Additional venous outflow from the left hemisphere was directed toward a large extracranial parietal vein via posterior frontal emissary channels.

HISTOPATHOLOGY (FIGURE 35.3, A–E)

Microscopic section showed hypercellular proliferation of intermediate sized cells with a vesicular chromatin pattern, small prominent nucleoli, and nuclear pseudoinclusions. The tumor cells were arranged in sheets with areas of prominent whorling pattern. Psammoma bodies and focal areas of pseudopapillary growth were seen admixed with multiple foci of tumor necrosis. Thick collagen bundles were interspersed between the tumor cells. Tumor cells invaded the brain parenchyma. Specimen showed PR positivity and MIB-1/Ki-67 immunostaining showed 8% proliferation index.

DIAGNOSIS: Recurrent atypical meningioma.

DISCUSSION

Meningiomas are usually benign tumors attached to the dura that account for 15% of intracranial primary brain tumors. They are the most common extra-axial tumors in the brain that originate from the mesodermal or meningeal layers. The most common locations of origin include:

- Parasagittal
- Sylvian fissure
- Sphenoid wing
- Spinal cord
- Olfactory groove
- Tuberculum sellae
- Occipital region

Meningiomas are at least 2 times more common in women than men between the ages of 40 and 70. The tumors have been found to have estrogen, progesterone, and androgen

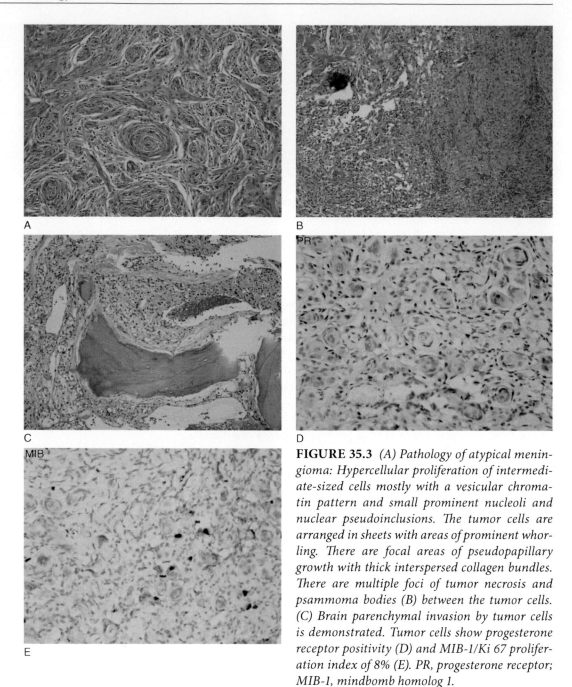

FIGURE 35.3 *(A) Pathology of atypical meningioma: Hypercellular proliferation of intermediate-sized cells mostly with a vesicular chromatin pattern and small prominent nucleoli and nuclear pseudoinclusions. The tumor cells are arranged in sheets with areas of prominent whorling. There are focal areas of pseudopapillary growth with thick interspersed collagen bundles. There are multiple foci of tumor necrosis and psammoma bodies (B) between the tumor cells. (C) Brain parenchymal invasion by tumor cells is demonstrated. Tumor cells show progesterone receptor positivity (D) and MIB-1/Ki 67 proliferation index of 8% (E). PR, progesterone receptor; MIB-1, mindbomb homolog 1.*

receptors in some cases. They can occur anywhere along the neuraxis, including intracranial, spinal, intraventricular, and extracranial sites. The established risk factors of meningioma include NF2 gene deletion on chromosome 22q, ionizing radiation, head injury, and hormonal receptors. The latency of developing meningiomas may be inversely related to the dose of radiation. Other etiologies include head trauma, viruses, and other genetic factors. At present, there is no convincing evidence to show association with the use of cell phones.

Meningiomas are extremely slowly growing tumors that may go unrecognized for years. Small tumors less than 2.0 cm are usually asymptomatic and are incidental findings at autopsy. Larger tumors can cause myriad of symptoms such as focal seizures, personality changes, memory loss, visual or hearing disturbances, anosmia, progressive spastic weakness in legs and incontinence, headaches, motor, sensory, or language disturbances, depending on the size and location (see Table 35.1). Increased intracranial pressure may occur, but is definitely less frequent than in gliomas. Our patient had left inferior quarantonopia and left sensory findings that indicate the possibility of right parietal lesion.

Plain skull radiograph may reveal hyperostosis and increased vascular markings of the skull, as well as intracranial calcifications. On noncontrast head CT scans, meningiomas are usually dural-based tumors that are isodense to slightly hyperdense. They enhance homogeneously and intensely after the injection of iodinated contrast material. On MRI, the tumor is typically iso- or hypointense on noncontrast T1WI, and iso- or hyperintense on T2WI. An enhancing tail involving the dura may be apparent. This is called "dural tail sign." There can be various variants of meningiomas. Although MRA and MRV have widely replaced the conventional angiography, the latter remains a powerful tool for planning surgery and sometimes providing useful information about the location of feeding arteries, draining veins, and degrees of tumor vascularity.

Atypical meningiomas account for between 4.7% and 7.2% of all meningiomas and represent an intermediate category of tumor that has a higher risk for relapse. Mortality and morbidity rates for meningiomas are difficult to assess. They may cause symptoms by irritating the underlying cortex, compressing the brain or the cranial nerves, producing hyperostosis and/or invading the overlying soft tissues, or inducing vascular injuries to the brain. They may cause seizures, headaches, stereotyped symptoms, and sometime hormonal imbalances. The WHO has recognized various variants of meningiomas as listed in Table 35.2. There is lot of overlap of pathology, and a clear distinction is not always easy.

TABLE 35.1 *Common Locations of Meningiomas and Their Symptoms*

Location of Meningioma	Symptoms
Convexity	~ 20% of meningiomas, asymptomatic but may exert symptoms depending on their location
Falcine and parasagittal	Contralateral leg weakness, bladder symptoms
Olfactory groove and planum sphenoidale	~10% of meningiomas, may cause anosmia and vision problems; Foster Kennedy syndrome (anosmia, ipsilateral optic atrophy and contralateral papilledema
Intraventricular	Headaches, nausea, vomiting if large enough to cause obstructive hydrocepahalus
Sphenoid wing	~ 20% of meningiomas, tumors growing in the inner wing (clinoidal) cause direct damage to the optic nerve (cecocentral scotoma, decreased visual acuity, afferent pupillary defect, progressive loss of color vision), proptosis and cavernous sinus syndrome if large enough

Posterior fossa
  Clival (medial origin)
  Petroclival (origin at the petrous tip medial to the V nerve)
  Sphenopetroclival (origin at Meckel's cave)
  Cerebellopontine angle
  Foramen magnum
	Symptoms vary based on their location:
	Cranial nerve deficits, facial hypesthesia, occipital headaches, upper cervical pain, unique progressive pattern of motor weakness with foramen magnum tumors (*unilateral arm sensory and motor deficits that progress to ipsilateral leg and then contralateral leg and finally contralateral arm,* sensory loss around C2 dermatome) and cranial nerve deficits with large tumors, ataxia, nystagmus

Suprasellar	Visual problems and pituitary dysfunction

TABLE 35.2 *WHO Classification of Meningiomas*

Meningothelial
Fibrous
Angiomatous
Transitional
Psammomatous
Microcystic
Secretory
Clear cell
Chordoid
Lymphoplasmacyte-rich
Metaplastic
Atypical meningioma (grade II)
Papillary meningioma (grade III)
Rhabdoid meningioma (grade III)
Anaplastic meningioma (grade III)

Atypical meningioma as defined by WHO criteria is a prognostically heterogeneous group with most patients living a long time (some of whom eventually fall victim to malignant transformation) and others surviving only a few years (5-year survival is 57%). Reports in the literature indicate that routine evaluation of proliferative potential and the cytogenetic pattern of resected tumors will eventually help to determine with more accuracy the prognosis for atypical meningiomas. Mayo clinic grading system emphasizes on three features:

- A patternless architecture or sheeting
- Prominent nucleoli
- Formation of small cells

The mitotic figures ≥ 4/10 high power field is considered one of the criteria for atypical meningioma. Brain invasion suggests more aggressive features and carries more malignant potential and high chance of recurrence. More than 75% of meningiomas express PRs. PR negativity carries a poorer prognosis. A combination of PR status and proliferation indices has been shown to predict recurrence reliably. Extracranial metastases can be present in only 5% of the cases.

As per WHO classification, atypical meningiomas are classified as grade II tumors. Histological features include increase in mitotic rate, high cellularity, sheeting of tumor cells with loss of typical histological pattern, prominent nucleoli, focal necrosis, and tumor invasion into cortex or bone. An accurate interpretation of the atypical meningioma is essential since these tumors are likely to recur much earlier than benign variants. Grade III anaplastic meningiomas are considered to have more malignant features than atypical meningiomas and abundant necrosis.

TREATMENT

Small benign meningiomas may be totally asymptomatic and require nothing more than observation. Total/partial surgical resection should be considered in large tumors causing symptoms and neurological deficits. Use of corticosteroids preoperatively and postoperatively has reduced the morbidity and mortality of these tumors. The prophylactic use of antiepileptics is recommended in supratentorial tumors. Levetiracetam (Keppra) is the most favored antiepileptic because it has no drug-to-drug interactions and one does not need to worry about the interactions with the corticosteroids or chemotherapeutic agents. Tegretol and Trileptal are other good choices for partial epilepsy, but these agents do induce cytochrome P-450 system. The chemotherapeutic agents such as Temodar, Hydroxyurea, and Interferon-alpha have not shown promising results. The recurrent atypical meningiomas are difficult to treat successfully. The recurrence rate of atypical meningioma, within 2 years, is 38% as compared to 9.3% for benign meningioma.

At the time of recurrence, radiation therapy with or without surgical resection is appropriate. However, radiation therapy can be given as primary treatment in some cases (optic nerve meningiomas and some unresectable tumors). Stereotactic radiosurgery has been shown to provide excellent local tumor control with minimal toxicity if tumor is small (<3 cm in diameter) residual or recurrent lesions when surgery is considered to carry a significantly high risk of morbidity such as meningiomas near the skull base and cavernous sinus.

SUGGESTED READING

Bruna J, Brell M, Ferrer I, Gimenez-Bonafe P, Tortosa A. Ki-67 proliferative index predicts clinical outcome in patients with atypical or anaplastic meningioma. *Neuropathology.* 2007;27:114–120.

Drummond KJ, Zhu JJ, Black PM. Meningiomas: Updating basic science, management, and outcome. *Neurologist.* 2004;10(3):113–130.

Kleihues P, Cavenee WK. *WHO Classification Tumours of the Central Nervous System.* Lyons, France: IACR; 2000:176–184.

Louis DN, Budka H, Von Deimling A, Meningiomas. Kleihues P, Cavenee WK. *World Health Organization Classification of Tumours. Pathology and Genetics of Tumours of the Nervous System.* Lyon, France: IARC Press; 1993:134–141.

Louis DN, Ohgaki H, Wiestler OD, Cavenee WK, Burger PC. The 2007 WHO classification of tumors of the central nervous system. *Acta Neuropathol.* 2007;114(5):547.

Petscavage JM, Fink JR, Chew FS. Cerebellopontine angle meningioma presenting with hearing loss. *Radiology Case Reports.* 2010;5:2.

Roser F, Nakamura M, Bellinzona M. The prognostic value of progesterone receptor status in meningiomas. *J Clin Pathol.* 2004;57:1033–1037. doi:10.1136/jcp.2004.018333.

Acute Onset of Double Vision

David Schick

CHIEF COMPLAINT: **I am seeing two of everything.**

HISTORY OF PRESENT ILLNESS

A 54-year-old, right-handed male with a history of uncontrolled diabetes and hypertension presented with acute-onset double vision upon awakening in the morning. He noticed that his double vision got worse on looking toward the right side; the two images were seen side by side. The double vision resolved when he tried to close either eye. He did not complain of any loss of vision. Patient denied any pain or redness in the eyes, headache, nausea, vomiting, fever, neck pain, or spinning sensation. Patient did not experience any weakness, loss of sensations, swallowing, or speech problems. There was no preceding head trauma or trauma to the eye. He was not diagnosed with any thyroid problems. He denied any swallowing or speech difficulties. He had no previous history of TIA/stroke.

PAST MEDICAL HISTORY

Diabetes mellitus type II (poorly controlled), hypertension (poorly controlled), lumbar disc herniation.

PAST SURGICAL HISTORY

L4 to L5 laminectomy.

MEDICATIONS

Lisinopril 5 mg PO once daily, Metformin 500 mg PO twice daily.

ALLERGIES

NKDA.

PERSONAL HISTORY

Born and raised in South India, but now lives in New York City; a construction worker. Denied smoking, alcohol, and drug use.

FAMILY HISTORY

Noncontributory.

PHYSICAL EXAMINATION

Overweight male in no acute distress.
Vital signs: Blood pressure, 164/102 mm Hg; pulse, 77/min, regular; respiratory rate, 18/min; afebrile.
HEENT: No Proptosis. No pharyngeal erythema or exudates. No sinus tenderness.
Neck: Supple, no carotid bruits, no lymphadenopathy, and thyroid not palpable.
Chest, CVS, abdomen, skin, and extremities: Normal.

NEUROLOGICAL EXAMINATION

Mental status: A&Ox 3, pleasant and cooperative, appropriately interactive with normal affect. Speech fluent with comprehension, repetition, and naming intact.

CNS

CN I: Not tested.

CN II: Pupils equal, round, and reactive to light. Visual acuity 20/50 bilaterally with glasses, visual fields intact, fundi normal. No afferent pupillary defect.

CN III, IV, and VI: Full conjugate left lateral gaze. On right lateral gaze, the patient's left eye cannot adduct past the midline; the right eye can fully abduct but there is mild nystagmus. Superior and inferior gaze were intact. No ptosis.

CN V: Sensation intact to LT/PP in V1 to V3 bilaterally. Masseters strong bilaterally.

CN VII: No facial asymmetry. Nasolabial folds equal bilaterally.

CN VIII: Hearing intact to finger rub and whispering bilaterally.

CN IX, X: Voice normal, palate elevation symmetrical, uvula midline.

CN XI: SCM and trapezii full strength bilaterally.

CN XII: Tongue protrusion midline, no atrophy or fasciculations.

Motor: Normal bulk and tone; no tremor, rigidity, or bradykinesia. No pronator drift. Strength 5/5 in all muscle groups, proximally and distally. Finger tapping intact.

Sensory: Decreased sensation to pin prick, temperature, vibration, and proprioception in the feet up to the midcalves bilaterally. The sensory findings were symmetric.

Reflexes: 2+ in the LUE, 3+ in the RUE except 4+ in the right brachioradialis. No Hoffman's; 2+ in bilateral lower extremities.

Plantars: Flexors.

Cerebellar: RAM, FNF, and HKS intact bilaterally.

Gait: Posture, stance, stride, and arm swing normal. No ataxia.

DIAGNOSTIC TEST RESULTS

HbA1c: 8.7; Total cholesterol: 279, LDL: 193.

MRI brain: Small punctuate focus of restricted diffusion and faintly bright T2/FLAIR hyperintensity in the periaqueductal gray centered to the left (see Figure 36.1), consistent with an acute infarction in the midbrain.

DIAGNOSIS: Internuclear ophthalmoplegia (INO).

DISCUSSION

The differential diagnosis of diplopia is fairly broad. It is important to make a distinction whether the diplopia is binocular or monocular. Binocular diplopia is present only if both eyes are open whereas monocular diplopia is present when one eye is covered. Monocular diplopia is always caused by an ophthalmological problem (caused by a distortion of light transmission to the retina) whereas binocular diplopia is usually caused by a neurological problem, most likely an ophthalmoplegia causing disconjugate alignment of the eyes.

Binocular diplopia can result from damage anywhere from the orbit itself to visual cortices. The orbit itself can be affected causing mechanical restriction of eye movements (as in trauma, Graves ophthalmopathy, and orbital tumor/pseudotumor). The extraocular muscles can themselves be affected in isolation, as in chronic progressive external ophthalmoplegia and Kearns–Sayre syndrome. Ophthalmoplegia can also result from diseases of the neuromuscular junction (as in myasthenia gravis). Damage to cranial nerves III, IV, or VI anywhere along their course is the most common cause of ophthalmopegia. Finally, it can also result from lesions in the brain stem or cortex. The white matter tracts in the brain stem are affected in internuclear ophthalmoplegia, and supranuclear structures are affected in progressive supranuclear palsy. Very rarely, lesions of the parietal cortex can

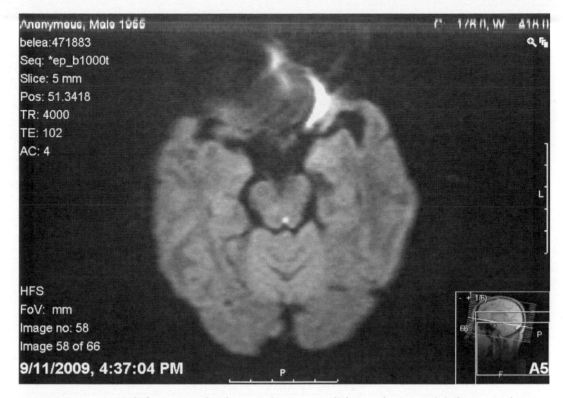

FIGURE 36.1 *MRI diffusion-weighted image showing small focus of restricted diffusion in the peri-aqueductal gray of the midbrain centered to the left.*

also cause ophthalmoparesis. Lastly, thiamine deficiency can cause ophthalmoparesis (as in Wernicke's encephalopathy) by an unknown mechanism.

The signs discovered on examination are classic findings in a patient with internuclear ophthalmoplegia. INO is caused by a lesion in the MLF. The MLF is part of the brain stem circuit responsible for the control of horizontal eye movements; it interconnects the oculomotor, trochlear, abducens, and vestibular nuclei. On lateral gaze, the ipsilateral abducens nucleus communicates with the contralateral oculomotor nucleus via the MLF. Thus, a lesion of the MLF interrupts the input to the medial rectus, and the eye ipsilateral to the lesion will be unable to fully adduct. For unknown reasons, there is also nystagmus in the contralateral eye that can be fully abducted. Even though eye adduction on the side of the lesion is impaired, in some cases, eye adduction can still be intact during convergence because it is thought that convergence is mediated by a different pathway that does not travel via the MLF.

INO has multiple etiologies, but the most common causes are infarction and multiple sclerosis (especially if it is a bilateral INO). Other less likely causes include trauma, infection, neoplasm, hemorrhage, and vasculitis. In the above case, the most likely etiology is acute infarction secondary to small vessel ischemic disease (usually seen in occlusion of the basilar artery or its paramedian branches) most likely due to uncontrolled diabetes and hypertension. In younger patients, the most likely etiology is multiple sclerosis whereas in older patients, INO is usually the result of ischemic vascular infarction.

An INO is managed by identifying and treating the underlying cause. The appropriate testing includes an MRI of the brain, VDRL, Lyme titer, fasting blood glucose, HbA1C, lipid profile, CBC with differential, blood pressure management, and a urine toxicology screen. The brain MRI should help determine the underlying cause, whether it be multiple sclerosis or an infarct, and the appropriate treatment should be chosen accordingly.

SUGGESTED READING

Kim JS. Internuclear ophthalmoplegia as an isolated or predominant symptom of brain stem infarction. *Neurology.* 2004;62(9):1491.

Martin JH. *Neuroanatomy Text and Atlas.* 3rd ed. McGraw-Hill Companies, New York; 2003.

Zee DS. Internuclear ophthalmoplegia: Pathophysiology and diagnosis. *Baillieres Clin Neurol.* 1992;1(2):455.

Right-Sided Headache

Mitchell Miglis and Jerome J. Graber

CHIEF COMPLAINT: **I have a bad headache on my right side.**

HISTORY OF PRESENT ILLNESS

A 37-year-old Asian male presented to the ER with subacute onset of right frontal headache. The headache was described as dull and throbbing in nature, 8/10 in severity. The headache came on slowly and gradually worsened over the past 3 days. His pain worsened with coughing and bending forward. He felt nauseous all day prior to coming to the ER and vomited once in the emergency room. He had never experienced similar headaches in the past. He denied any confusion, difficulty speaking, vision changes, photophobia, phonophobia, fever, or neck pain. He denied any weakness or loss of sensations in any extremities. He denied any bladder or bowel problems. He has no difficulty swallowing, slurring of speech, or balance problems.

PAST MEDICAL HISTORY

Acute lymphocytic leukemia with positive CSF cytology and had received intrathecal chemotherapy 2 months ago, cycle #1 of systemic L-asparaginase chemotherapy 4 days ago.

PAST SURGICAL HISTORY

None.

MEDICATIONS

Chemotherapy cycles with L-asparaginase.

ALLERGIES

NKDA.

PERSONAL HISTORY

Denied smoking, alcohol, or drug use.

FAMILY HISTORY

Noncontributory.

PHYSICAL EXAMINATION

Vitals: Blood pressure, 130/80; heart rate, 85/min; respiratory rate, 18/mm; temperature, 98.7°F.
General: Uncomfortable and in pain, was pressing his head with his hands.
HEENT: Atraumatic, no meningismus.
Negative Kernig and Brudzinski signs.
Pulmonary: Lungs clear to auscultation bilaterally.
Cardiovascular: Regular rate, no murmurs, rubs, or gallops.
Abdomen: Soft, nontender, nondistended.
Musculoskeletal: No joint pain or swelling.
Skin: No rashes.

NEUROLOGICAL EXAMINATION

Mental status: Alert and oriented to time, place, and person. Language intact. Able to spell the word "world" backwards without difficulty, registration and recall 3/3 after 5 minutes.

CNs II–XII: Fundoscopic examination revealed clear disc margins. Visual fields full to confrontation, visual acuity 20/20 bilaterally. Pupils 3 mm bilaterally and equally reactive to light. No facial asymmetry. Facial sensation intact to light touch. No facial droop. Hearing intact to finger rub and whispering. Tongue and palate midline. Shoulder shrug full bilaterally. Trapezii and sternocleidomastoid had good strength.

Motor: Normal bulk and tone in all four extremities without atrophy. Full strength 5/5 both upper and lower extremities.

Sensory: Intact to all modalities of sensations.

Reflexes: 2+ bilaterally and symmetric.

Plantars: Flexors.

Coordination: Finger-to-nose and heel-to-shin intact bilaterally, no tremors.

Romberg: Negative.

Gait: Normal, able to tandem without difficulty.

STOP AND THINK QUESTIONS

➢ What is the differential diagnoses of headache in a patient with a previous history of leukemia?

➢ How does the character of the headache aid us in narrowing down the differential?

➢ Does a nonfocal examination help exclude some diagnoses?

DIAGNOSTIC TEST RESULTS

Non-enhanced CT of the head (see Figure 37.1) revealed hyperintense signal of the right transverse sinus (A) extending into the jugular foramen. Contrast-enhanced image revealed non-visualization of the right transverse sinus (B) and jugular foramen consistent with venous sinus thrombosis.

DIAGNOSIS: Cerebral venous thrombosis (CVT).

DISCUSSION

CVT is variable in its clinical presentation, ranging from headache and impairment of consciousness to focal neurologic deficits, seizures, ischemic or hemorrhagic infarcts, and coma, depending on the degree of venous congestion and the vessel involved. Headache is common, though not specific, and can present as either a gradual worsening over several days or an acute thunderclap headache. Thombosis of the lateral sinus can mimic idiopathic intracranial hypertension.

The superior sagittal, cavernous, and lateral sinuses are most frequently affected. Females are more susceptible than males, and younger patients more so than older. Major risk factors include pregnancy, dehydration, infectious thrombophlebitis, and hypercoagulable states. Hypercoagulable states can be either primary (sickle cell disease, clotting factor abnormalities) or secondary (underlying malignancy, prothrombotic medications such as oral contraceptives or, as in this patient's case, L-asparaginase (see Table 37.1). L-asparaginase is believed to contribute to venous thrombosis due to inhibition of antithrombin and fibrinogen levels.

Intraparenchymal hemorrhage, either primary or secondary to conversion of an ischemic infarct, can also occur, and subarachnoid hemorrhage has been described. Cranial

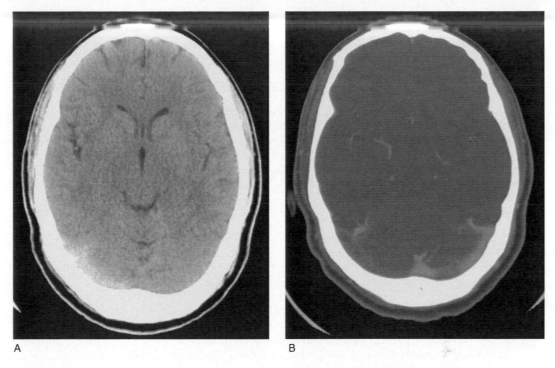

FIGURE 37.1 *Non-enhanced CT head axial image (A) showing hyperintense signal of the right transverse sinus extending into the jugular foramen; contrast enhanced image demonstrates non-visualization of the right transverse sinus (B) and jugular foramen consistent with venous sinus thrombosis.*

nerve palsies tend to occur with cavernous sinus thrombosis. In this patient, the thrombus extended to the jugular foramen. Extension of thrombus into the jugular bulb may cause unilateral paresis of 9th, 10th, and 11th cranial nerves, called *jugular foramen syndrome*. Superior sagittal thrombosis may also present as bilateral lower extremity weakness or paraplegia due to bilateral infarcts of the medial frontal lobe.

Thrombosis of the lateral and cavernous sinus is more often associated with disseminated infection, and positive blood cultures are isolated in approximately 50% of affected patients. CSF analysis often suggests aseptic meningitis secondary to meningeal irritation, and may cloud the correct diagnosis, as both can present with nonspecific headache. In comparison, superior sagittal sinus thrombosis occurs primarily in the absence of infection and can be seen in patients without any identifiable risk factors.

Diagnosis is established by imaging. MRI with MRV is most commonly utilized; however, CT venography is gaining acceptance and thought to have comparable sensitivity. Thrombosed sinuses are hyperintense on T1- and T2-weighted MR sequences, and hyperdense on head CT (as in our patient). MRV or CT venography demonstrates lack of flow in the involved sinus. Several nonspecific signs are described in the literature. The *cord sign* is a linear increase in signal intensity along the site of thrombosis, with filling defects often seen distal to the occluded vessel. The *empty delta sign* is seen on axial cuts of the sagittal sinus and represents the flow of contrast around the site of thrombosis.

Although there is limited data available on efficacy of treatment, most practitioners favor anticoagulation with low molecular weight heparin in the acute phase, with eventual bridge to oral anticoagulation. Duration of treatment is not established, though at least 6 months of oral anticoagulation with a target INR of 2 to 3 is usually recommended.

TABLE 37.1 *Risk Factors for Cerebral Venous Thrombosis*

Pregnancy and Puerperium Medications	Hypercoagulable States	Infections	Hematologic Conditions	Inflammatory Conditions	Nephrotic Syndrome Dehydration Mechanical
Oral contraceptives Corticosteroids L-asparaginase Thalidomide Erythropoietin Tamoxifen Epsilon amino caproic acid inhibitor (fibrinolytic inhibitor)	Protein C and protein S deficiency Antiphospholipid syndrome Lupus anticoagulant Leiden factor V mutation Antithrombin III deficiency Prothrombin mutation Hyperhomocystinemia	Otitis, mastoiditis, sinusitis, meningitis Disseminated infection	Paroxysmal nocturnal hemoglobinuria Polycythemia vera Sickle cell disease Thrombotic thrombocytopenic purpura	Behcet's syndrome Crohn's disease Lupus Ulcerative colitis Sacroidosis Wegener's granulomatosis	Trauma Lumbar puncture, lumbar drains.

Any precipitating factors such as underlying infection should be aggressively sought out and treated. There is insufficient evidence to support the use of either systemic or local thrombolysis in patients with CVT. Seizures and elevated ICP are common treatable complications.

SUGGESTED READING

Mashur F and Einhaupl K. Treatment of cerebral venous and sinus thrombosis. *Front Neurol Neurosci.* 2008;23:132–143.

Stam J. Thrombosis of the cerebral veins and sinuses. *N Engl J Med.* 2005;352:1791–1798.

Van den Berg et al. The spectrum of presentations of venous infarction caused by deep cerebral vein thrombosis. *Neurology.* 2005;65(2):192–196.

Transient Inversions of Visuospatial Field

Susan Shin, Rachael Oxman, Matt Morrison,
Qingliang Wang, and Lara V. Marcuse

CHIEF COMPLAINT: **I see the world upside down.**

HISTORY OF PRESENT ILLNESS

A 79-year-old, right-handed female was admitted for an elective hip replacement. Neurology was consulted on postoperative day 2 for a change in mental status. At that time she had been on narcotic analgesics and had transient hypotension to 70/30. The neurology consult service found her to be agitated and disoriented with an otherwise nonfocal neurological exam. An emergent noncontrast head CT did not reveal any acute stroke or hemorrhage; however, it did show a 1.7 cm calcified lesion in the left parietal lobe, most likely a cavernoma (Figure 38.1). She was treated with IV fluids and cessation of narcotic analgesic medication, and her neurological exam returned to normal.

Three days after the initial neurologic evaluation, the patient described multiple episodes of visual distortions. She felt that she was seeing her room "upside down." For example, the television that was attached to the ceiling appeared on the floor, and the floor tiles appeared as if they were on the ceiling. The patient experienced at least four discrete episodes, each lasting anywhere from 1 to 10 minutes. Family members who were present during the episodes did not report any change in the patient's mental status nor were there any speech difficulties during the episodes. The patient denied any persistence (palinopsia) of the inverted visual image when she turned her head.

She denied any double vision, vertigo, visual trailing of objects, photophobia, focal motor or sensory abnormalities, or headache. There was no history of prior seizures, strokes, migraines, or vestibular problems.

PAST MEDICAL HISTORY

Hypertension, hyperlipidemia, osteoarthritis.

PAST SURGICAL HISTORY

Left hip replacement.

MEDICATIONS

Metoprolol, albuterol, labetalol, lisinopril, simvastatin.

ALLERGIES

None.

PERSONAL HISTORY

No history of alcohol, drug, or tobacco use.

FAMILY HISTORY

Noncontributory.

PHYSICAL EXAMINATION

Blood pressure was 118/70, pulse 66 bpm, respiratory rate 14/min, temperature 98.4°F. Notable for an immobilized left hip.

NEUROLOGICAL EXAMINATION

Mental status: Alert, oriented, and able to follow simple and complex commands. Speech fluent, short-term memory 2/3, normal attention and concentration, judgment normal.
CNs II–XI: Normal.
Motor: 5/5 in all three extremities except the strength in the left lower extremity could not be assessed properly due to recent surgery.
Sensory: Intact to vibration, position, pin prick, and temperature, no neglect, normal cortical sensations.
Reflexes: Symmetrical 2+.
Plantars: Flexor.
Gait: Deferred.
Cerebellar: No dysmetria on finger-nose-finger.

STOP AND THINK QUESTIONS

➤ What is your differential diagnosis for the patient's visual distortions?

➤ What test(s) would you perform to confirm your clinical suspicion?

➤ What treatment can you offer her?

DIAGNOSTIC TEST RESULTS

Laboratory results: Vitamin B$_{12}$ 191 (low), Methylmalonic acid 456 (high), Homocysteine 21.5 (high), Hemoglobin A1c 5.6, Troponin I 0.0, Total Cholesterol 114, Triglycerides 93, HDL 34, LDL 61, TSH 1.93, Folate >20, CBC and chemistries were within normal limits.
MRI/MRA brain: Focal region of diffusion restriction in the right posterior centrum semi-ovale consistent with an acute infarct (Figure 38.2). Region of susceptibility with

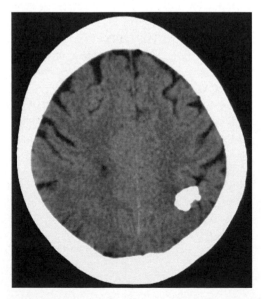

FIGURE 38.1 *Noncontrast head CT with a coarsely calcified left parietal intra-axial lesion with no surrounding edema.*

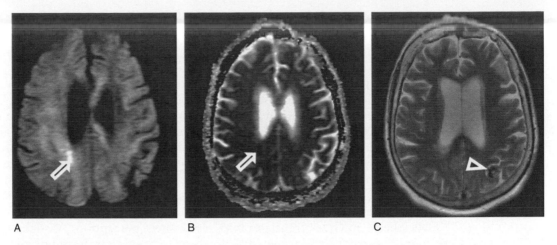

A   B   C

FIGURE 38.2 *MRI diffusion (A) and ADC (B) demonstrate an acute right parietal centrum semio-vale stroke (arrow). T2 MRI (C) with a mixed signal intensity left parieto-occipital lesion consistent with a cavernoma (carrot).*

peripheral enhancement in the left occipital lobe, likely a cavernoma. Unremarkable MRA of the head.

Carotid Doppler: No plaque at either carotid bifurcation. Normal vertebral arteries bilaterally.

Transthoracic ECHO: Hyperdynamic left ventricular systolic function. Mild concentric left ventricular hypertrophy. No thrombus. No atrial septal defect.

Electrocardiogram: Normal sinus rhythm, 66 beats per minute.

24-hour Holter Monitor: No arrhythmia or atrial fibrillation.

EEG: Well organized and reactive, 9 to 10 Hz posterior dominant rhythm. There was no generalized or focal slowing, and no epileptiform discharges were seen in either hemisphere.

DIAGNOSIS: Visual allesthesia secondary to an acute ischemic stroke.

DISCUSSION

Prior to the MRI brain, the differential for the patient's visual inversion included seizures secondary to the left parietal/occipital cavernoma, vestibular problems, or a new acute stroke. DWI confirmed the acute ischemic infarct in the right posterior centrum semiovale. The visual inversion was then attributed to the new parietal lobe stroke. The disturbance was paroxysmal, which suggests the possibility that the acute stroke was causing simple partial seizures characterized by complex visual distortions. The stroke, on MRI, shows only white matter involvement. However, it is possible that the penumbra affected surrounding cortical gray matter, causing the patient to have seizures. Given the normal EEG and the cessation of further episodes, anticonvulsant medication was not started.

The small stroke is in a watershed distribution. Watershed (border-zone) stroke is defined as ischemia/infarction caused by hypoperfusion of a distal territory between two (or more) arterial vascular supplies of brain parenchyma. Watershed strokes can be cortical between ACA and MCA or MCA and PCA. Internal watershed infarctions occur in the cerebral white matter between the vascular supply of the deep penetrating arteries of the ACA/MCA/PCA and the superficial pial medullary arteries. Classic imaging findings of watershed stroke include wedge-shaped infarcts between ACA/MCA, MCA/PCA. In the centrum semiovale, there can be multiple small infarcts lending an MRI appearance of "beads on a string." Most watershed infarcts are due to systemic hypotension often coupled with stenosis of extracranial and/or intracranial vessels.

Our patient does have risk factors for stroke, particularly her history of hypertension and hyperlipidemia. The authors postulate that the mechanism of her stroke was her systemic hypotension causing an infarct in a watershed border zone in the cerebral white matter. As there was only the single small stroke, it is likely that there was an area of small vessel disease that was particularly vulnerable to hypotension. For secondary stroke prevention, she was started on an aspirin. Her high homocysteine level likely secondary to low vitamin B_{12} can contribute to small vessel disease. Therefore, she was started on vitamin B_{12} supplementation. She was maintained on her antihypertensive agents, and she did not have any further episodes of hypotension when narcotic analgesics were discontinued.

Allesthesia, in Greek translates into "elsewhere + perception." Visual allesthesia is used to connote when the visual fields are transposed either vertically or horizontally. Abnormal visual perceptions are a common symptom in various neurologic and psychiatric conditions such as psychosis, delirium, epilepsy, migraines, and dementia. However, when they occur in isolation, they are known as positive spontaneous visual phenomena (PSVP). PSVP include *visual hallucinations, distortions, photopsias, phosphenes, kinetopsias, polyopia, palinopsia, and visual allesthesia* (see Table 38.1). Although the presence of these phenomena could help in anatomic localization in the nervous system, various case reports have shown that lesions in any part of the visual system from the retina to the occipital cortex can produce these symptoms. The pathophysiology of PSVP is complex and poorly understood.

The patient in our case experienced a transposition of objects between her upper and lower visual quadrants. This phenomenon is quite rare and only a handful of case reports have been published in the literature. Its presence is often diagnostically nonspecific. Visual allesthesia has been reported in various neurological conditions such as stroke, calcified cysticercosis, arteriole-venous malformation, meningioma, and traumatic brain injury following shunt placement. Most of these lesions were located in the parieto-occipital region, and predominantly in the nondominant hemisphere. Our patient had an acute ischemic stroke in her nondominant parietal lobe.

Visual allesthesia is a rare phenomenon whose pathophysiology is not known. In general, visuospatial perception is considered a multiorder, highly complex process that integrates visual, vestibular, and somatosensory stimuli.

TABLE 38.1 *Examples of PSVP*

Type of PSVP	Definition
Visual Allesthesia	Transposition of a visual image from one-half of the visual field to the other; it can occur either horizontally or vertically
Visual Distortion	Abnormal visual perception of objects and figures
Visual hallucination	Perception of an image in the absence of a visual stimulus; images may consist of unusual scenes, including inanimate objects, animals, and people. It can only be classified as a PSVP if it occurs in the absence of mental disturbance (i.e., delirium)
Palinopsia	A type of visual perseveration. Trailing of a visual image even after the stimulus is removed
Photopsias	Structured geometric shapes, like the fortification spectra of migraine with aura, usually recurs in a repetitive pattern
Phosphenes	Unstructured lights

It is known that visual stimuli are processed through a distinct primary visual cortex (Brodmann's area 17) and visual association areas (Brodmann's area 18 and 19) located within the occipital lobe. There are also postulations of a "vestibular cortex" located in the posterior parietal lobe (Broadmann's area 7), which may be important in integrating vestibular, visual, and somatosensory information. Given that patients with visual allesthesia frequently have lesions in the posterior parietal region, it may suggest that allesthesia could be the result of visual and vestibular stimuli mismatch or disruption. On the other hand, abnormal firing of cortical neurons (e.g., seizure) in the "vestibular cortex" may also lead to visual distortions and allesthesia.

SUGGESTED READING

Ardila A, Botero M, Gomez J. Palinopsia and visual allesthesia. *Int J Neurosci.* 1987;32(3–4):775–782.

Bogousslavsky J, Moulin T. Borderzone Infarcts. In Bogousslavsky J and Caplan L, eds. *Stroke Syndromes.* New York, NY, Cambridge University Press; 1995;358–365.

Brandt T, Dieterich M. The vestibular cortex: Its locations, functions, and disorders. *Annals of the New York Academy of Sciences* 1999;871:293–312.

Celesia GG. Positive Spontaneous Visual Phenomena. In: Celesia GG, ed. *Disorders of Visual Processing.* Vol. 5. Edinburgh: Elsevier, 2005: 353–370. Print.

Jacobs L. Visual allesthesia. *Neurology* 1980;30(10):1059–1063.

Mendez MF, Chen JWY. Epilepsy partialis continua with visual allesthesia. *J Neurol.* 2009;256(6): 1009–1011. Epub 2009 Feb 25.

Norton JW, Corbett JJ. Visual perceptual abnormalities: Hallucinations and illusions. *Semin Neurol.* 2000;20(1):111–121. Review.

Slow Onset Memory Problems With Aggressive Behavior

Michael Boffa

CHIEF COMPLAINT: He is losing all his memory, maybe he has Alzheimer's disease.

HISTORY OF PRESENT ILLNESS

Patient is a 65-year-old, right-handed male with a history of suspected Alzheimer's disease who was brought in by EMS after an episode of violent and inappropriate sexual behavior at home. Patient's wife reports that he threw a chair at their son today. She also reports progressive cognitive decline for the past 6 years. Specifically, she reports increasing short- and long-term memory loss, and an inability to recognize faces, read, or write. Patient is no longer able to bathe himself, she reports "he stands in the shower, staring at the soap, and doesn't know what to do." Additionally, his personality has changed, he has become increasingly violent and started using profanity profusely, which is all very atypical of him.

When the patient first started showing symptoms 6 years prior, he was brought to an outside hospital for evaluation where he had a head CT and laboratory work done. He was diagnosed with possible Alzheimer's disease. The family was resistant to long-term placement and brought him home on Namenda and Aricept. He has had no improvement in his cognition; on the contrary, he has become more violent and sexually disinhibited. The patient urinates freely wherever he wants, including on people, will masturbate wherever he pleases, and has made sexual advances on his daughters and granddaughters without recognizing them.

In the ED, patient was exceptionally violent and the family was frightened. He was given haldol for agitation.

PAST MEDICAL HISTORY

Patient has a history of a "nonspecific heart disease." More information was unavailable, but patient takes metoprolol for hypertension. Patient has no other medical history.

PAST SURGICAL HISTORY

None.

MEDICATIONS

Metoprolol 12.5 mg daily; aspirin, 81 mg daily; Seroquel, 25 mg qHS; Depakote, 250 mg qAM, 500 mg qHS; Namenda, 10mg bid; Aricept, 10 mg once daily.

ALLERGIES

Patient has no known allergies.

PERSONAL HISTORY

Patient was born and has lived in New York his whole life. He is the youngest of the six children, two of whom are still alive. Patient lives at home with his family and lived briefly in a nursing home. Patient has been married to one woman since 1969, and they have four children and multiple grandchildren. Patient does not use drugs or alcohol but is an active smoker.

FAMILY HISTORY

Patient's brother has ALS. Patient has no family history of Alzheimer's disease.

REVIEW OF SYSTEMS

General: Progressive weight loss over the past several years.
Skin: No rash, itching, or dryness.
HEENT: No pain, redness, tearing, or diplopia. No changes in hearing or earache. No changes in teeth or gums. No dysphagia.
Respiratory: No cough, dyspnea, or wheezing.
Cardiovascular: No chest pain or palpitations.
Gastrointestinal: No nausea or decreased appetite. No heartburn, vomiting, or abdominal pain. No diarrhea.
Musculoskeletal: No joint pain, swelling, or stiffness.
Genitourinary: No dysuria or frequency.
Neurological: See History of Present Illness.
Psychiatric: Recent increase in aggressive behavior. No changes in mood.

PHYSICAL EXAMINATION

Vital signs: Temperature, 96.9°F; pulse, 63; respiratory rate, 18/min; blood pressure, 111/70 mm Hg; O_2 saturation, 97% on room air, finger-stick glucose 117.
General: Patient is a healthy but disheveled appearing male, appearing his stated age, sitting comfortably in bed in no acute distress.
Skin: No rashes or irregularities noted.
HEENT: Normocephalic atraumatic, conjunctiva pink, sclerae anicteric. Pupils equal, round, reactive to light and accommodation. Pharynx noninjected. Tongue and buccal mucosa pink without lesions. Moist membranes.

NEUROLOGICAL EXAMINATION

Mental status: Patient is alert but oriented to his own first name and city only. He denies having a last name. MMSE score was 4/30. Patient was unable to repeat words, draw, or write. Patient was otherwise uncooperative or unable and would often answer "I don't know." Patient is unable to follow complicated or simple commands during the examination, and required repeated prompting. He could not name his own body parts and did not remember where he was born. He has severe comprehension difficulties, anomia, telegraphic speech, but no clear apraxia (can show how to throw a ball or brush his teeth). When asked what the expression "a hole in the wall" means, he says "a circle is a hole in the wall." Patient often perseverates and mumbles.
CNs: I Not tested.
   II Visual fields intact.
   III, IV, VI Extra ocular movements intact. No nystagmus.
   V Normal sensation on face, jaw clench.
   VII No weakness of facial muscles.
   VIII No hearing deficits.
   X Intact.
   XI Symmetric and intact trapezii and sternocleidomastoids strength.

XII Tongue midline.
Motor: Normal muscle tone/mass. Strength 5/5 throughout.
No rigidity or tremors.
Sensory: Intact to light touch and vibration.
Cerebellar: Rapid alternating movements and finger-to-nose intact.
Reflexes: right—biceps 2+, triceps 2+, brach 2+, knee 2+, ankle 2+, plantar downgoing; left—biceps 2+, triceps 2+, brach 2+, knee 2+, ankle 2+, plantar downgoing.
Gait: Normal, without Romberg's sign. No abnormal movements.
Glabellar sign: Closes eyes every time despite being asked to keep open.
Clapping: Mimics examiner incorrectly, doing two claps instead of three.
No meningeal signs; no myoclonus.

DIAGNOSTIC TEST RESULTS

CBC: WBC, 8.4; hemoglobin/hematocrit, 14.8/43.7; platelets, 204.
Electrolytes: Na, 142; K, 4.0; Cl, 106; CO_2, 31; BUN, 22; Cr, 1; Glu, 107; Ca, 10.3.
Liver Function Tests: AST, 24; ALT, 30; ALK, 105; Tail, 0.6; Dill, 0.2; TP, 7.5; Alb, 4.6.
Coagulation: PT, 13.9; INR, 1.18; PTT, 21.7.
RPR: Nonreactive HIV: negative TSH: wnl valproic acid level: 38.3 B_{12}: 616
Head CT without Contrast: Mild ventriculomegaly with sulcal prominence. Marked cerebral volume loss mostly concentrated in the frontal and temporal lobes (see Figure 39.1).

STOP AND THINK QUESTIONS

➢ What are the common causes of memory loss?

➢ What are treatable causes of dementia?

➢ What is typical about this case?

DIAGNOSIS: Frontotemporal dementia.

DISCUSSION

The patient's history of increasing aggression, lack of control, short-term memory loss, dysphasia, apraxia, agnosia, executive function loss, loss of ability to read/write, all without alteration of consciousness, suggest the diagnosis of dementia. Additionally, the patient had a steady decline from a previous level of functioning that was severe enough to interfere with daily function and independence. Therefore, all the criteria to make a diagnosis of dementia were met (1) but a specific dementia diagnosis would require further analysis. However, due to the extreme nature of the patient's violent and sexual tendency, a general approach to dementia and supportive care were administered while discussing the dementia diagnosis.

TREATMENT

1. Metroprolol 12.5 mg daily for blood pressure, check vitals q 4 h

2. Seroquel increased to 25 mg bid, additional 25 mg PRN for agitation

3. Head CT without contrast ordered (pt unable to have MRI)

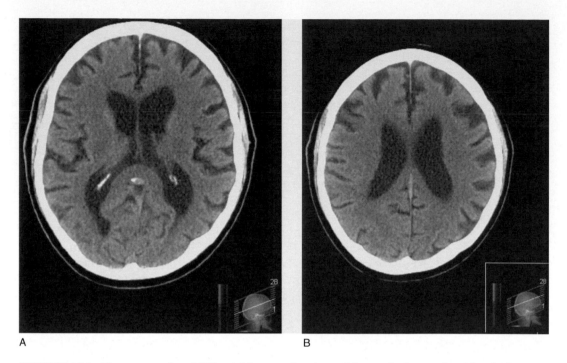

A   B

FIGURE 39.1 *Noncontrast head CT axial images showing mild ventriculomegaly with sulcal prominence and marked cerebral volume loss mostly concentrated in the frontal and temporal lobes.*

 4. Psychiatry consult ordered
 5. Patient on 1:1 watch for danger to self and others

DIFFERENTIAL DIAGNOSIS

There are many diagnoses to consider when working up dementia. Things important to consider are FTD, Alzheimer's disease, vascular dementia, dementia with Lewy bodies, Parkinson's disease with dementia, and to rule out reversible causes of dementia (see Table 39.1).

Statistically, the majority of patients with dementia have Alzheimer's disease, as it accounts for 60% to 80% of cases and affects more than 4 million Americans (2). Although the patient presented with a previous diagnosis of Alzheimer's disease, it was reconsidered due to the patient's age at diagnosis being 59, which is exceptionally young for Alzheimer's, which is rarely diagnosed before age 60. Additionally, on CT, the patient had no evidence of hippocampal volume loss, which has been shown to be a sign of Alzheimer's on scanning (3). Cognitive deficits appear the earliest in Alzheimer's and progress insidiously. The patient's problems had a sudden onset and rapidly progressed to his current presentation. Loss of memory of recent events is an essential feature of AD and is usually its first manifestation, which again is not how the patient presented. Other cognitive defects usually appear afterward, affecting things like language and visuospatial skills. Loss of executive function and apraxia often manifest significantly later in the disease, but the patient presented initially with them in this case. The patient's behavioral issues are consistent with the middle and late Alzheimer's stages, but the patient was initially diagnosed with them making Alzheimer's a good choice but more unlikely due to the order of symptomatology. Therefore, Alzheimer's disease is lower on the differential diagnosis (4).

Another type of dementia important to consider would be vascular dementia. Vascular dementia is a cognitive decline that occurs due to cerebrovascular disease. The presentation of a patient with vascular dementia is very distinct, especially early on. Even with mild memory impairments, the patient generally has significant deficits in executive functioning and can have severe disability. The patient in question did have early executive dysfunction but lacked key points of diagnosis for vascular dementia. Specifically, he had no history of stroke/TIA/vascular disease, where the onset of cognitive deficits in vascular dementia is associated with one of these. Additionally, on CT, there is no evidence of past strokes or infarcts, leading to the conclusion that the patient was not suffering from vascular dementia (5).

Dementia with Lewy bodies is another important dementia to consider. This dementia is the second most common dementia. It has a gradual onset and a very characteristic picture. The patient will have fluctuations in their cognitive function as well as consistent/specific visual hallucinations. Of note, Lewy body dementia is the dementia most commonly associated with parkinsonian symptoms. Additional features of dementia with Lewy bodies include syncope/falls, delusions, nonvisual hallucinations, parasomnias, and depression (6). The patient did not show any of the core features or demonstrate the supportive features so this was ruled out.

Other things to consider would be Parkinson's disease. Patients with Parkinson's disease have six times greater risk of becoming demented compared to people without Parkinson's (7). It can be distinguished however as the Parkinson's motor defects must be present at least 1 year before the onset of dementia rather than the dementia occurring before or with parkinsonism. In the patient described above, the motor deficits were very minimal, if any, and occurred after the cognitive decline, ruling out dementia secondary to Parkinson's disease.

There are many reversible causes of dementia that need to be assessed because if they are the cause, they can be remedied. Additionally, the quicker they are remedied, the more likely the patient will recover fully. This is the reason most hospitals have a laboratory screen for patients who present with altered mental status. Many of the things considered and assessed for were medication induced, such as analgesics, anticholinergics, psychotropic medications, sedative-hypnotics, and steroids. Alcohol related was less likely due to the time frame but intoxication or withdrawal has been shown to cause a dementia-like syndrome. Metabolic disorders such as thyroid problems, vitamin B_{12} deficiency, hyponatremia, hypercalcemia, hepatic, and renal dysfunction can also cause dementia. In this patient, all of the laboratory tests came back normal ruling these issues out. An additional important dementia to consider is pseudodementia. Depression can cause a pseudodementia state. In this case, a psychiatric evaluation came and reported there was no psychiatric diagnosis. Additionally, CNS neoplasms, chronic subdural hematomas, chronic meningitis, and normal pressure hydrocephalus can all cause dementia states. However, all these things were looked for on CT, and all came back negative. Therefore, after ruling out all other causes and lengthy discussion, the diagnosis of FTD was decided upon.

FRONTOTEMPORAL DEMENTIA

FTD is a neurodegenerative disorder that is mainly characterized by atrophy of the frontal and temporal lobes (8). Overall, FTD is the fourth most common dementia behind Alzheimer disease, vascular dementia, and dementia with Lewy bodies. The prevalence in people less than 65 years old is 15 per 100,000 (9). The age of onset is usually between age 50 and 70, with the average age on diagnosis being 58 years old (10). The prevalence of men and women with FTD is roughly equal, but some studies suggest a slight increase in males (10). Between 20% and 40% of patients with FTD have a family history of the disease (10).

However, a family history does not increase nor correlate with the age of presentation (11). FTD has had many names including Pick's disease, frontal lobe dementia, and Pick's complex, among other names. Generally, FTD is the preferred term. There are three subtypes of FTD, a behavioral variant—the most common, a progressive nonfluent aphasia variant, and semantic dementia variant. While all three have characteristic features, there is much overlap between them, namely they all have behavioral/personality changes as a major feature. Additionally, for all the variants, the onset is insidious and has a gradual progression, with memory loss generally spared until more advanced disease. The prognosis of FTD is not well studied. One retrospective study showed the median survival to be 8.7 years from the time of symptom onset (12).

The typical initial clinical presentation is personality changes and social behavior or language changes, which will progress to a global dementia. Often, patients may be misdiagnosed with a psychiatric illness (13). A small percentage of patients will also experience initial extrapyramidal symptoms or motor neuron involvement, but this is rare. Interestingly, patients with MND-associated FTD most often have an inherited condition; in a recent study, more than half of patients had a family history that was consistent with autosomal dominant inheritance pattern (14). Two genes on chromosome 17, and genes on chromosomes 3 and 9, have been linked to FTD (15). In 2008, TAR DNA binding protein 43 KDa (TDP-43) gene mutations were discovered in amyotrophic lateral sclerosis, indicating that TDP-43 protein abnormality is associated with neurodegeneration (21). Recently, it has been discovered that the same protein, TDP-43, has been identified in patients with FTD as well. Ubiquitin-positive, pathologic TDP-43 are hyper-phosphorylated, ubiquitinated, and cleaved to generate C-terminal fragments and have been recovered only from affected CNS regions, including hippocampus, neocortex, and spinal cord. TDP-43 represents the common pathologic substrate linking several neurodegenerative disorders. TDP-43 has been identified as the major component of the ubiquitin-positive inclusion bodies in ALS, FTLD, and FTLD with motor neuron disease. Due to this finding, the name TDP-43 proteinopathy has been proposed to lump together these diseases (21). TDP-43 has many conformations, over 30 in ALS alone, and has been found to differ between ALS and FTLD (22). However, the C-terminal band pattern is indistinguishable among brain regions and spinal cord in each individual patient, which suggests that abnormal TDP-43 produced in a cell may be transferred to different regions and propagated during disease progression (22). Even though a diagnosis is not made by MRI, there are some prominent changes that can be seen. However, the MRI may be normal early in the course of the disease (16). As the disease progresses, there is evidence of atrophy of the frontal and temporal lobes. Specific patterns of atrophy have been associated with the clinical syndrome in about 50% to 70% of patients (16). Usually, bifrontal atrophy first is the most common finding, later on, this usually progresses to include bitemporal atrophy as well. Right frontal atrophy correlates the most with the prominent behavioral manifestations.

The personality change that patients with this disease have can manifest in many ways. It can manifest as an apathy including social withdrawal, loss of spontaneity, and abulia, which is often mistaken for depression. Some patients do not show these symptoms, and some will instead show the more disinhibited and impulsive side of FTD. In the behavioral variant, patients show progressive change in both behavior and personality. The features can include abnormal social interactions, unusual eating patterns, loss of social skills, emotional blunting, loss of insight and ritualized behaviors. The lack of insight can result in inappropriate remarks and sexual/aggressive behavior. Common behaviors include sexual advances, roaming, hoarding, and childish behavior. Cognitive impairments appear later and are most prominent in tasks of executive function, judgment, and problem-solving. Disinhibition/impulsivity, which is the lack of restraint in motor, emotional, cognitive, and social

TABLE 39.1 Major Dementia Syndromes

	Presentation	Radiology	Pathology	Treatment	Notes
Frontotemporal dementia/Pick's disease	Significant changes in behavior and personality early in disease	Atrophy of the frontal and temporal lobes	Atrophy of the frontal and temporal lobes Pick bodies	Symptomatic. SSRI. Cholinesterase inhibitors Atypical Antipsychotics	See detailed discussion in text
Alzheimer's disease	Cortical dementia. Early- depression, insomnia, agitation, anxiety, excitability, mild forgetfulness, impaired judgment. Middle-short-term memory loss, fatigue, decrease in concentration, aphasia, acalculia, getting lost, difficulty following commands. Late-decreased interest, loss of language, confusion, psychosis, loss of functional independence	Cortical atrophy Wide ventricles	Neuronal loss in cerebral cortex, basal temporal lobe (hippocampus), temporoparietal regions. Paucity of cells. Neuritic plaques (senile)—focal dilated neuritic processes surrounding a central amyloid core and neurofibrillary tangles. Amyloid angiopathy present often. Diminished acetylcholine	Cholinesterase inhibitors (donepezil, rivastigmine, galantamine, tacrine). Memantine—an N-methyl-D-aspartate receptor antagonist. Symptom management-depression, psychosis, insomnia, agitation. Special care facilities. Training family members to assist in activities of daily living. Supplements controversial in efficacy. Vitamin E, ginkgo, lecithin may be beneficial. Avoid anticholinergics	Familial cases, chromosome 21q (amyloid precursor), 19q (Apo E) Associated with Down's syndrome. Survival 5 to 10 years. #4 cause of death in the US. Prevalence increases with age
Vascular dementia	Strikes patients with arterial hypertension, vascular risk factors like hyperlipidemia and diabetes History of TIAs/stroke Can arise suddenly, progressive in a stepwise manner Deficit depends on area of infarct Common is incontinence of affect	Multiple focal lesions, usually in the subcortical white matter	Multiple small infarcts	Vascular risk reduction. Treat underlying cause. Management of HTN, HLD, DM. Aspirin, clopidogrel for prophylaxis	Second most common form of dementia
Creutzfeldt-Jakob disease	Prion disease Extremely rare Spongiform encephalopathy Subacute dementia Ataxia, myoclonic jerks. Mental abnormalities, insomnia, fatiguability Pyramidal tract signs, cerebellar signs, abnormalities of muscle tone, fasciculation, and myoclonus. Rapid clinical decline	MRI with diffusion-weighted imaging Increased intensity in the putamen and the head of the caudate on T2 and Fluid-Attenuated Inversion Recovery	Spongy degeneration. Neuronal loss Astrocytic proliferation Protease resistant prion protein accumulates in brain	No current treatments. Rapidly progressive and fatal	Pyramidal signs and periodic sharp waves on EEG 1:1,000,000 cases per year

(continued)

TABLE 39.1 *(continued)*

	Presentation	Radiology	Pathology	Treatment	Notes
Dementia with Lewy bodies	Progressive dementia. Frequent visual hallucinations. Parkinsonian manifestations. Repeated falls, syncope, episodes of unconsciousness.	Large hippocampal and putamen atrophy.	Lewy bodies in neurons of cerebral cortex and brain stem.	Adverse effect to neuroleptics. Can tray selegiline, acetylcholinesterase inhibitors.	Required triad of diagnosis is fluctuation in cognition, parkinsonism, and hallucinations.

circumstances, is also a common feature of FTD. The patient has a clear lack of inhibition and may even begin activities such as shoplifting (17). Patients have been noted to act sentimental or even perform violent acts of aggression towards loved ones. Some patients have even been shown to alternate back and forth between the 2 types. The majority of patients with this disease are not aware of their deficits when first diagnosed, and all exhibit no insight within a few years. The patient is no longer aware of social norms in a way that does not agree at all with how they acted before becoming demented. The patient may make offensive remarks and behave inappropriately, including neglecting personal hygiene. Patients often become incontinent, voiding urine or feces in inappropriate places without concern. While inappropriate sexual comments are somewhat common in patients, hypersexual behavior is not as most patients have a decreased libido. Patients often will do repetitive movements such as pacing or counting. Additionally, patients may have changes in their eating patterns such as binge eating or drinking heavily. A loss of empathy is also a common change; the patient will no longer care about others and appear to be self centered. Lastly, patients can become very irritable and distractible, loosing most of their ability to concentrate.

The semantic and progressive nonfluent aphasia subtypes are less common and have specific presentations. Patients with the semantic variation have flowing speech that lacks substance or meaning. They use very general terms and gradually lose the meanings of words altogether. They will even begin to ask about the meaning of certain words and replace words they lost with other similar ones, for example instead of the word "dog," they would use the word "animal." (17) Additionally, they lose the ability to recognize familiar faces early on. In the nonfluent aphasia, variant speech becomes very difficult. Stuttering often, they are very hesitant to speak. They have problems naming objects and finding words. They lose the ability to read, repeat, and even speak. Comprehension also becomes an issue. Early on, however, the patient's behavior and social skills are spared. Eventually, these deteriorate as well (17). In both semantic and progressive nonfluent aphasia, the patient will have similar behavioral and social issues as in the behavioral variant.

Some patients with FTD have associated motor symptoms. There are three generally common motor variations. The first is MND. In patients with MND and FTD, the motor presentation is a progressive muscular atrophy. The bulbar muscles and upper extremities are generally affected worst. Symptoms may include both flaccidity and fasciculations. Upper motor neuron signs are less prominent. If a patient is going to develop MND with FTD, the onset of the two is usually within 2 years of one another. The association of MND also has a negative prognostic value, with most an increased progression towards death. Another type of motor involvement is called corticobasal degeneration. This is a syndrome of apraxia and rigidity, generally asymmetric (18). An interesting phenomenon with this type of motor neuron involvement is called alien limb. This is when the affected limb first goes rigid and then has uncontrolled spontaneous jerks. It is self-limiting but can be very distressing for the patient. Other important symptoms include dystonia, reflex myoclonus, and impaired cortical sensory loss. Problems with gait and supranuclear gaze palsy also can be associated. The third motor syndrome is progressive supranuclear palsy. This is a well-defined syndrome consisting of supranuclear vertical gaze palsy, axial dystonia, bradykinesia, rigidity, and falls (19). There is a clear link between FTD and these syndromes, but there has been evidence of both the motor syndromes preceding the behavioral issues and vice versa. It is currently unclear which, if either, may cause the other.

Unfortunately, there is no treatment for this disease at this time. The best thing for the patient is to be in an environment where constant monitoring and support can be given. The majority of the current treatment regime is symptom management and supportive care. Additionally, patients can be treated with atypical antipsychotics to help control the behavioral problems and outbursts. Also, SSRIs may be used to help with the disinhibition, depression, and repetitive behaviors (20). There is some evidence for using galantamine or acetylcholine esterase inhibitors in patients with the progressive nonfluent aphasia variant. However, it is important to remember that the nonpharmacologic treatments may be better in this disease. Patients and families should be given references to support groups and educated as to what the disease process will entail as it progresses. Preparation for cognitive decline is very important. Patients with FTD will need lots of care and help with activities of daily living. Social, legal, and financial issues are a major concern as well. The patient may need long-term placement to safely take care of them. Losing inhibition put the patient at risk to themselves and others. Lastly, helping to develop behavioral management strategies and interventions for behavioral disturbances can help the family and the patient deal with that major issue.

REFERENCES

1. American Psychiatric Association. *American Psychiatric Association Diagnostic and Statistical Manual.* 4th ed. Washington DC: APA Press; 1994.
2. Evans DA. Estimated prevalence of Alzheimer's disease in the United States. *Milbank Q.* 1990;68:267.
3. Barnes J, Whitwell JL, Frost C, et al. Measurements of the amygdala and hippocampus in pathologically confirmed Alzheimer disease and frontotemporal lobar degeneration. *Arch Neurol.* 2006;63:1434.
4. Juva K, Sulkava R, Erkinjuntti R, et al. Staging the severity of dementia: Comparison of clinical (CDR, DSM-III-R), functional (ADL, IADL) and cognitive (MMSE) scales. *Acta Neurol Scand.* 1994;90:293.
5. Chui HC, Mack W, Jackson E, et al. Clinical criteria for the diagnosis of vascular dementia. A multicenter study of comparability and interrater reliability. *Arch Neurol.* 2000;57:191.
6. McKeith LG, Galasko D, Kosaka K, et al. Consensus guidelines for the clinical and pathologic diagnosis of dementia withLewy bodies (DLB): Report of the consortium on DLB international workshop. *Neurology.* 1996;47:1113.
7. Aarsland D, Andersen K, Larsen JP, et al. Risk of dementia in Parkinson's disease. A community-based, prospective study. *Neurology.* 2001;56:730.
8. Clinical and neuropathological criteria for frontotemporal dementia. The Lund and Manchester Groups. *J Neurol Neurosurg Psychiatry.* 1994;57:416.
9. Ratnavalli E, Brayne C, Dawson K, Hodges JR. The prevalence of frontotemporal dementia. *Neurology.* 2002;58(11):1615–1621.
10. Johnson JK, Diehl J, Mendez MF, et al. Frontotemporal lobar degeneration: Demographic characteristics of 353 patients. *Arch Neurol.* 2005;62:925.
11. Piguet O, Brooks WS, Halliday GM, et al. Similar early clinical presentations in familial and non-familial frontotemporal dementia. *J Neurol Neurosurg Psychiatry.* 2004;75:1743.
12. Roberson ED, Hesse JH, Rose KD, et al: Frontotemporal dementia progresses to death faster than Alzheimer disease. *Neurology.* 2005;65(5):719–725.

13. McKhann GM, Albert MS, Grossman M, et al. Clinical and pathological diagnosis of frontotemporal dementia: Report of the Work Group on Frontotemporal Dementia and Pick's Disease. Work Group on Frontotemporal Dementia and Pick's Disease. *Arch Neurol.* 2001;58(11):1803–1809.

14. Goldman JS, Farmer JM, Wood EM, et al. Comparison of family histories in FTLD subtypes and related tauopathies. *Neurology.* 2005;65:1817.

15. Sikkink S, Rollinson S, Pickering-Brown SM. The genetics of frontotemporal lobar degeneration. *Curr Opin Neurol.* 2007;20(6):693–698.

16. Josephs KA. Frontotemporal lobar degeneration. *Neurol Clin.* 2007;25:683.

17. Neary D, Snowden JS, Gustafson L, et al. Frontotemporal lobar degeneration: A consensus on clinical diagnostic criteria. *Neurology.* 1998;51(6):1546–1554.

18. Boeve BF, Lang AE, and Litvan I. Corticobasal degeneration and its relationship to progressive supranuclear palsy and frontotemporal dementia. *Ann Neurol.* 2003;54(Suppl 5):S15–S19.

19. Litvan I, Campbell G, Mangone CA, et al. Which clinical features differentiate progressive supranuclear palsy (Steele-Richardson-Olszewski syndrome) from related disorders? A clinicopathological study. *Brain.* 1997;120(Pt 1):65–74.

20. Chow TW, Mendez MF. Goals in symptomatic pharmacologic management of frontotemporal lobar degeneration. *Am J Alzheimers Dis Other Demen.* 2002;17(5):267–272.

21. Tomohiko I, Yuko A, Atsushi S, et al. FTLD/ALS as TDP-43 proteinopathies. *Rinsho Shinkeigaku.* 2010;50: 1022–1024.

22. Masato H, Tetsuaki A, Takashi N, et al. Molecular dissection of TDP-43 in ALS and FTLD. *Rinsho Shinkeigaku.* 2010;50:937–939.

CHIEF COMPLAINT: **I feel scared sometimes.**

HISTORY OF PRESENT ILLNESS

A 13-year-old girl born with a left facial cutaneous vascular malformation was admitted directly from the pediatric neurology clinic with a complaint of frequent feelings of fear for the past 18 months. She was unable to describe the fear clearly, but felt that it was worsening and making life unbearable. Her mother reported that the fear would seem very intense for seconds to minutes, and then would seem to abate. She would often have up to 10 episodes in one day. During these episodes, she would be slightly less alert. Her mother had noticed some mouth movements during these spells. The patient had a history of seizures that began at the age of 10 months. These were described as grand mal seizures that would begin with right facial twitching and progress to a generalized tonic clonic convulsion lasting about 1 minute. In the past 6 months, she has had at least 4 such events when she would lose consciousness. Her mother also gave history of headaches occurring about once per month with subsequent difficulty seeing in her right visual field for hours after the resolution of headache. The headaches are bitemporal, 6/10 in intensity, and without any nausea or vomiting.

PAST MEDICAL HISTORY AND PAST SURGICAL HISTORY

Seizures, complicated migraine headaches, left eye glaucoma, left facial cutaneous vascular malformation, dyslexia, and mild developmental delay.

MEDICATIONS

Carbamezapine 200 mg qam and 300 mg qpm, aspirin 81 mg daily, ibuprofen 400 mg three times daily as needed for headaches, dorzolamide hydrochloride 2% and timolol 0.25% 1 drop to left eye 2 times daily.

ALLERGIES

No known medication allergies.

PERSONAL HISTORY

No history of alcohol, drug, or tobacco use. She lives with her parents. She had recently changed neighborhoods, and with the change in schools, she was getting bullied and had become fearful of attending school. She was in the 7th grade and attended special education classes.

FAMILY HISTORY

Noncontributory.

PHYSICAL EXAMINATION

Blood pressure, 128/88 mm Hg; pulse, 70 bpm; respiratory rate, 12/min; temperature, 98.7°F.

General physical examination revealed a left facial cutaneous vascular malformation in the first and second division of the fifth cranial nerve (V1 and V2). Her left globe was slightly enlarged and proptotic. There was no increase in ocular pressure using the digital palpation method.

NEUROLOGICAL EXAMINATION

Mental status: She was alert and oriented to time, place, and person. She was able to spell the word "cat" forwards and backwards, but could not spell any 4-letter words or do simple arithmetic. She had a flat affect, appeared withdrawn, and would often not initiate conversation. She had slow processing speed. She followed all simple commands. Short-term memory was 3/3 at 5 minutes.

CNs II–XII testing revealed blurring of the left optic disc margins and a pale left optic disc. Her visual acuity was 20/20 in the right eye and 20/200 in the left eye. Visual fields were full to finger counting, extraocular movements were intact, and there was no nystagmus. Her face was symmetric but showed PWS on the left side (V1 and V2), and her tongue appeared midline without any atrophy. The uvula moved symmetrically. Trapezii and SCMs showed normal strength.

Motor: Revealed a mild right pronator drift but strength was 5/5 in both upper and lower extremities.

Sensory: Intact to all modalities.

Reflexes: Asymmetric, 3+ DTRs right side, 2+ DTRs left side.

Plantars: Right plantar reflex extensor and left plantar reflex flexor.

Gait: Normal.

STOP AND THINK QUESTIONS

➢ What is your differential diagnosis for her experience of fear?

➢ What is your differential diagnosis for a left facial cutaneous vascular malformation, seizures, glaucoma, migraines, and developmental delay?

➢ What test(s) would you perform to narrow your differential?

➢ What treatment(s) can you offer her?

DIAGNOSTIC TEST RESULTS

CBC, chemistry, and LFTs were all within normal limits. Carbamazepine level was 6.8 (normal 4–11).

Video EEG: The interictal EEG showed frequent low to medium amplitude left parietooccipital sharp waves and spikes that were most prominent in sleep (Figure 40.1A). Seven episodes of fear were captured that revealed ictal onset from the left temporal region (Figure 40.1B). She was able to press the button or tell her mom that she was feeling scared. She would then have subtle chewing movements and was not fully responsive to commands. During one episode, she was asked by the nurse to remember the color red. When the event was over, she could not recall the color. The EEG showed rhythmic left temporal 8 Hz activity, which slowed down to diffuse 3 to 4 Hz delta but maximal in the left temporal region (Figure 40.1B).

Brain MRI: Brain MRI with and without gadolinium demonstrated prominent leptomeningeal enhancement in the left occipital and parietal lobes consistent with leptomeningeal angiomatosis (Figure 40.2). An enlarged regional transmedullary vein can be seen in the left hemisphere in Figure 40.3. This probably represents as an alternative pathway for venous drainage as blood is shunted to the deep intracerebral venous system.

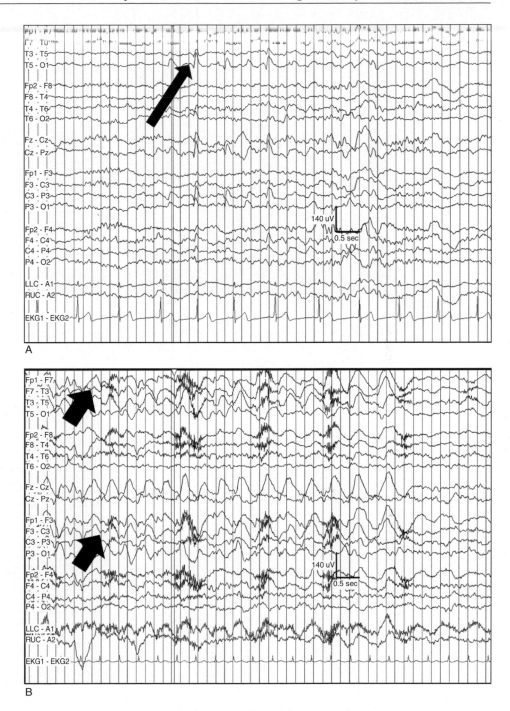

FIGURE 40.1 *Interictal EEG (A) demonstrating left occipital sharp waves (thin arrow). EEG during an episode of fear; (B) with rhythmic left hemisphere slowing, representing a seizure (thick arrows). The onset was in the left temporal lobe.*

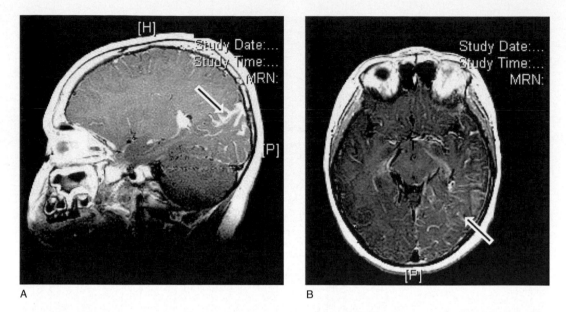

A B

FIGURE 40.2 *Gadolinium-enhanced MRI with a left-sided sagittal (A) and an axial (B) image demonstrating left parietal and occipital leptomeningeal enhnacement (arrow), signifying the patient's leptomeningeal angiomatosis.*

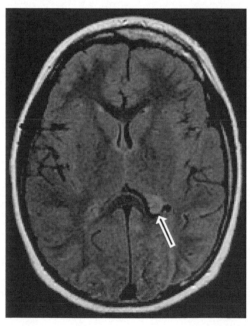

FIGURE 40.3 *Axial FLAIR MRI brain demonstrates an enlarged regional transmedullary vein (arrow) in the left hemisphere adjacent to the splenium of the corpus callosum. This image also shows very subtle left hemiatrophy caused by chronic hypoxia.*

DIAGNOSIS: Sturge-Weber syndrome (SWS), left-sided port-wine stain (PWS), an ipsilateral leptomeningeal angiomatosis, and left temporal seizures.

HOSPITAL COURSE

During the hospitalization, her carbamazepine dose was increased, and she was started on topiramate, with resolution of her electrographic seizures. She had two further episodes of fear that were without EEG correlate but could be surface negative simple partial seizures, or psychogenic events. A psychiatry consult was called to evaluate for a mood disorder and assist in helping the patient and the mother strategize regarding the bullying at school. The patient was discharged with follow-up with psychiatry and neurology.

DISCUSSION

SWS or encephalotrigeminal angiomatosis is a sporadic neurocutaneous syndrome affecting the cephalic venous microvasculature. Neurocutaneous disorders are also known as neurophakomatoses (Table 40.1) are characterized by a diverse set of symptoms that include both dermatologic and neurological manifestations, as well as the involvement of other organ systems. These disorders can have either a familial or sporadic inheritance pattern. In addition, neurocutaneous disorders are often associated with an increased risk of developing either benign or malignant neoplasms.

SWS is a rare (1 per 50,000 live births) neurocutaneous disorder that affects both sexes equally. There are no known prenatal or environmental risk factors. The disease is caused by a malformation of the embryonic vascular plexus that occurs within the cephalic mesenchyme. The abnormal vascular drainage leads to abnormal development of the face, eye, leptomeninges, and brain at 5 to 8 weeks of gestation. There is excessive proliferation of thin-walled vessels in the subarachnoid space. This arteriovenous malformation of the leptomeninges is referred to as "leptomeningeal angiomatosis," which steals blood supply from the adjacent brain parenchyma, causing ipsilateral cerebral atrophy.

The disease usually presents at birth with a facial cutaneous vascular malformation called a PWS over the area supplied by the first division of the fifth cranial nerve (V1). Interestingly, most children with a facial cutaneous vascular malformation do not have SWS. Rarely, some children with SWS do not have a PWS. There is altered fibronectin expression in the fibroblasts taken from PWS and the involved brain vasculature compared with normal tissue from controls. Fibronectin is believed to have effects on angiogenesis, vessel remodeling, and vessel innervation density, explaining the formation of cutaneous and cerebral angiomas.

Leptomeningeal angiomatosis develops primarily in the occipital and posterior parietal lobes, but it can affect any other lobe of the brain. It tends to be ipsilateral, but it can be bilateral. At birth, the leptomeningeal angioma is difficult to see, even with MRI. Over time, the meninges involved in the angioma thicken, and thick tortuous vessels develop. Underlying the abnormal meninges, the cortical vessels are thin and limited. This abnormal venous drainage causes chronic hypoperfusion and glucose hypometabolism, resulting in calcification, laminar cortical necrosis, and hemiatrophy. Overlying the cerebral hemiatrophy, the cranium can become hypertrophied. Enlarged centrally draining veins may develop (Figure 40.3) to compensate for poor superficial cortical drainage. Laminar cortical necrosis and calcification, not present in our patient, is best visualized by CT scan and is the cause of the characteristic "tram track" sign visible on X-ray of the skull. The syndrome of bilateral cortical calcifications related to celiac disease should be excluded in patients with bilateral angiomatoses. This syndrome can be distinguished from SWS by the bilateral and cortico-subcortical localization of the calcifications and by the absence of visible enhancement by gadolinium. Radiologic progression of SWS such as progressive cerebral atrophy and calcifications has been well documented.

SWS has complex symptomatology with seizures, glaucoma, headaches, mental retardation, stroke-like episodes, and behavioral disorders, such as ADHD. Developmentally, most children reach normal milestones in the first few months of life. The course then is variable and depends largely on the extent of neurological disease. Those with bilateral disease are more severely affected. The CNS involvement can be regional or hemispheric. Children with hemispheric SWS have an earlier and more severe clinical presentation.

TABLE 40.1 *Overview of Neurocutaneous Disorders*

Name of Disease	Inheritance Pattern	Genes/Protein	Incidence	Clinical Features
Sturge-Weber syndrome	Sporadic	Not applicable	1 in 50,000	Facial port-wine stain; glaucoma; choroid anima; headaches; seizures; leptomeningeal angiomatosis; intellectual disabilities; behavioral disorders; stroke-like episodes
Neurofibromatosis 1, Von Recklinghausen disease	50% are autosomal dominant, 50% are sporadic	NF1 gene (chromosome 17q 11.2)/ Neurofibromin	1 in 2,500 to 3,300	Café au lait spots; axillary or inguinal freckling; lisch nodules (iris hemartomas); neurofibromas; pheochromocytoma; optic nerve glioma; osseous lesions (e.g., sphenoid dysplasia or thinning of the cortex of long bones); learning disorders
Neurofibromatosis 2	50% are autosomal dominant; 50% are sporadic	NF2 (chromosome 22q12)/ merlin	1 in 25,000 to 40,000	Bilateral or unilateral vestibular schwannomas; glioma; meningioma; ependymoma; cataracts; café au lait spots are possible; neurofibromas
Tuberous sclerosis	50% are autosomal dominant; 50% are sporadic	TSC1 gene (chromosome 9q34)/ tuberin; TSC2 gene (chromosome 16p13)/ hemartin	1 in 6,000	Ash leaf spots; sebaceous adenoma; Shagreen patch; cortical tubers; seizures; mental retardation; subependymal nodules; subependymal giant cell astrocytomas; subungual fibromas; angiomyolipoma; rhabdomyoma; astrocytic hamartoma; lymphangioleiomyomatosis
Incontinentia pigmenti	X-linked dominant	NEMO gene (chromosome Xq28)	900 to 1,200 affected individuals have been reported	Lethal in males; characteristic skin lesions ("marble cake" hyperpigmentation); hypopigmented retina; seizures; mental retardation; spastic paralysis; strabismus; cataracts; retinal vascular changes
von Hippel-Lindau (VHL) syndrome	Autosomal dominant	VHL gene (chromosome 3p26)	1 in 36,000	Retinal hemangioblastoma; hemangioblastoma (commonly cerebellum, and spinal); renal cell carcinoma; pheochromocytoma
Hereditary hemorrhagic telangiectasia (Osler-Weber-Rendu syndrome)	Autosomal dominant	HHT1 gene (chromosome 9q34); HHT2 gene (chromosome 12q13)	1 in 5,000 to 10,000	Mucocutaneous telengiectasias; cerebral vascular malformations; ischemic stroke; epistaxis; gastrointestinal bleeding
Ataxia-telangiectasia	Autosomal recessive	ATM gene (chromosome 11q22)	1 in 40,000 to 100,000	Oculocutaneous telengiectasia; progressive ataxia; severe immune deficiencies; recurrent sinopulmonary infections; malignancy (most commonly non-Hodgkins lymphoma)
Xeroderma pigmentosum	Autosomal recessive	Genetically heterogenous	1 in 1,000,000	Photosensitivity; excessive freckling; developmental delay; ataxia; sensorineural hearing loss

Overall, 50% to 60% of those with SWS will have developmental delays, ADHD, learning disabilities, dyslexia, and intellectual disabilities are not uncommon.

Seizures are present in 75% to 90% of children with SWS and begin in infancy in the majority of cases (9). The seizures usually have an onset in the cortex underlying the leptomeningeal angiomatosis. Both clinical and subclinical seizures can occur. It is thought that seizures worsen neurological outcome, as the hypermetabolic state of a seizure intensifies the problem of limited superficial cortical venous drainage, leading to worsened hypoxia. Transcranial doppler and ictal SPECT studies have demonstrated that the usual hypermetabolism during a seizure is impaired in SWS. Clinically, there can be prolonged neurological deficits after seizures including homonymous hemianopia, hemiparesis, and hemisensory loss.

About 30% to 40% of patients will have migraine headaches, which are associated with frequent neurological deficits, particularly hemianopia and hemiparesis, which can last several hours after the headache has resolved. The etiology of migraine is thought to be secondary to the vasomotor disturbance within and around the angioma. Migraines have been described before and after both seizures and stroke-like episodes.

Stroke-like episodes with neurological deficits have been reported with varying temporal relationship to seizures and migraine headaches. The episodes have been described to last for hours to days and are postulated to be caused by venous thrombosis secondary to venous stasis. Vomiting, diarrhea, and fever can trigger stroke-like episodes, presumably by dehydration and a subsequent increased risk of thrombosis. Several studies have indicated that low-dose aspirin reduces the occurrence of these episodes.

If the PWS involves the eyelid, there may be ipsilateral ocular complications, the most common of which is glaucoma. Glaucoma is present in 30% to 70% of children with SWS and can be congenital or develops in the first 2 years of life. Neonates can have buphthalmos or "ox eye," which is characterized by enlargement of the eye and myopia as a result of glaucoma. Bilateral glaucoma can occur in 10% of the patients with bilateral leptomeningeal angiomatosis. The malformation of the anterior chamber angle, hypersecretion from a large choroid angioma, and elevated episcleral venous pressure are plausible explanations of increased intraocular pressure. Marked glaucomatous cupping may be seen in children with glaucoma. The normal choroidal vascular markings may not be visualized because of the presence of choroidal angioma. The choroidal angioma is diffuse and involves the posterior pole. The fundus findings are described as "Catsup" fundus as is seen in adults with choroid angiomas. Multiple dilated vessels and iris heterochromia, retinal, and choroid detachments are some other ocular findings.

In our patient, the interictal EEG has left occipital sharp waves, which is expected as the left occipital area underlies the leptomeningeal lesion. It is atypical to have ictal onset from the left medial temporal lobe. Regardless of etiology, having one area of the brain that is hyperexcitable and prone to seizures can over time "kindle" other distant areas of the brain. Seizures of the mesial temporal lobes can cause a variety of auras including sensations of déjà-vu, intense fear, euphoria, a rising sensation in the epigastrium, and a sense of being outside one's body (autoscopy). The sensations of intense emotions are thought to arise from the amygdala, which is part of the limbic system.

Her fear was not promptly diagnosed as seizure in part because she lacked the cognitive skills to describe it as brief, intense, and episodic. In addition, she was being bullied at school, and the fear was attributed to the bullying. When the seizures were captured in the epilepsy monitoring unit, it was clear that her sensorium was clouded during the event, making complex partial seizures. In simple partial seizures, there is no alteration in the

TABLE 40.2 *Treatment Options for Glaucoma*

Medical treatment	Beta blockers (Timolol), carbonic anhydrase inhibitors, brinzolamide and dorzolamide, sympathomimetics, propine and apraclonidine parasympathomimetics (pilocarpine); prostaglandin derivatives (xalatan)
Surgical	Goniotomy, trabeculotomy, trabeculectomy
Laser	Trabeculoplasty, sclerostomy, cycloablation

level of consciousness. Individuals with epilepsy sometimes are unaware of their auras and are amnestic for periods of unresponsiveness during seizures.

TREATMENT

Treatment for SWS includes regular monitoring for glaucoma, seizures, headache, and stroke-like episodes. Pulsed dye laser therapy of the facial nevus can prevent the development of soft tissue and bone overgrowth. Ophthalmology consultation is required for serial eye examinations. Congenital glaucoma may require geniotomy or trabeculotomy or trabeculectomy. Medical and surgical therapeutic options to treat glaucoma are listed in Table 40.2. Proton beam irradiation is used to control the growth of choroid angioma. Complete seizure control is the goal to limit neurological deterioration. As the syndrome is often comorbid with migraines, anti-epilepsy drugs that treat migraines, such as carbamazepine, valproate, gabapentin, oxcarbazepine, and topiramate, are often used.

Adequate seizure control can only be achieved in 40% of cases. Large epilepsy centers push for an early surgical intervention in patients with medically refractory seizures and progressive deficits. The first lobectomy for an angiomatous lesion was performed in 1936. Presurgical approaches and methods of surgery have advanced since then. Various approaches include:

- Resection of the pial angioma and removable of underlying cortex and calcification.
- Anatomic or functional hemispherectomy or hemispherotomy in patients with large hemispheric angiomatosis, progressive cerebral atrophy, and cognitive impairment or in children with previous hemiparesis.
- Corpus callosotomy for bilateral leptomeningeal disease, frequent tonic-clonic seizures or patients who cannot undergo hemispherectomy.

Prophylactic aspirin may reduce the rate of stroke-like episodes and may even decrease the frequency of seizures.

SUGGESTED READING

Bähr M, Schlagga BL. Chapter 70—Malformations and neurocutaneous disorders. In: *Neurological Disorders.* 2nd ed. 2003:947–969.

Comi AM, Weisz CJ, Highet BH. Sturge-Weber syndrome: Altered blood vessel fibronectin expression and morphology. *J Child Neurol.* 2005;20(7):572–527.

Hoffman HJ, Hendrick EB, Dennis M, et al., Hemispherectomy for Sturge-Weber syndrome. *Childs Brain.* 1979;5:233–248.

Jóźwiak S, Kotulska K. Gene table: Monogenic determined neurocutaneous disorders. *Eur J Paediatr Neurol.* 2010;14(5):449–451.

Kerrison, JB. Phacomatoses. In *Walsh and Hoyt's Clinical Neuro-ophthalmology.* 6th ed. Philadelphia, PA: Lippincott Williams & Wilkins, 2008; 1870–1878.

Kossoff, Eric H., Carol Buck, John M. Freeman. Outcomes of 32 hemispherectomies for Sturge-Weber syndrome worldwide. *Neurology.* 2002;59(11):1735–1738. *Neurology.org.* American Academy of Neurology. Web. 21 May 2011.

Kramer U, Kahana E, Shorer Z, Ben-Zeev B. Outcome of infants with unilateral Sturge-Weber syndrome and early onset seizures. *Dev Med Child Neurol.* 2000;42:756–759.

Maria BL, Neufeld JA, Rosainz LC, et al. Central nervous system structure and function in Sturge-Weber syndrome: Evidence of neurologic and radiologic progression. *J Child Neurol.* 1998;13(12):606–618.

Sujansky E, Conradi S. Sturge-Weber syndrome: Age of onset of seizures and glaucoma and the prognosis for affected children. Division of Genetics, University of Colorado School of Medicine, Children's Hospital, Denver 80218–1088, USA.

Thomas-Sohl KA, Vaslow DF, Maria BL. Sturge-Weber syndrome: A review. *Pediatric Neurology.* 2003;30(5):303–310.

Acute Left-Sided Weakness

Maria Philip, Vincci Ngan, and Anuradha Singh

CHIEF COMPLAINT: **Unresponsiveness and inability to use the left side of the body.**

HISTORY OF PRESENT ILLNESS

A 60-year-old, right-handed female who was witnessed to have fallen, unconscious, on the street and brought in by ambulance for further evaluation. The patient was given Narcan (Naloxone) by the EMS with no improvement. She remained lethargic in the ER and was only able to state that she felt dizzy before collapsing. She was noted to be looking only to the right and not moving her left arm and leg. A stroke alert was subsequently activated. The patient was evaluated by the stroke team at 1 hour 30 minutes after her symptom onset.

PAST MEDICAL HISTORY

Hypertension, osteoporosis.

PAST SURGICAL HISTORY

Remote cosmetic foot surgery, recent colonoscopy.

MEDICATIONS

None.

ALLERGIES

None.

PERSONAL HISTORY

No history of smoking or illicit drug use.

FAMILY HISTORY

Noncontributory.

PHYSICAL EXAMINATION

Vitals: Blood pressure, 130/84 mm Hg; pulse, 62/min; respiratory rate, 22/min; O_2 saturation, 99%; temperature, 98.3°F.
GPE: Thin-built female.
CVS, chest, abdomen: Unremarkable.
Peripheral pulses and skin: Normal.
Neck: No carotid bruits.

NEUROLOGICAL EXAMINATION

Mental status: Lethargic but arousable by voice or light touch; oriented to person, time, and place; follows simple commands.
CNs II–XII: Pupils are equal and reactive, forced deviation of the eyes to the right, unable to move eyes past midline; left visual field neglect; sensation intact to light touch in V1, V2, and V3 bilaterally; left facial droop; palate elevates symmetrically and uvula midline; shoulder shrug symmetric; tongue protrudes midline.

Motor: 5/5 in right upper and lower extremities; 0/5 in left upper extremity; 0/5 in distal left lower extremity and 2/5 in proximal left lower extremity.
Sensory: Left-sided extinction with double simultaneous stimulation to light touch.
Reflexes: 2+ symmetrical upper and lower extremities.
Plantars: Flexor on right, extensor on left.
Coordination: Not assessed.
Gait: Not assessed.

STOP AND THINK QUESTIONS

➤ What kinds of imaging results would give the most valuable information about a patient suspected of having an acute stroke?

➤ What is currently the only FDA-approved evidence-based treatment for a patient who has had an acute ischemic stroke?

DIAGNOSTIC TEST RESULTS

CBC, SMA-20, PT/PTT/INR normal.
CKMB 1.01 ng/ml; Troponin 0.016 ng/ml; hemoglobin A1C 6.0, serum cholesterol 213 mg/dl, LDL 131 mg/dl, HDL and triglycerides were normal.
EKG: Normal sinus rhythm.
Doppler lower extremities: No evidence of deep vein thrombosis.

DIAGNOSIS: Acute right MCA ischemic stroke.

HOSPITAL COURSE

Based on the clinical history and examination, a right MCA infarct was suspected. She was taken emergently to noncontrast head CT as well as a CT perfusion study. No hemorrhage was noted, but a hyperdense right MCA sign was seen (see Figure 41.1). Patient was initiated on IV tPA at approximately 2 hours 10 minutes after symptom onset and neuro-interventional service was contacted. However, given the lack of significant diffusion/perfusion mismatch (Figure 41.2A–D), no further interventional procedures were warranted. The patient was admitted to the stroke unit for monitoring and remained stable overnight. The following morning, the patient was noted to be more lethargic, had worsening left-sided weakness, and a dilated unreactive right pupil. An urgent CT was obtained showing no hemorrhage but worsening edema with 6 mm right-to-left midline shift (Figure 41.3). Mannitol was given while the patient was being prepped for the OR. The patient underwent emergent hemicraniectomy and expansile duraplasty (Figure 41.4). Her condition stabilized. She was able to communicate but she remained plegic in the left arm. Her gaze preference subsided.

DISCUSSION

Efficiency in diagnosis is crucial in the patient who is suspected of having an acute ischemic stroke, given the narrow therapeutic window for thrombolytics. The initial approach to the patient must include clinical stabilization of the patient, rapid neurological assessment, measurement of vital signs, fasting serum glucose, basic laboratory values, EKG recording as well a directed history of present illness and medical history. Of particular importance in these patients is the time of symptom onset, which is defined by the time the patient was last seen normal or symptom free. Information regarding the patient's risk factors for

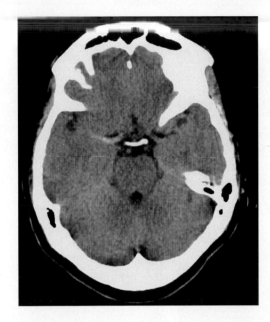

FIGURE 41.1 *NCHCT axial images showing "hyperdense MCA" sign; high attenuation expansion of the supraclinoid right internal carotid artery extending into the right M1 segment of the MCA.*

stroke as well as a previous history of medical conditions that could mimic stroke should be elicited from the patient or family members (Table 41.1).

Use of the NIHSS is helpful in quantifying the degree of neurological deficit as well as providing information regarding eligibility for therapeutic options and prognostic information (Table 41.2).

Certain diagnostic blood tests should routinely be performed in patients with suspected stroke that may help differentiate stroke from stroke mimics as well as providing important information necessary for therapeutic options. Vital signs and ABC should be assessed. These include blood glucose, electrolytes, CBC with platelet count, prothrombin time, activated partial thromboplastin time, international normalized ratio, and renal function studies. A 12-lead EKG and serum troponins should be done to rule out atrial fibrillation and myocardial infarction. Stroke team should be alerted. Serum lipid profile, ESR, thyroid function tests, and RPR should be sent to assess risk factors for stroke. Urinalysis, chest X-ray, urine h-CG (if child-bearing years) should be obtained in appropriate cases. The nursing staff should document height and weight of the patient and obtain neuro checks every 15 minutes in the acute phase.

A NCHCT should be performed soon after initial assessment to rule out intracranial hemorrhage which appears hyperdense (bright) on NCHCT. An ischemic stroke acutely may appear normal on NCHCT or may demonstrate early signs of ischemia such as a hyperdense MCA sign, loss of gray/white matter distinction, evidence of sulcal effacement, or loss of the insular ribbon.

The best imaging modality in the evaluation of ischemic stroke is MRI, which should routinely be done following the early management and treatment period. MRI has many advantages over CT including its ability to detect very small areas of infarct, providing more anatomical detail of the infarct and its vascular territory as well as its ability to distinguish acute from chronic cerebral infarctions. Brain stem strokes may be completely missed on the CT brain because of bony streak artifacts. The DWI and ADC sequences are especially useful in determining an acute stroke. Acute ischemic stroke appears

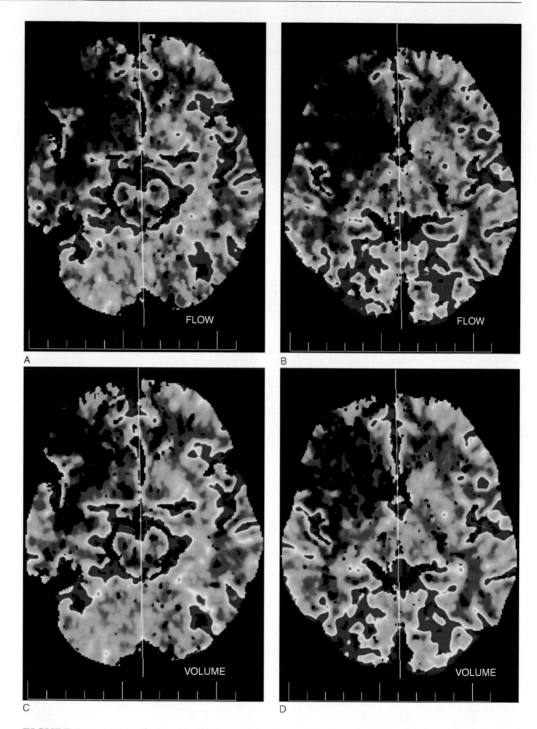

FIGURE 41.2 *CT perfusion (A–D) demonstrates matched cerebral blood volume and cerebral blood flow defects encompassing the entire right MCA territory. Mean transit time and time to peak maps also demonstrate corresponding areas of hypoperfusion, consistent with core area of infarction.*

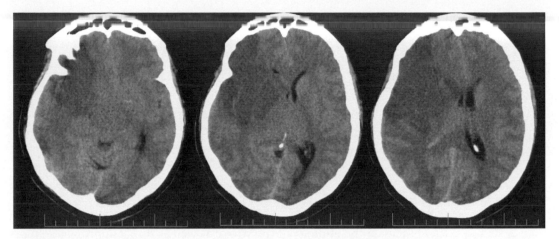

FIGURE 41.3 *Axial NCHCT showing evolution of the ischemic right MCA stroke with increasing cytotoxic edema and midline shift.*

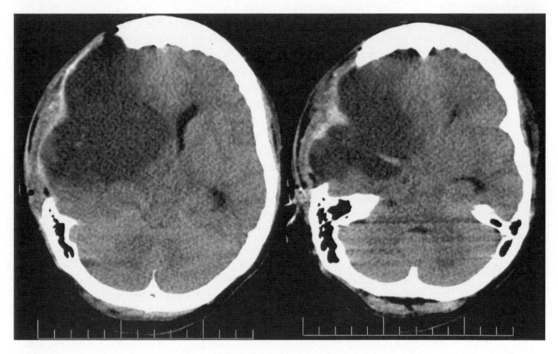

FIGURE 41.4 *Postoperative NCHCT axial images after right hemicraniectomy. The right cerebral hemisphere mildly bulges through the craniectomy defect.*

hyperintense (bright) on DWI and hypointense (dark) on ADC sequences. An important disadvantage of MRI is the time required for the study, which is why the relatively quick NCHCT is the primary imaging modality recommended for patients with suspected acute ischemic stroke so that therapeutic options may be quickly determined and administered if not otherwise contraindicated.

TABLE 41.1 *Stroke Mimics*

Nonthrombotic Causes of Neurological Deficits

Conversion disorder
Hepatic encephalopathy
Hyperglycemia
Hypoglycemia
Hyponatremia
Mass lesions
Migraines
Postictal states

Following early management and treatment, other diagnostic tests are necessary to further elucidate the etiology of the stroke as well as direct appropriate interventions for secondary stroke prevention.

TREATMENT

The treatment for patients with acute ischemic stroke who present within 3 hours of symptom onset is intravenous thrombolysis with tissue plasminogen activator, tPA (Table 41.3). TPA binds to fibrin and converts tissue plasminogen to plasmin, thus promoting fibrinolysis. The concept behind thrombolytic therapy is that cerebral hypoperfusion leads to a central area of irreversibly infarcted brain tissue surrounded by a presumably salvageable area of ischemic brain tissue known as the "penumbra." Therefore, tPA acts to reperfuse the penumbra by clot lysis.

Intravenous administration of tPA is the only FDA-approved medical treatment for patients with acute ischemic stroke. An important study contributing to its implementation was the NINDS study, which demonstrated that IV-tPA when given within 3 hours of symptom onset was 30% more likely to have minimal or no disability at 3 months as compared to placebo. Interestingly, there was no significant difference in clinical improvement at 24 hours of treatment between treatment and placebo groups. Therefore, it is important to keep in mind that the use of tPA in acute ischemic stroke is instituted because of the improvement seen in long term rather than early recovery. Another important study is the ECASS III study which looked specifically at the expansion of the treatment time window from 3 to 4.5 hours. This study demonstrated a favorable outcome at 90 days for patients treated with IV tPA as compared to placebo despite being treated 3 to 4.5 hours after symptom onset. The American Heart Association and American Stroke Association guidelines for the early management of acute ischemic stroke have not yet reflected the results of the ECASS III study and at this point only recommend IV tPA given within the 3 hours of symptom onset. The most important complication of IV tPA is intracranial hemorrhage. Symptomatic intracranial hemorrhage occurred in 6.4% of treated patients in the NINDS trial as compared to 0.6% of the placebo group.

Other treatment modalities are available for certain patients with acute ischemic stroke depending on their presentation and also the availability of therapeutic options at the stroke center. This includes administration of intra-arterial tPA, which is an option for patients presenting within 6 hours of symptoms onset with evidence of an MCA infarction. Other endovascular interventions such as mechanical clot disruption, clot extraction, and angioplasty and stenting require further studies to establish them as treatment

TABLE 41.2 *National Institute of Health Stroke Scale*

Tested Item	Title	Responses and Scores
1A	Level of consciousness	0—alert 1—drowsy 2—obtunded 3—coma/unresponsive
1B	Orientation questions (2)	0—answers both correctly 1—answers one correctly 2—answers neither correctly
1C	Response to commands (2)	0—performs both tasks correctly 1—performs one task correctly 2—performs neither
2	Gaze	0—normal horizontal movements 1—partial gaze palsy 2—complete gaze palsy
3	Visual fields	0—no visual field defect 1—partial hemianopia 2—complete hemianopia 3—bilateral hemianopia
4	Facial movement	0—normal 1—minor facial weakness 2—partial facial weakness 3—complete unilateral palsy
5	Motor function (arm) a. Left b. Right	0—no drift 1—drift before 5 seconds 2—falls before 10 seconds 3—no effort against gravity 4—no movement
6	Motor function (leg) a. Left b. Right	0—no drift 1—drift before 5 seconds 2—falls before 10 seconds 3—no effort against gravity 4—no movement
7	Limb ataxia	0—no ataxia 1—ataxia in 1 limb 2—ataxia in 2 limbs
8	Sensory	0—no sensory loss 1—mild sensory loss 2—severe sensory loss
9	Language	0—normal 1—mild aphasia 2—severe aphasia 3—mute or global aphasia
10	Articulation	0—normal 1—mild dysarthria 2—severe dysarthria
11	Extinction	0—absent 1—mild (loss 1 sensory modality) 2—severe (loss 2 modalities)

TABLE 41.3 *t-PA Indications*

Characteristics of patients with ischemic stroke who could be treated with tPA

No evidence of intracranial hemorrhage or suggestive of subarachnoid hemorrhage
Diagnosis of ischemic stroke causing measurable neurological deficit
Neurological signs should not be minor or clearing spontaneously
Caution should be exercised in treating a patient with major deficits.
Onset of symptoms <3 hours before beginning treatment
No head trauma or prior stroke in previous 3 months
No myocardial infarction in the previous 3 months
No gastrointestinal or urinary tract hemorrhage in previous 21 days
No major surgery in the previous 14 days
No arterial puncture at a noncompressible site in the previous 7 days
No history of previous intracranial hemorrhage
Blood pressure not elevated (systolic <185 mm Hg and diastolic <110 mm Hg)
No evidence of active bleeding or acute trauma (fracture) on examination
Not taking an oral anticoagulant or, if anticoagulant being taken, INR ≤ 1.7
If receiving heparin in previous 48 hours, aPTT must be in normal range
Platelet count ≥100,000 mm^3
Blood glucose concentration ≥50 mg/dL (2.7 mmol/L)
No seizure with postictal residual neurological impairments
CT does not show a multilobar infarction (hypodensity >1/3 cerebral hemisphere).
The patient or family members understand the potential risks and benefits from treatment

TABLE 41.4 *Vascular Risk Factors of Stroke*

High blood pressure	Smoking
Atrial fibrillation	Obesity
Diabetes mellitus	Physical inactivity
Myocardial infarction	Heavy alcohol use
Carotid artery disease	Hyperhomocystinemia
High cholesterol	

options. Ultimately, the experience of a stroke center in its ability to provide these alternative treatments is most important in offering it as a treatment option.

Vascular risk factors should be identified and modified (Table 41.4). With stroke, "time is brain." Management of acute stroke is a true emergency. Stroke care units with specially trained neurologists in stroke and supporting staff show improved outcomes. Comorbid medical problems need to be addressed. Assessments of swallow function prior to the reinstitution of oral feeding are recommended. Patients should receive deep venous thrombosis prophylaxis, although the timing of institution of this therapy is unknown. Table 41.5 enlists the management of acute stroke and prevention of complications. Transient ischemic attacks should be recognized and worked up in a timely manner. Failure to perform a timely assessment for stroke risk factors or administer t-PA when indicated can expose neurologists to medical litigations. Neurologists should initiate primary and secondary stroke prevention to reduce undue risk of stroke in the future.

TABLE 41.5 *Management of Stroke Patients in the Acute and Chronic Phase*

ABCs; adequate oxygenation, 2L nasal O_2
Treat hypotension
Avoid over hydration
Avoid hyperglycemia (↑ blood sugar increases the size of infarction and reduces functional outcome)
Monitor input and output
Avoid hypermetabolic states such as fever or hyperglycemia
Avoid and treat hypotension
Hypothermia may reduce mortality
Treat BP first if BP> 185/110 mm Hg if patient is a candidate for fibrinolytics; BP in the range of 180–230/110–140 mm Hg should be treated.
Treat increased intracranial pressure: head elevation up to 30°, mannitol, diuretics, barbiturates, neurosurgical decompression (especially young patients and non-dominant side), maintain $PaCO_2$ of 30 mm Hg.
Management of seizures: anticonvulsants (Keppra preferred because of least drug-to-drug interactions with coumadin or statins, other choices include trileptal or tegretol, lamictal)
Prevention of complications
  —prevent aspiration by withholding oral feeding until intact swallowing is demonstrated. Nasogastric or percutaneous enteral gastrostomy
  —frequent changes of the patient's position
  —pulmonary physical therapy
  —recognition of early symptoms and signs of UTI and early treatment
  —DVT and PE prevention: good hydration, low-dose low molecular weight heparin
  —prevent falls: ensure good bone health, orthotic, and assistive device
Prevention of recurrent stroke (modifications of risk factors, use of antiplatelet therapy {aspirin, Persantine, Aggrenox, Plavix}, Coumadin, Dabigatran)
Supportive treatment (physical and occupational therapy; speech therapy and cognitive therapy
Depression and behavioral disorders (psychotherapy, cognitive behavioral therapy, antidepressant).

SUGGESTED READING

Adams H, Del Zoppo G, Alberts M, et al. Guidelines for the early management of adults with ischemic stroke: A guideline from the American Hearth Association/American Stroke Association Stroke Council, Clinical Cardiology Council, Cardiovascular Radiology and Intervention Council, and the Atherosclerotic Peripheral Vascular Disease and Quality of CAre Outcomes in Research Interdisciplinary Working Groups. *Stroke.* 2007;38:1655–1711.

Hacke W, Kaste M, Bluhmki E, et al. Thrombolysis with alteplase 3 to 4.5 hours after acute ischemic stroke. *N Engl J Med.* 2008;359:1317–1329.

The National Institute of Neurological Disorders and Stroke rt-PA Stroke Study Group. Tissue plasminogen activator for acute ischemic stroke. *N Engl J Med.* 1995;333:1581–1587.

Left-Sided Neck Pain Followed by Difficulty Reading, Performing Motor Tasks, and Speaking

Jonathan H. Howard

CHIEF COMPLAINT: **I am having difficulty moving and speaking.**

HISTORY OF PRESENT ILLNESS

Patient was a 45-year-old, right-handed man who was in his usual state of health until 2 days before admission when he developed left-sided neck pain after carrying luggage at the airport. The patient said the pain felt like a small knife in his neck, but he did not seek medical attention. On the day of admission, he noticed that he had difficulty reading a newspaper, saying that he could only read the left half of a line of text before his eyes would move to the next line. The patient went to make a cup of coffee to "perk himself up." Though he did not feel weak, he had great difficulty with this task. He found himself unable to properly operate his coffee machine or even adequately pour milk into his cup. He tried to ask his wife for help, but she noticed that he was having difficulty forming words properly and called 911. When the ambulance arrived, the patient had difficulty answering basic questions about himself. He understood the questions being asked of him, and he knew the answers to the questions he was being asked, but was unable to say more than one or two words in response. When asked where he worked, for example, the patient was only able to say "computers." By the time the patient arrived to the emergency room 30 minutes later, both he and his wife felt that he had returned to normal.

PAST MEDICAL HISTORY

None

MEDICATIONS

None

ALLERGIES

None

PERSONAL HISTORY

No history of smoking and recreational drug abuse, and drinks socially.

FAMILY HISTORY

Noncontributory.

PHYSICAL EXAMINATION

Blood pressure, 128/78 mm Hg; pulse, 78/min, regular; no carotid bruits.
Chest, CVS, abdomen, skin, and musculoskeletal examination was unremarkable.

NEUROLOGICAL EXAMINATION

Higher mental functions: On examination in the emergency room, the patient was awake and alert and appeared comfortable. His spontaneous speech was fluent; he could follow

301

complex commands and repeat complex phrases. Naming was intact. He could read and write well.

Cranial nerves II–XII: Patient's left pupil was pin point, even in a dark room, though it was reactive to light, and his left eyelid was droopy. His visual acuity and visual fields were intact. Rest of the cranial nerve examination was normal.

Motor: Patient had a mild right pronator drift with his fingertips curling on his right hand. This disappeared by the time the patient reached the floor several hours later. He was able to perform complex motor tasks.

Sensory: Intact to all modalities of sensations.

Reflexes: Symmetrical.

Plantars: Down on both sides.

Romberg's: Negative.

Cerebellar: Negative.

STOP AND THINK QUESTIONS

➢ Where could the lesion be in this patient?

➢ What are the risk factors for this type of injury?

➢ What is the significance of the eye findings in this patient?

➢ How does the injury explain the patient's transient symptoms?

DIAGNOSTIC TEST RESULTS

MRI of the brain showed scattered T2 hyperintensities in the subcortical/frontal white matter bilaterally. There was no restricted diffusion to suggest an acute stroke.

MRA of the head with contrast was unremarkable.

CTA brain axial images showed dissected left ICA (Figure 42.1A); CTA neck revealed severe stenosis of the ascending cervical segment of the left ICA (Figure 42.1B).

Cerebral angiogram demonstrated the dissection of the left ICA. Contrast flowed throughout the left ICA showing the artery was not entirely occluded. Injection of the right ICA, however, showed that all significant blood flow to the left cerebral hemisphere came through the circle of Willis and the posterior circulation. There was no evidence of disease in any other vessel.

DIAGNOSIS: Left internal carotid artery (ICA) dissection.

DISCUSSION

Blood is carried from the heart to the brain by paired carotid and vertebral arteries. A CAD occurs when there is a tear in the tunica intima or between the tunica media and tunica adventitia of an artery such that blood flows between layers of the blood vessel rather than through the lumen of the artery. In the vast majority of cases, the ICA is affected extracranially, 2 cm after the bifurcation of the common carotid artery.

A CAD can create an intramural hematoma, which can result in narrowing of the carotid artery or an aneurysmal dilatation. This, is turn, may lead to focal neurological symptoms by emboli traveling through the vessel to the brain, or less commonly via hypoperfusion from stenosis of the vessel. Ischemic events occur in 30% to 80% of cases of CAD as either TIA or completed strokes. In one series of 78 patients with CAD, 71% presented with a completed stroke, 13% presented with a TIA, and 17% presented with symptoms directly referable to the ICA itself. In patients with a traumatic CAD, strokes tend to occur at the

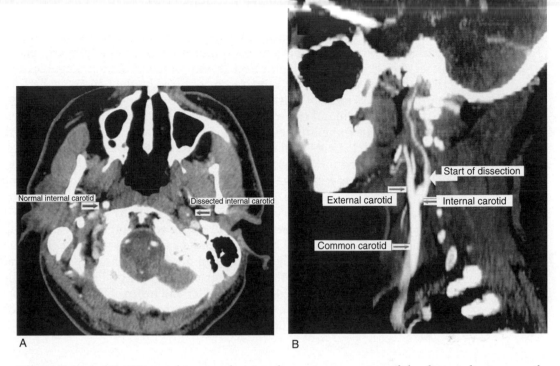

FIGURE 42.1 *(A) CTA axial images showing the severe narrowing of the dissected artery on the left. (B) CTA shows severe narrowing of the internal carotid artery (white arrow) shortly after the bifurcation of the common carotid artery. A thin flow of blood is visible in the artery, termed the "string sign."*

time of the trauma, though there can be a delay by several days. Overall, CAD is a relatively uncommon cause of stroke or TIA with incidence estimated to be 2.6 to 2.9 per 100,000. Unlike other causes of stroke, however, dissections occur far more commonly in otherwise young (younger than 50), healthy people. CAD accounts for up to 25% of ischemic strokes in these patients.

Most often, the presenting complaint in a patient with CAD is a vascular event. This may be transient monocular blindness due to an embolus to the ophthalmic artery. Other patients, such as the patient in this case, present with a cerebral vascular syndrome. The patient suffered a TIA that manifested itself as a right homonymous hemianopsia (he could not read his newspaper), an apraxia (he could not make himself a cup of coffee), and eventually an expressive aphasia such that he could not answer questions properly. The likely etiology of these symptoms was a thrombus through the narrowed (though not occluded) carotid artery traveling to the left hemisphere. The patient was quite fortunate he did not suffer from any permanent neurological damage.

A second presenting complaint in patients with CAD is ipsilateral neck pain or headache. The pain is often quite stabbing and sharp and may localize to the anterior part of the neck. Such pain is seen in only half of patients with CAD, however, and is more characteristic of VAD than of CAD. Another characteristic of CAD is a partial Horner's syndrome (ptosis and miosis) due to disruption of the sympathetic fibers that travel along with the ICA. A Horner's syndrome is present in approximately 40% of patients. Other signs of a CAD include an absent carotid pulse, a carotid bruit, pulsatile tinnitus, or lower cranial nerve defects, the hypoglossal nerve in particular, if mass effect develops from an ICA aneurysm.

Risk factors for CAD include conditions that weaken the walls of blood vessels. Fibromuscular dysplasia is the most common of these, but illnesses such as Marfan's syndrome and Ehlers-Danlos syndrome are risks as well. Other risk factors include dyslipidemia, smoking, or taking oral contraceptives. Additionally, many people with carotid dissection are able to recall some neck trauma or manipulation that preceded the dissection. This "trauma" may be quite mild and recognized by the patient at the time. Chiropractic manipulation is more of a risk factor for VAD than for CAD.

There is a 1% annual risk of recurrent CAD, and the greatest risk seems to be in the first month after the initial dissection. Previously unaffected vessels are at greater risk than the original vessel. Patients with extracranial CAD typically have a good prognosis, with 70% of patients having mild or no residual neurological deficits. There is a 5% mortality rate, usually in patients with large hemispheric strokes. Patients with intracranial CAD have a worse prognosis.

Imaging is necessary to confirm the diagnosis of any dissection. The "gold standard" for diagnosis remains conventional four-vessel angiography. The pathognomonic finding is an intimal flap, or double lumen, secondary to an intramural hematoma. Additionally, as with our patient, a so-called string sign may be seen as only a small trail of contrast is able to travel through the lumen of the artery. Because of the time, cost, and 1% complication rate associated with angiography, MRA and helical CTA are being increasingly used. Indications of a CAD on MRA also include an intramural hematoma or a double lumen. A CTA, as in this case, will show a marked narrowing of the ICA lumen.

TREATMENT

Anticoagulation with intravenous heparin followed by warfarin is generally accepted as the treatment of choice for CAD. Patients are typically kept on anticoagulation with a target INR of 2 to 3 for 3 to 6 months, and imaging studies are repeated in this time frame to evaluate for recanalization of the vessel. Most patients with CAD heal spontaneously, and if there is evidence of recanalization, the patient can be taken off all medicines or switched to antiplatelet agents. There is no evidence base to support this practice, however, and a meta-analysis of over 286 patients found that initial treatment with antiplatelet agents seems to be just as effective as anticoagulation. Further investigations are needed to clarify optimal treatment.

Surgical or endovascular stenting of the ICA can be considered for those few patients who remain symptomatic while on anticoagulation. Ligation of the ICA is an option for treating refractory patients who have a patent ICA, yet have no meaningful cerebral blood flow through the artery as determined by a conventional angiogram. This procedure prevents thrombi from traveling to the brain from the ICA without compromising blood flow.

SUGGESTED READING

Dziewas R, Konrad C, Drager B, et al. Cervical artery dissection—clinical features, risk factors, therapy and outcome in 126 patients. *J Neurol.* 2003;250(10):1179–1184.

Georgiadis D, Caso V, Baumgartner RW. Acute therapy and prevention of stroke in spontaneous carotid dissection. *Clin Exp Hypertens.* 2006;28(3–4):365–370.

Schievink WI. Spontaneous dissection of the carotid and vertebral arteries. *N Engl J Med.* 2001;344(12): 898–906.

CHIEF COMPLAINT: **My father has been falling a lot.**

HISTORY OF PRESENT ILLNESS

The patient is a 64-year-old, right-handed male who was seen in the neurobehavioral clinic for management of PD. The patient's symptoms reportedly began at age 56 when he noted a left-hand tremor. Gradually, he started noticing slowness in his physical activities and increased difficulty walking. He was formally evaluated and diagnosed with PD at age 58 at an outside hospital and was started on Sinemet with some improvement in his symptoms. However, his gait difficulties have progressed to the point that the patient required a cane for ambulation by age 60, a walker by age 62, and has been using a wheelchair for the past 6 months.

He reported that his most distressing symptoms have been difficulty with ambulation and trouble with his speech. His symptoms fluctuate depending on the timing of his medications; he had wearing-off effects 3 hours after taking Sinemet. During his "off" periods, he experiences worsening of his tremor, decreased movements, and low speech volume. He also noted having abnormal movements within a short period of taking each Sinemet dose, which interfere with his ADL, such as eating and dressing himself. He reported that these movements had improved since the recent addition of amantadine to his medication regimen. However, given the severity of his symptoms and worsening quality of life, he indicated interest in undergoing evaluation for DBS.

He denied experiencing nightmares, visual or other hallucinations, obsessional thinking, or compulsive behaviors. He denied having any significant cognitive or affective symptoms including loss of attention or memory, depression, or any negative thoughts. He denied having problems related to sleep but endorsed some mild daytime sleepiness. He endorsed intermittent urinary urgency, necessitating the use of diapers. He reported experiencing lightheadedness upon standing but denied loss of consciousness. He endorsed a decreased sense of smell, intermittent constipation and a weight loss of 15 pounds in the past year that he attributed to dental issues resulting in difficulty with chewing and swallowing. He reported increasing falls, drooling, and difficulty using his hands.

PAST MEDICAL HISTORY

PD, diet-controlled diabetes mellitus type II, restrictive lung disease.

PAST SURGICAL HISTORY

None.

MEDICATIONS

Pramipexole 1.25 mg: PO TID
Entacapone 200 mg: PO at 8 a.m., 11 a.m., 3 p.m., 7 p.m.
Carbidopa/Levodopa 25/100 mg: 2 tabs at 8 a.m., 2 tabs at 11 a.m., 2 tabs at 3 p.m., 1 tab at 7 p.m.
Amantadine 100 mg: BID

ALLERGIES

None.

PHYSICAL EXAMINATION

Vital signs: Temperature, 98.6°F; O_2 saturation, 98% RA; respiratory rate, 15 breaths/min.
Supine: Blood pressure, 116/89 mm Hg; pulse, 68.
Standing: Blood pressure 108/85 mm Hg; pulse, 76.
General: Well-appearing African American man, sitting in wheelchair, notable dyskinetic movements of left arm and trunk at rest.

PERSONAL HISTORY

Smoked 1 pack per day for 20 years but quit 18 years ago. Does not use alcohol and has no history of illicit drug use. Lives with spouse.

FAMILY HISTORY

Patient was adopted and thus does not know if he has a history of movement disorders.

NEUROLOGICAL EXAMINATION

Mental status: Alert, oriented to conversation. Mini-mental state examination (refer to Appendix 43.I) with 24/30; losing points for cube copy, reverse digit span, serial sevens (3/5), verbal fluency (seven words), recall (4/5), and orientation (date only).
CNs I–XII: Anosmia, PERRL, EOMI without nystagmus, normal smooth pursuits, visual fields full, no facial asymmetry, masked facies, hearing intact bilaterally to finger rub, tongue and palate midline, SCM equal, shrug with slower activation of left side.
Motor: Strength 5/5 throughout but with slowed activation of left side compared to right side.
Sensory: Intact to light touch, pin prick, temperature, position and vibration throughout.
Reflexes: 2+ symmetrical biceps, triceps, brachioradialis, patellar, ankle jerks bilaterally.
Plantars: Flexor responses bilaterally.
Frontal lobe signs: Negative.
Cerebellar: Finger-to-nose slow but without dysmetria.
Romberg's sign: Negative.
Movement disorder examination: Masked facies, moderate hypomimia and hypophonia. Negative Myerson's sign. Rigidity in both arms and intermittent cogwheeling with contralateral activation (more notable on the left side compared to right). Moderate bradykinesia in the left arm on rapid alternating movements, more mild on the right. Moderate full body Bradykinesia. Moderate–severe dyskinesias of trunk, head/neck, and extremities. Dyskinesias were more remarkable in arms than legs (L>R), worsening with voluntary movements. There were no tremors at rest or action. Postural reflexes were intact on formal pull test. Gait showed stooped posture, short stride length but not festinating gait, notable dyskinesias of legs with ambulation, decreased arm swing bilaterally (L>R), and turning en bloc. He was unable to tandem, toe walk, or heel walk.

Unified Parkinson's Disease Rating Scale (see Appendix 43.II):

I. Behavior:
Mentation 2
Thought Disorder 0
Depression 1
Motivation 1
TOTAL I = 4

II. ADL.
Speech 2
Salivation 2
Swallowing 1
Handwriting 1
Cutting food 1
Dressing 3
Hygiene 1
Turning in Bed 1
Falling 2
Freezing 2
Walking 3
Tremor 1
Sensory Symptoms 0
TOTAL II = 20

III. Motor:
Speech 3
Facial Expression 1
Tremor at rest:
Face 0, Right hand 0, Left hand 0, Right foot 0, Left foot 0
Action tremor:
Right hand 0, Left hand 0
Rigidity:
Neck 1, Right hand 1, Left hand 1, Right leg 2, Left leg 2
Finger Taps:
Right 2, Left 3
Hand grips:
Right 1, Left 1
Hand pronate/supine:
Right 2, Left 2
Leg Agility
Right 3, Left 3
Arise from chair 0
Posture 1
Gait 3
Postural Stability 2
Body Bradykinesia 2
TOTAL III = 36

SUM TOTAL = 60

DIAGNOSTIC TEST RESULTS

CBC, BMP, LFTs, TSH, RPR, Vitamin B_{12} unremarkable.
MRI brain without gadolinium: Mild microvascular disease.

DIAGNOSIS: **Parkinson's disease (PD) (Hoehn and Yahr Stage: 4.0, see Appendix 43.III). Schwab and England ADL: 60% (see Appendix 43.IV).**

DISCUSSION

PD is a progressive neurodegenerative disorder that is characterized by four cardinal features: Bradykinesia, rest tremor, rigidity, and postural instability. The "premotor" symptoms, symptoms that typically develop in patients prior to the onset of motor difficulties, include loss of smell (anosmia), constipation, anxiety/depression, sleep disorders, and dysautonomia. The peak age of onset is in the early 60s (range 35–85 years), and the course of the illness ranges between 10 and 25 years. PD accounts for ~75% of all cases of parkinsonism. A diagnosis of PD can be made with some confidence in patients who present with at least two of the three cardinal signs—rest tremor, rigidity, and bradykinesia. Tremor is present in 85% of patients with PD; a diagnosis of PD is difficult and often alternate diagnosed are entertained when tremor is absent. A unilateral and gradual onset of symptoms further supports the diagnosis.

MOTOR FEATURES

Bradykinesia (slowness of movement) causes decreased manual dexterity and micrographia (small handwriting). Soft speech (hypophonia), masked facies (hypomimia), and sialorrhea are the manifestations of bulbar bradykinesia. Masked facies, decreased eye blinking, micrographia, hypophonia, stooped posture, and decreased arm swing are some of the commonly encountered clinical findings on examination.

Rest tremor, at a frequency of 4–6 Hz, often has a "pill-rolling" character and is most evident in the hands and wrists. Tremor typically starts on one side before appearing on the other side after a year or more. It may appear later in the lips, tongue, and jaw but usually spares the neck.

Rigidity is felt as a uniform resistance to passive movement around a joint throughout the full range of motion. "Cogwheeling" occurs due to regular brief interruptions of resistance due to subclinical tremor, and although is a classic feature, is often not present on examination. Dystonia of the distal extremities may occur early in the disease, unrelated to treatment, especially in younger patients. It can also be provoked by antiparkinsonian drug therapy.

Gait disturbance with short shuffling steps and a tendency to turn en bloc is a prominent feature of PD. Festinating gait results from the combination of flexed posture and loss of postural reflexes, which cause the patient to accelerate in an effort to "catch up" with the body's center of gravity. Freezing of gait, a feature of more advanced PD, is common at the onset of locomotion (start hesitation), when attempting to change direction or turn around, and upon entering a crowded room or narrow space.

Abnormalities of balance and posture tend to increase as the disease progresses. Flexion of the head, stooping and tilting of the upper trunk, and a tendency to hold the arm in a flexed posture while walking are common. Postural instability is a very disabling feature of advanced PD, contributing to falls and injuries and leading to major morbidity and mortality. It can be tested in the office with the "pull test," in which the examiner stands behind the patient and asks the patient to maintain their balance when pulled backwards. The examiner pulls back briskly to assess the patient's ability to recover. While performing this test, extreme caution should be taken to prevent any falls.

In patients with advancing disease the phenomenon of motor fluctuations can develop. These patients fluctuate between periods of time during which their medications work and they are "on," and periods of time during which their medications do not work and they are "off." Frequently, the "on" time may be accompanied by Sinemet-induced dyskinesias or extra abnormal movements.

NONMOTOR FEATURES

Depression, anxiety, cognitive impairment, sleep disturbances, sensory abnormalities and pain, anosmia, and disturbances of autonomic function are common in PD. Some of these nonmotor disturbances may be present long before the onset of motor signs. Sleep disorders, sleep apnea, and impaired daytime alertness are common in PD. Restless leg syndrome and

REM (rapid eye movement) behavioral sleep disorder can precede the onset of motor signs of PD. REM behavior sleep disorder refers to a condition in which patients are not paralyzed during their dreams and therefore act them out, with potentially violent behavior and screaming. Vivid dreams and hallucinations may be related to dopaminergic therapy. Autonomic dysfunction can include orthostatic hypotension, constipation, urinary urgency and frequency, sexual dysfunction, excessive sweating, and seborrhea. Paroxysms of drenching sweats occur in advanced PD possibly due to "wearing-off" effects of anti-parkinsonian medications. Sensory symptoms, which manifest as a distressing sensation of inner restlessness or akathisia, can also occur during "off" periods. Pain and discomfort in the extremities can occur in the initial stages of disease or as a "wearing-off" effect in late disease. Subjective shortness of breath in the absence of any underlying cardiorespiratory pathology is also reported.

Neuropsychiatric symptoms such as changes in mood, cognition, and behavior are very common in PD. Depression affects approximately half of patients with PD and its recognition and early treatment is important to improve quality of life for PD patients. Anxiety is also very common. This can be an "off" phenomenon, provoked by under treatment of motor symptoms. In severe cases, the "offs" may mimic panic attacks.

Cognitive abnormalities are very common in PD and the incidence of significant dementia is six times higher than age-matched controls. Executive function is usually affected, with cognitive arenas such as language and simple mathematical skills, relatively spared. Predictors

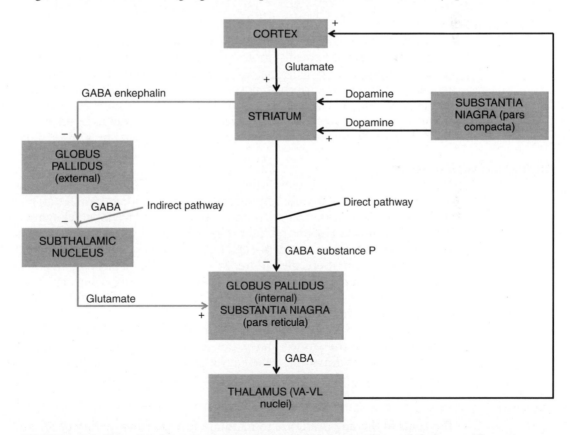

FIGURE 43.1 *Functional circuitry between the cortex, basal ganglia, and thalamus. The major neurotransmitters are indicated. In PD, there is degeneration of the pars compacta of the substantia nigra, leading to overactivity in the indirect pathway (gray) and increased glutamatergic activity by the subthalamic nucleus.*

of dementia include late age of onset, akinetic-rigid phenotype, and presence of severe depression, persistent hallucinations, and advanced stages of disease. Psychotic symptoms affect up to 40% of patients with PD. Dopaminergic drug therapy can contribute to psychotic symptoms.

ICDs, such as pathologic gambling, hypersexuality, compulsive shopping, and compulsive eating, are seen in PD and are often associated with the use of dopaminergic agents. Punding or stereotypical motor behavior that manifests as repetitive handling and examining of mechanical objects, such as picking at oneself, taking apart watches and radios, or sorting and arranging common objects, is common in PD as well.

PATHOPHYSIOLOGY

Gross examination of the brain shows mild frontal atrophy with loss of melanin in the midbrain. Microscopically, there is degeneration of the dopaminergic cells. In addition, Lewy bodies, the pathological hallmark of the disease, which represents abnormal accumulation of alpha-synuclein, are present in the remaining neurons and processes of the SNpc, other brain stem nuclei, and cortex. The pathology appears first in the anterior olfactory nuclei and lower brain stem, after which it ascends through the brain stem to the amygdala, SNpc, thalamus, and cortex. Involvement of these extranigral areas is postulated to play a role in the nonmotor and levodopa-unresponsive motor aspects of PD. Figure 43.1 details the functional circuitry between the cortex, basal ganglia, and thalamus.

NATURAL HISTORY

In patients with newly diagnosed PD, older age at onset and rigidity/hypokinesia as an initial symptom can be used to predict more rapid rate of motor progression and earlier development of cognitive decline and dementia. The presence of associated comorbidities (stroke, auditory deficits, and visual impairments), postural instability and gait disorder (PIGD), and male sex may be used to predict faster rates of motor progression. Tremor as a presenting symptom may predict a more benign course and longer therapeutic benefit to levodopa. Older age at onset, dementia, and decreased dopamine responsiveness are poor prognostic indicators.

DIFFERENTIAL DIAGNOSIS

The differential diagnosis of parkinsonism is listed in Table 43.1. The following clinical features in early stages of disease help suggest a diagnosis other than PD: (a) falls at presentation and early in the disease course, (b) poor response to levodopa, (c) symmetry at onset, (d) rapid progression to Hoehn and Yahr stage 3 in 3 years, (e) lack of tremor, and (f) dysautonomia (urinary urgency/incontinence and fecal incontinence, urinary retention requiring catheterization, persistent erectile failure, or symptomatic orthostatic hypotension). Levodopa and apomorphine challenge can be considered for confirmation when the diagnosis of PD is in doubt; however, it is unclear if it has any advantage over clinical criteria. Olfaction testing should be considered to differentiate PD from PSP and CBD, but not PD from MSA.

DaT SCAN, a SPECT imaging modality that has been in use in Europe and was just FDA approved in the United States, images the dopamine transporter. This test can reliably determine if a dopamine deficiency is present, but cannot distinguish between PD and Parkinson plus syndromes, all of which have a dopamine deficiency.

TREATMENT

The goals of therapy in PD are to maintain function and quality of life and to avoid drug-induced complications. Patients should be treated as soon as symptoms begin to interfere with function.

The aim of all dopaminomimetic strategies is to restore dopamine transmission in the striatum. This is accomplished by stimulating postsynaptic receptors (directly with

TABLE 43.1 *Differential Diagnosis of Parkinsonism*

I. Primary Parkinsonism
Genetically based PD
Idiopathic ("sporadic") PD (most common form)
Other neurodegenerative disorders
    Disorders associated with alpha-synuclein pathology
    Multiple system atrophies (glial and neuronal inclusions)
        Striatonigral degeneration
        Sporadic olivopontocerebellar atrophy
        Shy-Drager syndrome
    Motor neuron disease with PD features
    Dementia with Lewy bodies (cortical and brain stem neuronal inclusions)
    Disorders associated with primary tau pathology ("tauopathies")
        Progressive supranuclear palsy
        Corticobasal degeneration
        Frontotemporal dementia
    Disorders associated with primary amyloid pathology ("amyloidopathies")
        Alzheimer's disease with parkinsonism
Genetically mediated disorders with occasional Parkinsonian features:
    Wilson's disease
    Hallervorden-Spatz disease
    Chédiak-Hagashi syndrome
    SCA-3 spinocerebellar ataxia
    X-linked dystonia-parkinsonism (DYT3)
    Fragile X premutation associated ataxia-tremor-parkinsonism syndrome
    Huntington's disease (Westphal variant)
    Prion disease
Miscellaneous acquired conditions
    Vascular parkinsonism
    Normal pressure hydrocephalus
    Cerebral palsy
    Catatonia
II. Secondary Parkinsonism
    Repeated head trauma ("Dementia pugilistica" with Parkinsonian features)
    Infectious and postinfectious diseases
    Postencephalitic PD
    Neurosyphillis
    Metabolic conditions: Hypoparathyroidism or pseudohypoparathyroidism with basal ganglia calcifications
    Non-Wilsonian hepatolenticular degeneration
    Drugs: Neuroleptics (e.g., haloperidol), antiemetics (e.g., metoclopramide), dopamine-depleting agents
       (reserpine, tetrabenazine), methyldopa, lithium carbonate, valproic acid
    Toxins: MPTP, Manganese, Cyanide, Methanol, Carbon monoxide, Carbon disulfide, Hexane

dopamine agonists), increasing dopamine precursor availability (levodopa), blocking the metabolism of levodopa in the periphery and in the brain, and blocking the catabolism of dopamine at the synapse. Table 43.2 lists commonly used anti-parkinsonian therapy, their dosages, and frequent side effects.

INITIATION OF THERAPY

The ideal first-line agent is a dopamine agonist, a levodopa preparation, or one of the MAO-B inhibitors. In early PD, dopamine agonist monotherapy is well tolerated, significantly improves motor function and disability, and has an approximately 50% lower risk of dyskinesias and 25% lower risk of motor fluctuations compared to levodopa-treated patients. Once a levadopa preparation is added, however, dyskinesias and motor fluctuations can begin to emerge, suggesting that dopamine agonists delay the onset but do not prevent the development of these problems. In fact, about two-thirds of patients on agonist mono-therapy require levodopa therapy by year 5 in order to maintain motor function.

Motor fluctuations, also known as "on–off" phenomena, are experienced by many patients between doses of antiparkinsonian medications and worsen as disease progresses. *Dyskinesias* refer to choreiform and/or dystonic movements that can occur as a peak dose effect or at the beginning or end of the dose (diphasic dyskinesias). More than 50% of patients with PD treated over 5 years with levodopa will develop these complications.

Older patients and those with the akinetic rigid forms of PD have a lower risk of motor complications and dyskinesias compared to the average PD patient.

TABLE 43.2 *Common Medications Used in the Treatment of Motor Symptoms of Parkinson's Disease*

Generic Medication Name (Trade-Name)	Initial Dose Ranges	Titration Schedule		Common Side Effects
Levodopa Formulations				
Carbidopa/Levodopa (Sinemet IR, Parcopa)	25/100 mg PO TID	Increase by 1 tablet every 1–2 days as indicated.	Maximum dosage of 200 mg of carbidopa and 2000 mg of levodopa	Nausea, somnolence, dizziness, headache, confusion, hallucinations, delusions, agitation osteoporosis, motor fluctuations
Sustained-release Carbidopa/Levodopa (Sinemet CR)	50/200 mg PO BID	May adjust every three days	Maximum dosage of 200 mg of carbidopa and 2000 mg of levodopa	Same as immediate release but possibly decrease in motor fluctuations
Carbidopa-Levodopa-Entacapone (Stalevo 50, 100, 150, 200)	1 tablet TID; may start higher if known response to levodopa	Replace each levodopa dose up to maximum of 1600 mg per day of levodopa	Maximum dosage of 1600 mg per day of entacapone or 1600 mg per day of levodopa	Same as immediate release carbidopa/levodopa and entacapone
Dopamine Agonists				
Pramipexole (Mirapex)	0.125 mg PO TID	7-week titration to maximum daily dose of 4.5 mg PO qdaily	Maximum dosage of 1.5 mg PO TID	Somnolence, sleep attacks, nausea, vomiting, orthostatic hypotension, confusion, hallucinations, pedal edema, mood changes, compulsive behaviors
Pramipexole extended-release (Mirapex ER)	0.375 mg PO qdaily	7-week titration to maximum daily dose of 4.5 mg PO qdaily	Maximum dosage of 4.5 mg PO qdaily	Same as immediate release
Ropinirole (Requip)	0.25 mg PO TID	8-week titration to 3.0 mg PO TID	Maximum dosage of 8.0 mg PO TID	Same as pramipexole
Ropinirole XL (Requip XL)	1–2 mg PO q daily	Weekly upwards titration by 2 mg as indicated	Maximum dosage of 24 mg PO q daily	Same as pramipexole
Bromocriptine (Parlodel)	1.25 mg PO BID	Increase by 2.5 mg per day in 2–4 week intervals	Maximum dosage of 100 mg PO q daily	Same as pramipexole in addition to ergot-induced fibrosis

(continued)

TABLE 43.1 *(continued)*

Generic Medication Name (Trade-Name)	Initial Dose Ranges	Titration Schedule		Common Side Effects
Apomorphine (Apokyn)	2 mg SC test dose	If patient responds, increase by 1 mg increments every few days	Maximum total daily dosage of 20mg SC	Same as pramipexole in addition to cutaneous reactions and severe nausea/vomiting.
MAO-B Inhibitors Rasagiline (Azilect)	0.5 mg PO q daily	As indicated	1 mg PO q daily	Dyskinesia, nausea, weight loss, constipation, postural hypotension, vomiting, dry mouth, rash, somnolence
Selegiline (Eldepryl)	5 mg q daily	As indicated	5 mg PO BID	Insomnia, nausea, dizziness, confusion, hallucinations, constipation, orthostatic hypotension, dry mouth, dyskinesia
Orally dissolving Selegiline (Zelapar)	1.25 mg PO q daily	Increase to 2.5mg PO q daily after 6 weeks	2.5 mg PO q daily	Dizziness, dyskinesia, hallucinations, headache, dyspepsia
COMT Inhibitors Entacapone (Comtan)	200 mg PO q daily	200mg dose up to 8 times daily with each dose of levodopa	1600 mg PO q daily	Dyskinesia, hallucinations, confusion, nausea, orthostatic hypotension, diarrhea, orange discoloration of urine
Tolcapone (Tasmar)	100 mg PO TID	As indicated	200 mg PO TID	Same as Entacapone with addition of hepatotoxicity
Amantadine Amantadine (Symmetrel)	100 mg PO qdaily	As indicated	Maximum total daily dosage of 400 mg in divided doses	Dizziness, insomnia, anxiety, nausea, vomiting, pedal edema, livedo reticularis
Anticholinergics Trihexyphenidyl (Artane)	1 mg PO q daily	Increase by 2 mg increments every 3–5 days	Maximum total daily dosage of 15 mg in divided doses	Confusion, hallucinations, dry mouth, blurred vision, constipation, nausea, urinary retention, tachycardia
Benztropine (Cogentin)	0.5 mg PO BID	Increase by 0.5 mg increments every 5–6 days	Maximum total daily dosage of 6 mg in divided doses	Same as trihexyphenidyl

THERAPY FOR NONMOTOR SYMPTOMS

Frequent nighttime awakenings due to nocturnal akinesia or tremor, restless leg syndrome, or nocturnal urinary urgency can respond to supplemental doses of carbidopa/levodopa at night. Sometimes, a dose of Carbidopa/Levodopa CR is used for this purpose. REM behavior sleep disorder responds well to small doses of clonazepam.

Depression typically responds to antidepressants (either TCAs or SSRIs) or ECT.

For psychotic symptoms or confusion, anticholinergics and amantadine should be eliminated first. Following this, MAO-B inhibitors and dopamine agonists should be reduced or discontinued as needed to control symptoms. If symptoms persist, gradual reductions in nocturnal and then daytime doses of Sinemet CR, and finally carbidopa/levodopa. If in the process parkinsonian symptoms worsen, atypical antipsychotics that have a low incidence of extrapyramidal side effects should be considered. Clozapine (12.5–100 mg/d) is the best established agent for treatment of psychotic symptoms in PD. Quetiapine (12.5–100 mg) is sometimes used first because it lacks the small risk of agranulocytosis associated with clozapine, and therefore does not need weekly blood monitoring. Clozapine and quetiapine are limited by dose-dependent sedation, orthostatic hypotension, dizziness, and confusion. Other atypical antipsychotics such as risperidone, olanzapine, and aripiprazole are not well tolerated due to a higher incidence of DIP and akathisia.

Centrally acting acetylcholinesterase inhibitors like Rivastigmine and Donepezil can improve dementia symptoms in PD and may be useful for treatment of psychotic symptoms such as hallucinations and delusions. Sildenafil citrate may be considered in patients with erectile dysfunction. Isosmotic macrogol (polyethylene glycol) may be considered to treat constipation in PD. Methylphenidate and modafinil may be considered in patients

TABLE 43.3 *Common Medications Used in the Treatment of Motor Symptoms of Parkinson's Disease*

Symptom	Medication Type or Name	Recommended Dosage Ranges	Common Side Effects
Cognitive changes Dementia	Rivastigmine	1.5 mg to 6 mg PO BID	Dizziness, headache, nausea, vomiting, diarrhea, anorexia
	Donepezil	5 mg to 10 mg PO q daily	Insomnia, nausea, diarrhea, headache, dizziness, weight loss
Mood Changes Depression and Anxiety	Selective Serotonin Reuptake Inhibitors (e.g., Fluoxetine, Paroxetine, Sertraline, Citalopram)	Adjust based on specific medication	Sexual dysfunction, weight changes, mild sedation, nausea, vomiting, dizziness, headache
	Tricyclic Antidepressants (eg., Amytriptyline, Doxepin, Nortryptyline)	Adjust based on specific medication	Sedation, orthostatic hypotension, cognitive impairment, weight gain, urinary retention, constipation, cardiac conduction changes
	Serotonin-Norepinephrine Reuptake Inhibitor (e.g., Venlafaxine, Duloxetine)	Adjust based on specific medication	Sexual dysfunction, weight changes, mild sedation, nausea, vomiting, headache
Sleep disturbances Restless leg Syndrome and Periodic leg movements during sleep	Iron and folate supplementation; dopamine agonist, neurontin, Levodopa	Adjust based on specific medication	See previous table for side-effects of dopamine agonists
REM sleep behavior disorder	Clonazepem	0.5 to 2.0 mg PO q hs	Drowsiness, psychomotor agitation, cognitive impairment, withdrawal-related symptoms
Excessive daytime sedation	Methylphenidate	5 mg PO q daily	Nervousness, insomnia, appetite suppression, headache, nausea, dizziness, palpitations
	Amantadine	100 mg PO BID	Dizziness, insomnia, anxiety, nausea, vomiting, pedal edema, livedo reticularis
	Modafanil	50 to 100 mg PO q daily	Nervousness, insomnia, dizziness, headache, nausea, hypersensitivity reactions
Hallucinations	Quetiapine, clozapine	12.5 mg to 50 mg q hs	Sedation, fatigue, constipation, dizziness, orthostatic hypotension, weight gain
Other symptoms Urinary frequency	Oxybutynin	5 mg TID/QID	Dry mouth, constipation, blurred vision, confusion, dizziness, nausea, vomiting
	Tolterodine	2 mg PO BID	Dry mouth, constipation, blurred vision, headache, nausea, vomiting, dizziness

(continued)

TABLE 43.3 *(continued)*

Symptom	Medication Type or Name	Recommended Dosage Ranges	Common Side Effects
Urinary retention	Terazosin	1 mg PO q h	Dizziness, sedation, headache, constipation, weight changes, sexual dysfunction
	Tamsulosin	0.4 to 0.8 mg PO q daily	Dizziness, sedation, insomnia, blurred vision, hypotension, sexual dysfunction
	Bethanechol chloride	10 to 50 mg PO QID	Dizziness, hypotension, flushing, headache, nausea, abdominal discomfort, diarrhea
Constipation	Docusate sodium	50 mg PO q daily to 100 mg PO TID	Diarrhea, abdominal cramping, throat irritation
	Bisacodyl	10 to 15 mg PO q daily OR 10 mg per rectum q daily	Stomach pain, diarrhea, electrolyte or fluid imbalances
	Polyethylene glycol 3350 (Miralax)	17 g powder dissolved in 4–8 oz beverage q daily	Abdominal bloating, cramping, diarrhea, urticaria, electrolyte or fluid imbalances
	Lactulose	10 to 20 g PO q daily	Abdominal discomfort, diarrhea, flatulence, electrolyte or fluid imbalances
Erectile dysfunction	Sildenafil	50 to 100 mg PO prior to activity	Orthostatic hypotension, headache, flushing, blurred vision, priapism, palpitations, ventricular arrhythmias (rare), sudden hearing loss (rare)
	Vardenafil	5 to 20 mg PO prior to activity	Orthostatic hypotension, nausea, blurred vision, priapism, palpitations, ventricular arrhythmias (rare), sudden hearing loss (rare)
	Yohimbine	5 to 10 mg PO TID	Anxiety, palpitations, hypertension, insomnia, headaches, dizziness
Orthostatic hypotension	Midodrine	5 to 10 mg PO TID	Hypertension, piloerection, pruritis, urinary urgency or retention, paresthesias, abdominal pain
	Ephedrine	25 to 50 mg PO q4h as needed	Hypertension, palpitations, agitation, dizziness, headache, insomnia, anorexia, nausea, vomiting, tremor, dyspnea
	Fludrocortisone	0.05 to 0.2 mg PO q daily	Dizziness, headache, acne, hyperglycemia, peptic ulcer, congestive heart failure, cataracts, weakness
Excessive salivation	Benztropine	0.5 to 1.0 mg TID	Confusion, hallucinations, dry mouth, blurred vision, constipation, nausea, urinary retention, tachycardia
	Trihexyphenidyl	2 to 5 mg PO TID	Confusion, hallucinations, dry mouth, blurred vision, constipation, nausea, urinary retention, tachycardia
	Atropine 1% ophthalmic solution	1 drop sublingually BID	Confusion, hallucinations
	Glycopyrrolate	1 to 2 mg TID	Dizziness, confusion, insomnia, constipation, nausea, palpitations, blurred vision, arrhythmias, urinary hesitancy
Diaphoresis	Propranolol	40 mg PO BID	Hypotension, bradycardia, confusion, dyspnea, dizziness, fatigue, hypoglycemia
	Clonidine	0.1 mg PO q daily	Lightheadedness, dry mouth, constipation, hypotension

with fatigue. Exercise therapy can sometimes improve motor function. Speech therapy is useful to improve speech volume, in PD patient with dysarthria. Table 43.3 lists frequently encountered nonmotor symptoms of PD, medications that may be used to treat these symptoms, and recommended dosages and common side-effects of these medications.

NEUROPROTECTIVE THERAPY

Slowing the progression of PD through neuroprotective or restorative therapy is a major focus of research. Epidemiologic studies suggest that the chronic use of nonsteroidal anti-inflammatory agents, caffeine, nicotine, or the use of estrogen replacement in postmenopausal women may delay or prevent the onset of PD through yet-unclear mechanisms. None of these agents have enough data behind them for them to be used clinically yet.

DATATOP study showed that selegiline monotherapy delayed the need for levodopa therapy by 9 to 12 months in newly diagnosed patients and the patients who remained on selegiline for 7 years experienced slower motor decline compared to those who were changed to placebo after 5 years. The recently completed ADAGIO study compared the use of rasagiline in an "early start" and "delayed start" group. The "delayed start" group did not catch up to the "early start" group suggesting that rasagiline is neuroprotective.

There is insufficient evidence to support (Level U) or refute the use of riluzole, pramipexole, ropinirole, rasagiline, amantadine, thalamotomy, M prurians, creatine, acetyl levocarnitine, high-dose vitamin E, or acupuncture for neuroprotection. There was an ongoing trial conducted by NIH for high dose Coenzyme Q10 as a neuroprotective agent that was very recently stopped as no benefit was shown.

Other promising agents include nitric oxide synthetase inhibitors and antiapoptotic agents such as N-terminal kinase inhibitors and desmethylselegiline (selegiline metabolite).

SURGICAL TREATMENTS

DBS is the surgery of choice for PD today. The most common indications for surgery in PD are intractable tremor and drug-induced motor fluctuations or dyskinesias. The best candidates are patients with clear levodopa-responsive parkinsonism who are free of significant dementia or psychiatric comorbidities. In general, patients with atypical parkinsonism or dementia benefit little, or not at all. Currently the subthalamic nucleus is the preferred target, but controlled clinical trials comparing the pallidal and subthalamic targets are nearing completion. DBS is most often performed bilaterally and simultaneously, but unilateral DBS can be highly effective for asymmetric cases. DBS in these areas alleviates parkinsonian motor signs, particularly during "off" periods, and reduces troublesome dyskinesias, dystonias, and motor fluctuations that result from drug administration. Signs and symptoms not responsive to levodopa, such as postural instability and falling, hypophonia, micrographia, drooling, and autonomic dysfunction, are unlikely to benefit from surgery.

Other approaches: Trials with stem cell transplantation or direct infusion of glial cell-derived neurotrophic factor to the putamen have not shown any significant benefits. AAV2-GAD gene therapy for advanced PD has been recently studied in a double-blind, sham-surgery controlled, randomized trial. The demonstrated efficacy and safety of bilateral infusion of AAV2-GAD in the subthalamic nucleus support its further development for PD and show the promise for gene therapy for neurological disorders. Continuous infusion of carbidopa/levodopa via an intestinal pump is a strategy already approved in Europe and currently undergoing clinical trial in the United States.

SUGGESTED READING

DeLong Mahlon R, Juncos Jorge L. "Chapter 366. Parkinson's Disease and Other Extrapyramidal Movement Disorders" (Chapter). In Fauci AS, Braunwald E, Kasper DL, et al. *Harrison's Principles of Internal Medicine*, 17th ed. New York: Mcgraw-Hill Professional; 2008.

Fahn S, Elton RL, UPDRS Development Committee. Unified Parkinson's disease Rating Scale. In: Fahn S, Marsden CD, Calne DB, Goldstein M, eds. *Recent Developments in Parkinson's Disease.* Florham Park, NJ: Macmillan; 1987:153–163.

Gillingham FJ, Donaldson MC, eds., Third Symposium of Parkinson's Disease. Edinburgh, Scotland, E&S Livingstone; 1969:152–157.

Goetz CG, Poewe W, Rascol O, Sampaio C. Evidence-based medical review update: Pharmacological and surgical treatments of Parkinson's disease: 2001 to 2004. *Movement Disorders.* 2005;20(5):523–539.

Hoehn MM, Yahr MD. Parkinsonism: Onset, progression and mortality. *Neurology.* 1967;17:427.

Horstink M, Tolosa E, Bonuccelli U, et al. Review of the therapeutic management of Parkinson's disease. Report of a joint task force of the European Federation of Neurological Societies and the Movement Disorder Society-European Section. Part I: early (uncomplicated) Parkinson's disease. *Eur J Neurol.* 2006;13(11):1170–1185.

Horstink M, Tolosa E, Bonuccelli U, et al. Review of the therapeutic management of Parkinson's disease. Report of a joint task force of the European Federation of Neurological Societies and the Movement Disorder Society-European Section. Part II: late (complicated) Parkinson's disease. *Eur J Neurol.* 2006;13(11):1186–1202.

LeWitt PA, Rezai AR, Leehey MA. AAV2-GAD gene therapy for advanced Parkinson's disease: A double-blind, sham-surgery controlled, randomised trial. *Lancet Neurol.* 2011;10(4):309–319.

Olanow CW, Watts RL, Koller WC. An algorithm (decision tree) for the management of Parkinson's disease (2001): Treatment guidelines. *Neurology* 2001;56(11 suppl 5):S1–S88.

Pahwa R, Factor SA, Lyons KE, et al. Practice parameter: Treatment of Parkinson disease with motor fluctuations and dyskinesia (an evidence-based review): Report of the Quality Standards Subcommittee of the American Academy of Neurology. *Neurology.* 2006;66(7):983–995.

Pathak A, Senard JM. Blood pressure disorders during Parkinson's disease: Epidemiology, pathophysiology and management. *Expert Rev Neurother.* 2006;6(8):1173–1180.

Rascol O, Fitzer-Attas CJ, Hauser R. A double-blind, delayed-start trial of rasagiline in Parkinson's disease (the ADAGIO study): Prespecified and post-hoc analyses of the need for additional therapies, changes in UPDRS scores, and non-motor outcomes. *Lancet Neurol.* 2011 May;10(5):415–423. Epub 2011.

Sanders-Bush E, Hazelwood L. Chapter 13. 5-Hydroxytryptamine (Serotonin) and Dopamine (Chapter). In Brunton LL, Chabner BA, Knollmann BC, eds. *Goodman & Gilman's The Pharmacological Basis of Therapeutics,* 12e: http://www.accessmedicine.com/content.aspx?aID=16662305

Shulman LM, Taback RL, Rabinstein AA, Weiner WJ. Non-recognition of depression and other non-motor symptoms in Parkinson's disease. *Parkinsonism Related Disorders.* 2002;8(3):193–197.

Suchowersky O, Gronseth G, Perlmutter J, Reich S, Zesiewicz T, Weiner W. Practice parameter: Neuroprotective strategies and alternative therapies for Parkinson disease (an evidence-based review): Report of the Quality Standards Subcommittee of the American Academy of Neurology. *Neurology.* 2006;66:976–982.

Suchowersky O, Reich S, Perlmutter J, Zesiewicz T, Gronseth G, Weiner W. Practice parameter: Diagnosis and prognosis of new onset Parkinson disease (an evidence based review): Report of the Quality Standards Subcommittee of the American Academy of Neurology. *Neurology.* 2006;66:968–975.

Thorpy MJ, Adler CH. Parkinson's disease and sleep. *Neurol Clin.* 2005;23:1187–1208.

Zesiewicz TA, Sullivan KL, Arnulf I, et al. Practice parameter: treatment of nonmotor symptoms of Parkinson disease: Report of the Quality Standards Subcommittee of the American Academy of Neurology. *Neurology.* 2010;74:924–931.

Appendix 43.I *Mini-Mental State Examination (MMSE)*

Maximum	Category	How to Test
	Orientation	
5	To time	What is the (year) (season) (date) (day) (month)?
5	To place	Where are we (state) (country) (town) (hospital) (floor)?
3	Registration	Name 3 objects: 1 second to say each. Then ask the patient all 3 after you have said them. Give 1 point for each correct answer. Then repeat them until he/she learns all 3. Count trials and record.
5	Attention and calculation	Serial 7's. 1 point for each correct answer. Stop after 5 answers. Alternatively, spell "world" backward.
3	Recall	Ask for the 3 objects repeated above. Give 1 point for each correct answer.
2	Language	Name a pencil and watch.
1		Repeat the following "No ifs, ands, or buts."
3		Follow a 3-stage command: "Take a paper in your hand, fold it in half, and put it on the floor."
1		Read and obey the following: CLOSE YOUR EYES.
1		Write a sentence.
1		Copy the design shown.

Total score 30

Appendix 43.II *The Unified Parkinson's Disease Rating Scale (UPDRS)*

Part I Mentation, Behavior, and Mood

Intellectual impairment	0 = none
	1 = mild (consistent forgetfulness with partial recollection of events with no other difficulties)
	2 = moderate memory loss with disorientation and moderate difficulty handling complex problems
	3 = severe memory loss with disorientation to time and often place, severe impairment with problems
	4 = severe memory loss with orientation only to person, unable to make judgments or solve problems
Thought disorder	0 = none
	1 = vivid dreaming
	2 = "benign" hallucination with insight retained
	3 = occasional to frequent hallucination or delusions without insight, could interfere with daily activities
	4 = persistent hallucination, delusions, or florid psychosis
Depression	0 = not present
	1 = periods of sadness or guilt greater than normal, never sustained for more than a few days or a week
	2 = sustained depression for >1 week
	3 = vegetative symptoms (insomnia, anorexia, abulia, weight loss)
	4 = vegetative symptoms with suicidality

(continued)

APPENDIX 43 II *(continued)*

Motivation/initiative	0 = normal
	1 = less of assertive, more passive
	2 = loss of initiative or disinterest in elective activities
	3 = loss of initiative or disinterest in day to say (routine) activities
	4 = withdrawn, complete loss of motivation

Part II Activities of Daily Living

Speech	0 = normal
	1 = mildly affected, no difficulty being understood
	2 = moderately affected, may be asked to repeat
	3 = severely affected, frequently asked to repeat
	4 = unintelligible most of time
Salivation	0 = normal
	1 = slight but noticeable increase, may have nighttime drooling
	2 = moderately excessive saliva, may have minimal drooling
	3 = marked drooling
Swallowing	0 = normal
	1 = rare choking
	2 = occasional choking
	3 = requires soft food
	4 = requires NG tube or G-tube
Handwriting	0 = normal
	1 = slightly small or slow
	2 = all words small but legible
	3 = severely affected, not all words legible
	4 = majority illegible
Cutting food/handling utensils	0 = normal
	1 = somewhat slow and clumsy but no help needed
	2 = can cut most foods, some help needed
	3 = food must be cut, but can feed self
	4 = needs to be fed
Dressing	0 = normal
	1 = somewhat slow, no help needed
	2 = occasional help with buttons or arms in sleeves
	3 = considerable help required but can do something alone
	4 = helpless
Hygiene	0 = normal
	1 = somewhat slow but no help needed
	2 = needs help with shower or bath or very slow in hygienic care
	3 = requires assistance for washing, brushing teeth, going to bathroom
	4 = helpless
Turning in bed/adjusting bed clothes	0 = normal
	1 = somewhat slow no help needed
	2 = can turn alone or adjust sheets but with great difficulty
	3 = can initiate but not turn or adjust alone
	4 = helpless
Falling—unrelated to freezing	0 = none
	1 = rare falls
	2 = occasional, less than one per day
	3 = average of once per day
	4 = more than one per day

(continued)

APPENDIX 43.II *(continued)*

Freezing when walking	0 = normal
	1 = rare, may have start hesitation
	2 = occasional falls from freezing
	3 = frequent freezing, occasional falls
	4 = frequent falls from freezing
Walking	0 = normal
	1 = mild difficulty, day drag legs or decrease arm swing
	2 = moderate difficultly requires no assist
	3 = severe disturbance requires assistance
	4 = cannot walk at all even with assist
Tremor	0 = absent
	1 = slight and infrequent, not bothersome to patient
	2 = moderate, bothersome to patient
	3 = severe, interfere with many activities
	4 = marked, interferes with many activities
Sensory complaints related to Parkinsonism	0 = none
	1= occasionally has numbness, tingling, and mild aching
	2 = frequent, but not distressing
	3 = frequent painful sensation
	4 = excruciating pain

Part III Motor Exam

Speech	0 = normal
	1 = slight loss of expression, diction, volume
	2 = monotone, slurred but understandable, moderately impaired
	3 = marked impairment, difficult to understand
	4 = unintelligible
Facial expression	0 = normal
	1 = slight hypomimia, could be poker face
	2 = slight but definite abnormal diminution in expression
	3 = moderate hypomimia, lips parted some of time
	4 = masked or fixed face, lips parted 1/4 of inch or more with complete loss of expression
Tremor at rest (face)	0 = absent
	1 = slight and infrequent
	2 = mild and present most of time
	3 = moderate and present most of time
	4 = marked and present most of time
Tremor at rest (right upper extremity)	0 = absent
	1 = slight and infrequent
	2 = mild and present most of time
	3 = moderate and present most of time
	4 = marked and present most of time
Tremor at rest (left upper extremity)	0 = absent
	1 = slight and infrequent
	2 = mild and present most of time
	3 = moderate and present most of time
	4 = marked and present most of time
Tremor at rest (right lower extremity)	0 = absent
	1 = slight and infrequent
	2 = mild and present most of time
	3 = moderate and present most of time
	4 = marked and present most of time

(continued)

APPENDIX 43.11 *(continued)*

Tremor at rest (left lower extremity)	0 = absent 1 = slight and infrequent 2 = mild and present most of time 3 = moderate and present most of time 4 = marked and present most of time
Action or postural tremor (right upper extremity)	0 = absent 1 = slight, present with action 2 = moderate, present with action 3 = moderate present with action and posture holding 4 = marked, interferes with feeding
Action or postural tremor (left upper extremity)	0 = absent 1 = slight, present with action 2 = moderate, present with action 3 = moderate present with action and posture holding 4 = marked, interferes with feeding
Rigidity (neck)	0 = absent 1 = slight or only with activation 2 = mild/moderate 3 = marked, full range of motion 4 = severe
Rigidity (right upper extremity)	0 = absent 1 = slight or only with activation 2 = mild/moderate 3 = marked, full range of motion 4 = severe
Rigidity (left upper extremity)	0 = absent 1 = slight or only with activation 2 = mild/moderate 3 = marked, full range of motion 4 = severe
Rigidity (right lower extremity)	0 = absent 1 = slight or only with activation 2 = mild/moderate 3 = marked, full range of motion 4 = severe
Rigidity (left lower extremity)	0 = absent 1 = slight or only with activation 2 = mild/moderate 3 = marked, full range of motion 4 = severe
Finger taps (right)	0 = normal 1 = mild slowing, and/or reduction in amplitude. 2 = moderate impaired. Definite and early fatiguing, may have occasional arrests 3 = severely impaired. Frequent hesitations and arrests. 4 = can barely perform
Finger taps (left)	0 = normal 1 = mild slowing and/or reduction in amplitude. 2 = moderate impaired. Definite and early fatiguing, may have occasional arrests 3 = severely impaired. Frequent hesitations and arrests. 4 = can barely perform

(continued)

APPENDIX 43.II *(continued)*

Hand movements (right)	0 = normal
	1 = mild slowing, and/or reduction in amplitude.
	2 = moderate impaired. Definite and early fatiguing, may have occasional arrests.
	3 = severely impaired. Frequent hesitations and arrests.
	4 = can barely perform
Hand movements (left)	0 = normal
	1 = mild slowing, and/or reduction in amplitude.
	2 = moderate impaired. Definite and early fatiguing, may have occasional arrests.
	3 = severely impaired. Frequent hesitations and arrests.
	4 = can barely perform.
Rapid alternating movements (right)	0 = normal.
	1 = mild slowing, and/or reduction in amplitude.
	2 = moderate impaired. Definite and early fatiguing, may have occasional arrests.
	3 = severely impaired. Frequent hesitations and arrests.
	4 = can barely perform.
Rapid alternating movements (left)	0 = normal.
	1 = mild slowing, and/or reduction in amplitude.
	2 = moderate impaired. Definite and early fatiguing, may have occasional arrests.
	3 = severely impaired. Frequent hesitations and arrests.
	4 = can barely perform.
Leg agility (right)	0 = normal.
	1 = mild slowing, and/or reduction in amplitude.
	2 = moderate impaired. Definite and early fatiguing, may have occasional arrests.
	3 = severely impaired. Frequent hesitations and arrests.
	4 = can barely perform.
Leg agility (left)	0 = normal.
	1 = mild slowing, and/or reduction in amplitude.
	2 = moderate impaired. Definite and early fatiguing, may have occasional arrests
	3 = severely impaired. Frequent hesitations and arrests.
	4 = can barely perform
Arising from chair	0 = normal.
	1 = slow, may need more than one attempt.
	2 = pushes self up from arms or seat.
	3 = tends to fall back, may need multiple tries but can arise without assistance.
	4 = unable to arise without help.
Posture	0 = normal erect
	1 = slightly stooped, could be normal for older person
	2 = definitely abnormal, moderately stooped, may lean to one side
	3 = severely stooped with kyphosis
	4 = marked flexion with extreme abnormality of posture
Gait	0 = normal
	1 = walks slowly, may shuffle with short steps, no festination or propulsion
	2 = walks with difficulty, little or no assistance, some festination, short steps or propulsion
	3 = severe disturbance, frequent assistance
	4 = cannot walk

(continued)

APPENDIX 43.11 *(continued)*

Postural instability	0 = normal
	1 = recovers unaided
	2 = would fall if not caught
	3 = falls spontaneously
	4 = unable to stand
Body bradykinesia and hypokinsia	0 = none.
	1 = minimal slowness, could be normal, deliberate character.
	2 = mild slowness and poverty of movement, definitely abnormal, or decreased amplitude of movement.
	3 = moderate slowness, poverty, or small amplitude.
	4 = marked slowness, poverty, or amplitude.

Part IV Complications of Therapy

Dyskinesias (duration)	0 = None
	1 = 1–25% of day
	2 = 26–50% of day
	3 = 51–75% of day
	4 = 76–100% of day
Dyskinesias (disability)	0 = Not disabling
	1 = Mildly disabling
	2 = Moderately disabling
	3 = Severely disabling
	4 = Completely disabled
Painful dyskinesia	0 = No painful dyskinesias
	1 = Slight
	2 = Moderate
	3 = Severe
	4 = Marked
Presence of early morning dystonia	0 = No
	1 = Yes
Are "off" periods predictable?	0 = No
	1 = Yes
Are "off" periods unpredictable?	0 = No
	1 = Yes
Do "off" periods come on suddenly?	0 = No
	1 = Yes
What proportion of the waking day is "off" phase on average?	0 = None
	1 = 1–25% of day
	2 = 26–50% of day
	3 = 51–75% of day
	4 = 76–100% of day
Presence of anorexia, nausea, or vomiting?	0 = No
	1 = Yes
Any sleep disturbances, such as insomnia or hypersomnolence?	0 = No
	1 = Yes
Presence of symptomatic orthostasis	0 = No
	1 = Yes

(continued)

Appendix 43.III *Hoehn and Yahr Scale*

Stages	Symptoms
Stage 1: Unilateral involvement only, usually with minimal or no functional disability	1. Signs and symptoms on one side only 2. Symptoms mild 3. Symptoms inconvenient but not disabling 4. Usually presents with tremor of one limb 5. Friends have noticed changes in posture, locomotion, and facial expression
Stage 2: Bilateral or midline involvement without impairment of balance	1. Symptoms are bilateral 2. Minimal disability 3. Posture and gait affected
Stage 3: Bilateral disease; mild to moderate disability with impaired postural reflexes; physically independent	1. Significant slowing of body movements 2. Early impairment of equilibrium on walking or standing 3. Generalized dysfunction that is moderately severe
Stage 4: Severely disabling disease; still able to walk or stand unassisted	1. Severe symptoms 2. Can still walk to a limited extent 3. Rigidity and bradykinesia 4. No longer able to live alone 5. Tremor may be less than earlier stages
Stage 5: Confinement to bed or wheelchair unless aided	1. Cachectic stage 2. Invalidism complete 3. Cannot stand or walk 4. Requires constant nursing care

Appendix 43.IV *Schwab and England Activities of Daily Living*

Percentage	Symptoms
100%	Completely independent. Able to do all chores without slowness, difficulty, or impairment.
90%	Completely independent. Able to do all chores with some slowness, difficulty, or impairment. May take twice as long.
80%	Independent in most chores. Takes twice as long. Conscious of difficulty and slowing.
70%	Not completely independent. More difficulty with chores. Three to four times along on chores for some. May take large part of day for chores.
60%	Some dependency. Can do most chores, but very slowly and with much effort. Errors, some impossible.
50%	More dependant. Help with half of chores. Difficulty with everything
40%	Very dependant. Can assist with all chores but few alone.
30%	With effort, now and then does a few chores alone of begins alone. Much help needed.
20%	Nothing alone. Can do some slight help with some chores. Severe invalid.
10%	Totally dependant, helpless.
0%	Vegetative functions such as swallowing, bladder, and bowel function are not functioning. Bedridden.

Irfan Oh and Abhinav J. Rodrigues

CHIEF COMPLAINT: **My wife tells me that I snore heavily.**

HISTORY OF PRESENT ILLNESS

A 40-year-old man presents to the sleep clinic with snoring and excessive daytime sleepiness.

The patient has been snoring for many years, but recently it has become louder. He can be heard snoring outside his room with the door closed. His wife has mentioned that he stops breathing at night. He is aware of snort arousals, and his favorite sleep position is on his back. He wakes up with a dry mouth since he sleeps with his mouth open. There was no reference of morning headaches.

He goes to bed at 10 p.m. and has no problems falling asleep. He usually wakes up at 6 a.m. with help of an alarm clock. He feels tired and sleepy during the day. He has gained over 25 pounds during the past 2 years. He works as a teacher and he has found himself falling asleep in the class. His ESS is 13/24.

PAST MEDICAL HISTORY

Hypertension.

PAST SURGICAL HISTORY

Appendectomy.

MEDICATIONS

Hydrochlorothiazide 50 mg once daily.

ALLERGIES

NKDA.

PERSONAL HISTORY

He drinks four to six cups/coffee a day to stay awake. He drinks alcohol socially. He does not smoke or use drugs.

PHYSICAL EXAMINATION

Blood pressure, 150/90 mm Hg; respiratory rate, 12 per min; pulse, 72 per min, regular; height, 5′7″; weight, 240 lbs; body mass index (BMI), 37.6.

Eyes: Pupils and irises normal. Conjunctivae and lids normal.

Ears, nose, mouth, and throat: Narrow oropharynx. Low lying soft palate and uvula. Mild retrognathia. Enlarged base of the tongue. Teeth indentation in the tongue. Normal nasal mucosa, septum and turbinates. Congested nares, left more than right. External inspection of ears and nose normal. Hearing normal.

Neck: Normal; thyroid gland not enlarged, neck circumference 19 inches.

Respiratory: Normal.

Cardiovascular examination: Normal heart sounds; no murmurs.

NEUROLOGICAL EXAMINATION

Mental status: Alert and oriented; Language: normal; normal attention and concentration; Fund of knowledge adequate and normal judgment. Memory 3/3.
CNs II–XII: No abnormality detected.
Motor and sensory examination was normal.
Reflexes: 2+ and symmetrical.
Plantars: down.
Cerebellar: negative.
Gait: normal.

STOP AND THINK QUESTIONS

➢ What is the significance of snoring during sleep?

➢ What is a Polysomnogram?

➢ How will you treat patient's symptoms?

DIAGNOSTIC TEST RESULTS

The patient was ordered a diagnostic PSG. The diagnostic PSG (see Figure 44.1) showed a sleep efficiency of 74.0% with a sleep latency of 5 minutes. The total AHI was 34.5. The respiratory events were not positional. There was loud persistent snoring heard in all positions. The minimal oxygen saturation was 72%. The total arousal index was 84.0.

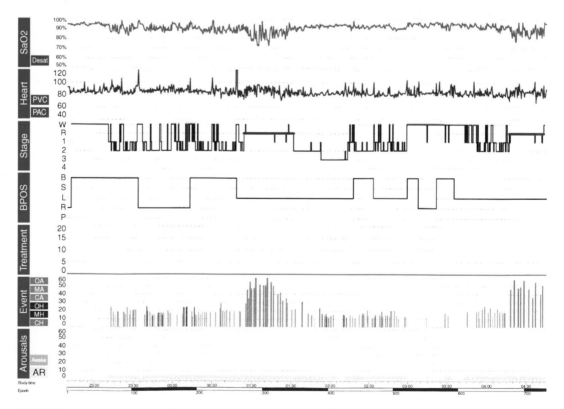

FIGURE 44.1 *Hypnogram shows the oxygen saturation (blue, first row); heart rate (second row in red); sleep stages (third row, REM sleep stage in red); body position (fourth row); different respiratory events (fifth row): obstructive apneas in green, obstructive hypopneas in red and respiratory effort-related arousals in blue; and arousals (sixth row in yellow).*

DIAGNOSIS. **Obstructive sleep apnea–hypopnea syndrome (OSAHS).**

DISCUSSION

The patient was recommended to use CPAP machine and return in six weeks. He was asked to see a nutritionist to encourage weight loss. Polysomnogram is useful in diagnosing various sleep-related disorders. The PSG measures multiple physiological variables, including, EEG, respiratory flow (via a nasal canula and a nasal and oral canula), respiratory effort (via elastic bands), oxygen saturation, EKG, and limb movements. It is beyond the scope of this book to describe various sleep disorders in detail. However, a brief introduction to various sleep-related breathing disorders is given below.

SLEEP-RELATED BREATHING DISORDERS

I. Central Sleep Apnea
Primary central apnea

Central sleep apnea due to Cheyne stokes breathing pattern

Central sleep apnea due to high-altitude periodic breathing

Central sleep apnea due to medical condition, not Cheyne stokes

Central sleep apnea due to drug or substance abuse

Primary sleep apnea of infancy

II. Obstructive Sleep Apnea Syndromes
Obstructive sleep apnea, adult

Obstructive sleep apnea, pediatric

III. Sleep-Related Hypoventilation/Hypoxemic Syndromes
Sleep-related nonobstructive alveolar hypoventilation, idiopathic

Congenital central alveolar hypoventilation syndrome

Sleep-related hypoventilation/hypoxemia due to medical condition

    Sleep-related hypoventilation/hypoxemia due to pulmonary parenchymal or vascular pathology

    Sleep-related hypoventilation/hypoxemia due to lower airways obstruction

    Sleep-related hypoventilation/hypoxemia due to neuromuscular and chest wall disorders

The OSAHS is characterized by repetitive episodes of breathing pauses during sleep. The obstruction occurs in the upper airway. Apnea is defined by a total cessation of breathing for 10 or more seconds, and hypopnea is defined as a drop in airflow by ≥ 30% of baseline and ≥ 4% desaturation lasting at least 10 seconds (Table 44.1). The apneic episodes are obstructive

TABLE 44.1 *Definitions Used in Sleep-Related Breathing Disorders*

Apnea	Total cessation of breathing for 10 or more seconds. Obstructive if effort, central if no effort to breathe
Hypopnea	Drop in flow by ≥ 30% of baseline and a ≥ 4% desaturation lasting at least 10 seconds
RERAs	Increased respiratory effort or flattening of the nasal pressure wave form leading to an arousal for at least 10 seconds
AHI	Total apneas + total hypopneas/total sleep time. Normal if < 5
RDI	Total apneas + total hypopneas + total RERAs/total sleep time. Normal if < 5

if the patient is making an effort to breathe. However, if there is no effort to breathe, apnea is referred as central apnea. The mixed category has features of both central and obstructive apnea. The OSAHS is closely related to weight and has a prevalence of 2% to 4% in the general population. OSAHS besides causing sleep fragmentation and subsequent sleepiness leads to an increased risk of hypertension and cardiovascular events, including CAD and strokes.

The AHI is defined as the total number of apneas and hypopneas during the night divided by the total sleep time in hours. A total AHI of less than 5 is considered normal, 5–15 is considered mild OSA, 15–30 is moderate OSA, and greater than 30 is considered severe OSA (Table 44.1).

The treatment of OSAHS is aimed to open the upper airway (Table 44.2). For cases that are mild to moderate, upper airway surgery, including removal of the soft palate and tonsils (if enlarged), may help. This procedure is called UPP surgery. Oral appliances, which are mouth guards that advance the mandible forward at night, are also indicated for mild to moderate cases or patients that cannot tolerate CPAP. CPAP is a device that acts as a pneumatic splint pushing compressed air though the upper airway. CPAP masks (Figure 44.2A and 44.2B) are

TABLE 44.2 *Treatment of OSA*

Mild OSA, AHI 5–15	Weight loss, positional therapy, oral appliances, uvulopalatopharyngoplasty surgery, CPAP
Moderate OSA, AHI 15–30	Weight loss, positional therapy, oral appliances, uvulopalatopharyngoplasty surgery, CPAP
Severe OSA, AHI ≥ 30	Bariatric surgery, maxilo-mandibular advancement surgery, CPAP/bi-level PAP

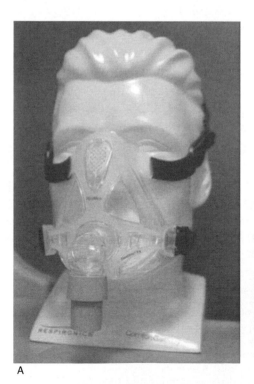
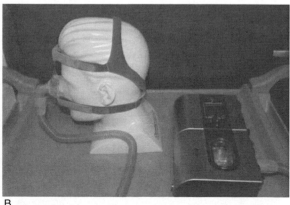

A   B

FIGURE 44.2 *(A,B) Various facial masks attached to the CPAP machine.*

worn on the face and attached with headgear. They receive air through a tube that is attached to a CPAP machine.

Other measures include bariatric surgery for morbid obesity, MMA surgery in patients that cannot tolerate CPAP or are not candidates for this device. MMA advances the mandible and maxilla, which opens up the upper airway. Lastly, tracheostomy will bypass the upper airway and essentially skip the site of obstruction. Lifestyles modifications should be part of the treatment of OSAHS, including weight loss, positional therapy (in cases with a positional component), and avoiding alcohol or sedatives, which can worsen OSAHS.

There is a group of patients that continue to be sleepy, even after properly treated for OSAHS. The cause of this problem is unknown. Modafinil at doses of 200 to 400 mg and armodafinil (longer acting enantiomer) at 150 to 250 mg are indicated for excessive daytime sleepiness. The clinician should be careful and try to rule out other sleep disorders or medications that can contribute to sleepiness in these patients.

SUGGESTED READING

Grunstein R. Continuous positive airway pressure treatment for obstructive sleep apnea–hypopnea syndrome. In: Kryger MH, Roth T, Dement WC, eds. *Principles and Practice of Sleep Medicine.* 4th ed. Philadelphia, PA: Elsevier Saunders; 2005:1066–1080.

Guilleminault C, Bassiri A. Clinical features and evaluation of obstructive sleep apnea–hypopnea syndrome and upper airway resistance syndrome. In: Kryger MH, Roth T, Dement WC, eds. *Principles and Practice of Sleep Medicine.* 4th ed. Philadelphia, PA: Elsevier Saunders; 2005:1043–1052.

Kushida CA, Littner MR, Hirshkowitz M, et al. Practice parameters for the use of continuous and bilevel positive airway pressure devices to treat adult patients with sleep-related breathing disorders. *Sleep.* 2006;29(3):375–380.

Morgenthaler TI, Kapen S, Lee-Chiong T. Practice parameters for the medical therapy of obstructive sleep apnea. *Sleep.* 2006;29(8):1031–1035.

Strollo PJ, Atwood CW, Sanders MH. Medical therapy for obstructive sleep apnea–hypopnea syndrome. In: Kryger MH, Roth T, Dement WC, eds. *Principles and Practice of Sleep Medicine.* 4th ed. Philadelphia, PA: Elsevier Saunders; 2005:1053–1065.

Young T, Palta M, Dempsey J, Skatrud J, Weber S, Badr S. The occurrence of sleep-disordered breathing among middle-aged adults. *N Engl J Med.* 1993;328:1230–1235.

Excessive Daytime Sleepiness and Recurrent Episodes of Sleep Paralysis

Alcibiades J. Rodriguez, Irina Ok, and Sonia Anand

CHIEF COMPLAINT: **I sleep too much.**

HISTORY OF PRESENT ILLNESS

A 25-year-old female was referred to our sleep clinic for EDS. She stated that she was in her usual state of health until her senior year of high school when she noted that she would become increasingly sleepy even during the daytime. The patient mentioned that she gets at least 10 to 12 hours of sleep at night but even then would fall asleep during her class sessions. Upon returning home from school, she has to take short naps. During the naps, she has been experiencing vivid dreams of images and faces. The patient would wake up in the early morning hours between 3 and 5 a.m. with inability to move for several seconds. These episodes were exacerbated by sleep deprivation. On further questioning, the patient mentioned episodes of knee buckling triggered by emotional outbursts, such as laughter.

Her sleep–wake cycle consisted of going to bed at 8 p.m. and waking up at 6 a.m. during the weekdays and between 8 p.m. and 10 a.m. during the weekends. She endorsed frequent movements of her legs during sleep and was told that she "kicks" her legs at night. However, she denied snoring or other abnormal night-time behavior.

The patient denied any past medical history and was not taking any medications. She denied any history of head trauma or infections in the past. Her ESS was 18/24.

PHYSICAL EXAMINATION

Patient's height is 5′6″ and she weighs about 130 pounds.
Vital signs: Blood pressure, 110/70 mm Hg; heart rate, 72; respiratory rate, 12.
Both the general and neurological examinations were unremarkable.
The patient underwent a diagnostic PSG followed by an MSLT.

STOP AND THINK QUESTIONS

➢ What is Polysomnography?

➢ What is Multiple Sleep Latency Test?

➢ What is the treatment for excessive daytime sleepiness?

DIAGNOSTIC TEST RESULTS

The PSG showed a sleep efficiency of 84% with a total sleep time of 510 minutes. The sleep latency was 5 minutes with an REM sleep latency of 25 minutes. There was no evidence of sleep disordered breathing. The PLMS was 25.0. There were PLMS also during REM sleep, but not definite increased muscle tone during REM sleep stage (Table 45.1). The MSLT showed a sleep latency of 2.5 minutes with four out of five naps with SOREMPs.

TABLE 45.1 *Results of Patient's PSG in Comparison to Normal Values*

Category in PSG	Total Sleep Time (min)	Sleep Efficiency (%)	Sleep Latency (min)	REM Sleep Latency (min)	PLMS Index (episodes/h)
Normal	450 to 480	85 to 100	15	90	< 5
Patient	510	84	5	25	25

TABLE 45.2 *Normal Stages of Sleep*

Stages of Sleep	Description of Stage	Time Spent in Stage (% total sleep time)
Non-REM I	Initiation of sleep cycle; light stage of sleep, transition between wakefulness and sleep; high amplitude theta waves	4 to 5
Non-REM II	Bursts of rapid rhythmic high frequency sleep spindles; decrease in body temperature and heart rate	45 to 55
Non-REM III	Deep, slow high amplitude delta waves begin to appear along with theta frequency; >20% of delta	20 to 25
REM	Salient feature is the presence of dreaming; characterized by eye movements, muscle atonia, low frequency EEG, alpha and beta frequency, increased respiratory rate and brain activity	20 to 25

DIAGNOSIS: **Narcolepsy and cataplexy.**

DISCUSSION

Sleep goes through a series of stages in which different brain wave patterns are displayed. There are two main types of sleep, active and quiet sleep. Active or paradoxical sleep is also known as REM sleep. Quiet sleep is often referred as NREM. The description of the different stages of sleep is represented below in Table 45.2.

The diagnosis of narcolepsy usually requires, besides the clinical manifestations, a PSG followed by a MSLT. PSG is derived from the Greek words, *poly:* multiple and *somnos:* sleep. It means the measure of multiple physiological variables during sleep. During this test, the variables measured include EEG, eye movements, respiratory flow, respiratory effort, limb movements, oxygen, and EKG. MSLT is an objective test to measure sleepiness. It consists of five 20-minute naps separated by 2-hour intervals. The sleep and REM sleep latency are measured. The PSG in patients with narcolepsy is done the night before to be sure that the patient sleeps enough time before a MSLT is performed the day after. The American Academy of Sleep Medicine requires a minimum of 6 hours of total sleep time in the PSG preceding the MSLT. These patients also may have RBD and increased PLMS Index, including in REM sleep stage. The MSLT criteria for narcolepsy require an average sleep latency of ≤ 5 minutes and at least 2 episodes of SOREMPs. SOREMPs are defined as REM sleep stage onset in less than 15 minutes.

Narcolepsy is a neurological sleep disorder characterized by clinical symptoms that are summarized in Table 45.3.

EDS is the irresistible urge to sleep, even during unusual situations, as for example, talking to other persons or driving. The ESS is a subjective test to measure sleepiness. The test consists of eight questions asking the patient the chances of dozing off during sedentary situations (0 – no chance to 3 – high chance). The values range from 0 to 24. A value of 10 or more is considered a possible indicator of EDS.

- Sitting and reading
- Watching TV
- Sitting, inactive in a public place (e.g., a car, theater, or a meeting)
- As a passenger in a car for an hour, without a break
- Lying down to rest in the afternoon, when circumstances permit
- Sitting and talking to someone
- Sitting quietly after a lunch without alcohol
- In a car, while stopped for a few minutes in traffic

There are other scales like the KSS, but the ESS is the most widely used scale in everyday clinical practice. The differential diagnosis of EDS include other conditions such as chronic sleep deprivation, OSA, idiopathic or related to brain injuries, coexisting medical disorders, and concomitant use of medications. It is important to remember that many patients may describe fatigue as sleepiness.

TABLE 45.3 *Clinical Characteristics of Narcolepsy*

Symptoms of Narcolepsy	Clinical Correlation	Prevalence Among Narcoleptics (%)
Excessive daytime sleepiness	Difficulty maintaining wakefulness during the day resulting in tendency to fall sleep	100
Hypnagogic/Hypnopompic hallucinations	Vivid images occurring either during sleep onset or upon awakening, respectively	66
Cataplexy	Sudden diminishment of muscle tone and absent reflexes resulting in muscle weakness, paralysis, or postural collapse; Exacerbated by emotional outbursts	60 to 100
Sleep paralysis	Inability to move during sleep onset or upon awakening	60
Fragmented sleep	Frequent arousals lasting from seconds to several hours	60 to 90

TABLE 45.4 *Diagnostic Tests for Narcolepsy*

Test	Description	Benefits	Limitations
PSG	Performed night prior to MSLT	Employed for initial evaluation of narcolepsy; confirms fragmented sleep patterns; Rule out other sleep d/o	Sleep time for PSG can differ from pt usual sleep time thereby results can be misleading; Environmental noise and other factors may confound PSG results
MSLT	Consists of five 20-minute naps separated by 2-hour intervals. Sleep and REM latency are measured. It must be performed the morning after the PSG	Essential to diagnosis of narcolepsy: diagnosis made with a mean sleep latency of ≤ 8 minutes and ≥ 2 SOREMPs:	Validity of test dependent on patient's total sleep time at least 6 hours prior night; must have at least two SOREMPs otherwise diagnosis less reliable
CSF hypocretin levels	Levels ≤110 pg/ml or one third of mean normal control values	It is positive in more than 90% of patients with narcolepsy and cataplexy	Not as useful in patients with narcolepsy without cataplexy
HLA testing	Supplementary tool for diagnosis	Can aid in diagnosis if results inconclusive	Lacks specificity for diagnosis

TABLE 45.5 *Medication Therapy for Narcolepsy*

Medication	Brand Name	Method of Action	Symptom Treated	Benefits	Side Effects
Sodium Oxybate	Xyrem	γ Hydroxybutyrate	EDS; Cataplexy	Short duration of action; anticatapletic effects during daytime	Habit forming; functional impairment due to sedative potential
Modafinil	Provigil	Nonsympathomimetic wakefulness promoting agent	EDS	Fewer sympathomimetic side effects; lower potency than amphetamines	Allergic reaction; diarrhea; back pain; headache
Armodafinil	Nuvigil	Nonsympathomimetic wakefulness promoting agent	EDS	Fewer sympathomimetic side effects; lower potency than amphetamines	Allergic reaction; diarrhea; dry mouth; headache
Methylphenidate	Concerta; Ritalin	Stimulant	EDS	Short duration of action	Dizziness; drowsiness; headache
Dextroamphetamine	Dexedrine	Stimulant	EDS	Variable duration of action	Heart palpitations; tremor; hallucinations
Methamphetamine	Desoxyn	Stimulant	EDS	Better central versus peripheral distribution; more effective than amphetamines	Constipation; diarrhea; headache; tremor
Dextroamphetamine/ Amphetamine salts	Adderall	Stimulant	EDS	Variable duration of action	Constipation; diarrhea; headache; Tremor
Nortriptyline	Pamelor	TCA	Cataplexy	Well tolerated	Dizziness; dry mouth; weight fluctuations
Fluoxetine	Prozac	SSRI	Cataplexy	Well tolerated; less weight gain	Anxiety; sexual dysfunction; diarrhea
Venlafaxine	Effexor	SNRI	EDS; Cataplexy	Acts on both serotoninergic and adrenergic systems	Anxiety; blurred vision; sexual dysfunction
Atomoxetine	Strattera	SNRI	EDS; Cataplexy	Well tolerated; less addictive potential	Constipation; coughing; sexual dysfunction
Selegilline	Eldepryl	MAO-B inhibitor	EDS; Cataplexy	Variable mechanism of action; less addictive potential	Dizziness; dry mouth; vivid dreams

Cataplexy is the sudden onset of muscle atonia (characteristic of REM sleep) during wakefulness. It is present in 60% to 100% of patients with narcolepsy. It is usually triggered by strong emotional outbursts, such as laughter or anger. *Sleep paralysis* is when despite waking up the patient is unable to move for several seconds to minutes secondary to persistent muscle atonia of REM sleep. Sleep paralysis is often accompanied by *hypnagogic and hypnopompic hallucinations*. Hallucinations are the intrusions of REM sleep imagery into wakefulness. These are often visual, but may include sensory or auditory experiences. The hallucinations may occur just prior to sleep onset (hypnagogic) or upon awakening (hypnopompic). Moreover, patients with narcolepsy have very fragmented sleep and other sleep disorders may coexist, including RBD, OSA, and PLMS.

Almost all patients with narcolepsy are positive for the HLA DQB1*0602. Interestingly, monozygotic twins are only approximately 25% to 31% concordant for narcolepsy, suggesting that environmental factors may play a role in the pathophysiology of the disease. There is evidence that infections, such as streptococcal throat infection, can trigger the onset of narcolepsy. Research studies have shown that hypocretin, a neuropeptide manufactured by cells in the hypothalamus to help control sleep, levels are low in patients with narcolepsy and cataplexy. Therefore, it is possible that an autoimmune process may trigger the disease in genetically susceptible individuals.

Patients who have narcolepsy with cataplexy also have very low levels of hypocretin in the CSF, which is an acceptable test used to confirm the diagnosis (Table 45.4).

The treatment for narcolepsy is directed towards managing its symptoms. EDS is treated with stimulants. Modafinil 200 to 400 mg daily divided into two doses is approved for the treatment of EDS in patients with narcolepsy. More recently, a longer acting enantiomer of modafinil has been used. Armodafinil 150 to 250 mg once daily is also approved for this purpose. If these two medications are not enough to help EDS, then amphetamine-based stimulants are used, including methylphenidate and dextroamphetamine. These medications come in short and long acting versions. There are a variety of other methods that can be employed for treating EDS, such as naps and improved sleep hygiene techniques (Table 45.5).

Sodium oxybate is the only medication approved for the treatment of cataplexy. Sodium oxybate in combination with modafinil helps to decrease sleepiness more than either drug alone. Before sodium oxybate, tricyclic antidepressants and SSRIs were used to treat cataplexy. Venlafaxine, an SNRI , also seems to be effective. The AASM has suggested the use of sodium oxybate for sleep paralysis and disrupted sleep in patients with narcolepsy. RBD can be treated with long acting benzodiazepines, such as clonazepam.

SUGGESTED READING

AASM. *International Classification of Sleep Disorders. Diagnostic and Coding Manual.* 2nd ed. Westchester, Illinois: American Academy of Sleep Medicine; 2005.

Aldrich MS. The clinical spectrum of narcolepsy and idiopathic hypersomnia. *Neurology.* 1996;46:393–401.

Nishino S, Mignot E. Narcolepsy and cataplexy. *Handb Clin Neurol.* 2011;99:783–814.

Zaharna M, Dimitriu A, Guilleminault C. Expert opinion on pharmacotherapy of narcolepsy. *Expert Opin Pharmacother.* 2010;11:1633–1645.

CHIEF COMPLAINT: **Right side is weak and cannot hear well.**

HISTORY OF PRESENT ILLNESS

This is a 21-year-old, left-handed male with a history of right-sided weakness and progressive hearing loss. Patient reported that he first experienced weakness in his right arm and leg at the age of 8 years. A brain MRI scan was performed, disclosing several lesions in the skull base, including bilateral vestibular schwannomas. As these lesions did not account for his symptoms, an MRI scan of his cervical and thoracic spine was done, showing an extensive intra- and extradural tumor at C4–C6, deforming his spinal cord. He underwent a partial surgical resection of the tumor and his weakness improved considerably. He was clinically diagnosed with NF 2 and he was then followed expectantly on a yearly basis with serial MRI scans and hearing assessments. His vestibular schwannomas have gradually increased and caused hearing loss. He received a course of hypofractionated stereotactic radiation therapy in five fractions for a total of 20 Gray at the age of 12 years for his left vestibular schwannoma, and a year later to the right vestibular schwannoma. Following such treatment, he became deaf in his right ear and had stable impaired hearing in his left ear until recently. Over the past few years, he has been losing hearing in the higher frequencies. He has also developed multiple cranial nerve schwannomas, predominantly on the right side, as well as some convexity meningiomas, with a larger in the right parasagittal frontal region. All of these tumors have been growing slowly. He underwent a partial resection of a large left cerebellopontine angle meningioma, distinct from his known vestibular schwannoma, at 19 years of age. Following this surgery, he noticed transient left facial numbness and worsening in his right arm weakness. He was told that he had some gradual recurrence and enlargement of the cervical and upper thoracic schwannomas. He has developed multiple subcutaneous neurofibromas, some of which have been removed. He denied any back pain, dysphagia, voice change, bladder symptoms, headache, seizure, or numbness in any of the four extremities. He does have balance difficulties, tinnitus, and mild persistent right-sided weakness.

PAST MEDICAL HISTORY

NF type 2 with multiple intracranial and intraspinal tumors.

PAST SURGICAL HISTORY

Partial resection of his cervical spinal schwannoma and left cerebellopontine angle meningioma; resection of several subcutaneous neurofibromas.

MEDICATIONS

None.

ALLERGIES

None.

PERSONAL HISTORY

Denied any smoking, drugs, and alcohol.

FAMILY HISTORY

No other family member with NF type 2.

GENERAL PHYSICAL EXAMINATION

Well-appearing male in no distress. No scoliosis. Well-healed craniotomies and cervical scars. Multiple small subcutaneous and cutaneous neurofi bromas. No café au lait spots.

NEUROLOGICAL EXAMINATION

Higher mental functions: Alert and oriented to time, place and person; affect showing emotional disengagement, attention and concentration, and judgment were normal; his immediate recall −3/3 and recall of three objects after 5 minutes was 3/3. Comprehension, expression (fluency), repetition, reading, and writing were normal.

CNs II–XII: OU 20/20 with corrective glasses, pupils equal and reactive, fundi normal, visual fields full by confrontation method, facial sensation normal and symmetrical, mild right-sided lower motor-neuron facial weakness; deaf in his right ear, could hear finger rubbing and whispering with his left ear, uvula moved symmetrically, tongue midline, no tongue atrophy, no tongue fasciculations, sternocleidomastoids and trapezii muscles showed normal strength.

Motor: Normal tone, strength proximally and distally in the left upper and lower extremities was normal and was 5/5, but decreased to 4/5 in his right upper extremity more than his lower extremity, both slightly worse distally than proximally.

Sensory: Intact to LT, PP, temperature, vibration, and position sense. There was no agraphesthesia.

Reflexes: Biceps, triceps, brachioradialis, patellar, and ankle jerks were 2+ on the left and 3+ on the right; there was no ankle clonus or Hoffman's.

Plantars: Flexor on the left, extensor on the right.

Romberg: Negative.

Cerebellar: Finger-to-nose and knee-shin-heel were normal on the left, but showed dysmetria on the right.

Gait: Normal, but significant difficulty with tandem.

DIAGNOSTIC TEST RESULTS

Labs: CBC and diff, SMA-20: unremarkable.

MRI brain and spine: Multiple intracranial and intraspinal tumors, including several meningiomas, the largest of which in the right parasagittal frontal region (see Figure 46.1), bilateral vestibular schwannomas (see Figure 46.2), multiple cranial and spinal schwannomas (see Figure 46.3).

Hearing test: Severe sensorineural hearing loss from 250 to 8000 Hz on the right, moderate sensorineural hearing loss from 200 to 1000 Hz and above 4000 Hz on the left.

DIAGNOSIS: Neurofibromatosis (NF) type 2.

DISCUSSION

NF types 1 and 2 do fall under the spectrum of neurophacomatosis, which are unique clinical syndromes with skin manifestations and neurological impairment (see Table 46.1). Phacos comes from the Greek word meaning mole or freckle. Neurological abnormalities are encountered with skin, multi-organ, and retinal pigmented lesions that can be explained by their common neural crest origin.

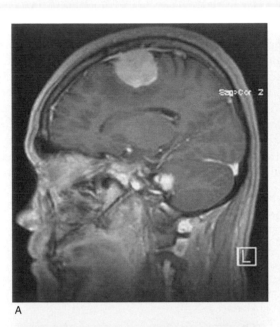

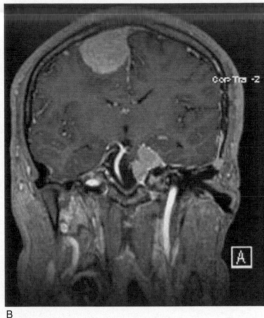

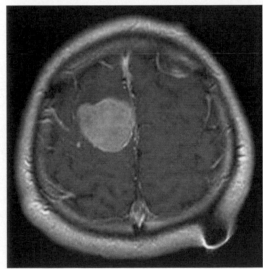

FIGURE 46.1 *MRI brain with Gd: sagittal (A), coronal (B), and axial (C) T1WI post gadolinium showing dural-based right frontal meningioma with surrounding mass effect, most evident in the sagittal image.*

Neurofibromatoses are genetic disorders that predispose people to form tumors on nerve tissue. These tumors can occur anywhere in the nervous system, including the brain, spinal cord, and large and small nerves. Neurofibromatoses comprise three autosomal dominant disorders: NF1 (also known as von Recklinghausen's disease), NF2, and schwannomatosis. Although NF1 is the most common of the neurofibromatoses, this discussion will focus primarily on NF type 2.

PATHOGENESIS

NF type 2 is linked with abnormalities in the *NF2* gene, located on chromosome 22q12. This gene normally acts as a tumor suppressor through inhibition of the ras oncogene pathway by producing merlin, also known as schwannomin. Merlin is a cell-membrane-related protein that interacts with actin and surface proteins to regulate cell proliferation and adhesion, although its exact function remains yet to be elucidated. NF2 is an autosomal dominant disorder, meaning only one copy of the mutated gene needs to be inherited to pass the disorder. A germ line mutation in the *NF2* gene makes its tumor suppressing properties dysfunctional. The development of tumors requires inactivation of both *NF2* alleles. Individuals with NF2 may inherit an abnormal allele from a parent or de novo mutations may take place

TABLE 46.1 *Common Types of Neurophacomatoses*

NF types 1 and 2
Tuberous sclerosis
Sturge-Weber syndrome
Von-Hippel Lindau
Klippel-Trenaunay-Weber syndrome
Ataxia telangiectasia
Incontinentia pigmenti
Hypomelanosis of Ito
Epidermal Nevus syndrome

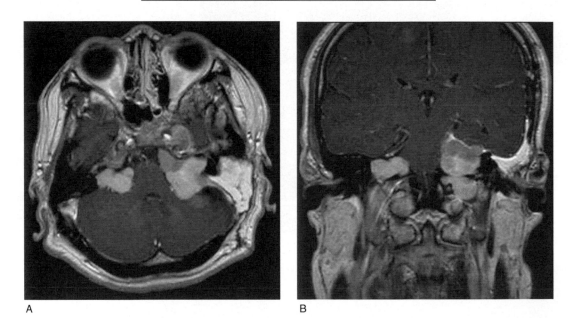

A   B

FIGURE 46.2 *MRI brain axial T1WI with Gd (A) showing enhancing bilateral vestibular schwannomas filling and expanding the internal auditory canals, with the left exerting moderate mass effect on the brain stem, cerebellum, and middle cerebral peduncle; MR T1WI with Gd, coronal plane (B) attention internal auditory canal demonstrating again the enhancing tumors, in association with fat packing within the left mastoidectomy defect from prior surgery. The large left complex lobulated mass represents a combination of lower cranial nerve, eighth nerve, and fifth nerve schwannomas and tentorial meningioma.*

after fertilization. With the latter, two separate cell lineages arise, and germline mosaicism occurs. Indeed, depending on the timing of the mutation during the embryological development, a small to large proportion of the cells constituting the entire body will harbor the mutation. It can lead to the appearance of segmental disease (only affecting one part of the body) and to a false leading negative serum molecular genetic testing, although mutation can be detected by testing directly the tumor specimen. In these cases, the risk of transmission to an offspring is consequently less than 50%. However, their offspring, if affected, may harbor a more severe phenotype as all of their cells will carry the mutation.

In familial cases, the expressivity of the disorder can be variable but the penetrance is 100%. Although questioned in certain studies and with documented phenotypic variability within families with the same mutation, a genotypic–phenotypic correlation has been suggested. More precisely, frameshift or nonsense mutations cause truncated protein expression and have been found to be associated with more severe disease manifestations (younger age at presentation, higher number of tumors, and greater disease-related mortality), whereas missense or inframe deletions seem to be associated with a milder phenotype. A somewhat earlier age of onset and slightly more severe course when the disease is inherited from the mother rather than from the father has raised the possibility of maternal imprinting affecting the *NF2* gene. Mutations of the *NF2* gene have been found in both NF2-related and sporadic unilateral vestibular schwannomas, although point mutations constitute the majority of mutations in the former, whereas small deletions account for the majority in the latter.

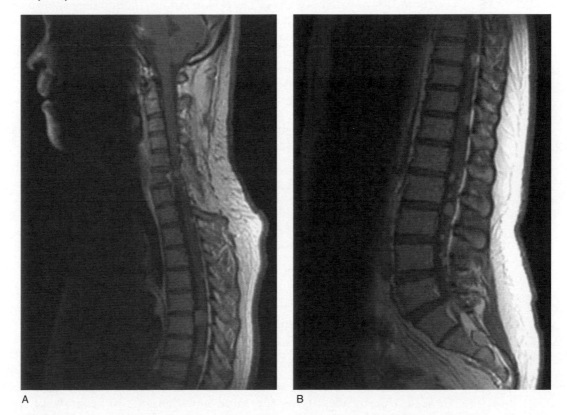

A B

FIGURE 46.3 *MRI sagittal spine T1WI with Gd: cervical and thoracic spine (A) showing an extensive intra and extradural tumor at C4–C6, deforming his spinal cord. Multiple intraspinal and extradural tumors were seen throughout the lower thoracic and lumbosacral spine (B).*

EPIDEMIOLOGY

The frequency of NF2 is about 1 in 40,000 to 50,000. It is much less common than NF1, which has a frequency of 1 in 3000. Now, NF2 is more readily identified than it was originally due to the recognition that greater than one half of cases represent de novo mutations and can occur in the absence of positive family history.

CLINICAL MANIFESTATIONS

Patients with NF2 typically present around 20 years of age. The clinical features include neurological, eye, and skin lesions.

Bilateral vestibular schwannomas are the hallmark of NF2, generally occurring by age 30 and developing in 90% to 95% of cases. They typically cause tinnitus, profound hearing loss, and balance dysfunction. Although they are nearly always benign, if left untreated, they can extend medially and cause brain stem compression and hydrocephalus. Schwannomas also occur on other cranial nerves and in the spinal cord. They are the most common spinal tumor in patients with NF2, though others include meningiomas in the extramedullary space and ependymomas in the intramedullary space. Meningiomas occur in the brain and spinal cord and are often multiple. Figure 46.1 shows meningiomas typically seen in NF2. Neuropathies can manifest in various ways, sometimes as a mononeuropathy involving the facial nerve or less commonly as a severe polyneuropathy.

Ophthalmic lesions of NF2 typically manifest as cataracts. Other manifestations include optic nerve meningiomas, retinal hamartomas, and epiretinal membranes.

About 70% of patients with NF2 have skin lesions, though they are typically not as abundant as in those with NF1. People can have plaque-like lesions that are slightly raised and may be hyperpigmented or associated with increased hair. Subcutaneous nodules can exist along the course of peripheral nerves; they are palpable and represent swelling of the nerve. Finally, patients can have intracutaneous tumors. In NF1, these typically represent neurofibromas whereas in NF2, these can represent schwannomas.

CRITICAL CRITERIA

Clinical criteria for the diagnosis of NF2 (the Manchester criteria) are based on the presence of one of the following criteria:

- Bilateral vestibular schwannomas
- A first-degree relative with NF2 AND
  - Unilateral vestibular schwannoma OR
  - Any two of the following: meningioma, schwannoma, glioma, neurofibroma, posterior subcapsular lenticular opacities
- Unilateral vestibular schwannoma AND
  - Any two of: meningioma, schwannoma, glioma, neurofibroma, posterior subcapsular lenticular opacities
- Multiple meningiomas AND
  - Unilateral vestibular schwannoma OR
  - Any two of: schwannoma, glioma, neurofibroma, cataract

The clinical diagnosis can be confirmed by identifying a pathogenic mutation of NF2 in serum or by identifying the same mutation in two separate tumors in the same individual.

There are certain individuals who do not fully meet the diagnostic criteria for NF2, yet screening is indicated to identify NF2 and help minimize complications of disease manifestations. Screening is done by testing for gene mutation in the patient's serum. When a specific mutation has been identified in the index case, this serves as a 100% specific marker to test other family members. Prenatal testing is possible where a known mutation exists. Individuals in whom screening is indicated include:

- Those with a first-degree relative with NF2
- Those with multiple spinal tumors
- Those with cutaneous schwannomas
- Those with a vestibular schwannoma less than 30 years of age or a spinal tumor or meningioma less than 20 years of age

If screening identifies an NF2 mutation, certain follow-up examinations are recommended including: annual hearing evaluations with brain stem auditory evoked response, ophthalmologic evaluation, skin examination, and craniospinal MRI beginning at age 10 and repeated every 3 to 5 years after age 20 years. If lesions are found, then testing should be performed annually.

MANAGEMENT

The management of patients with NF2 is aimed at treating the various lesions that arise and their complications. Vestibular schwannomas do not always warrant treatment, though it is generally indicated when there is a risk of brain stem compression, deterioration of hearing, or facial nerve dysfunction. Surgical resection is the usual treatment, though stereotactic radiosurgery and stereotactic radiotherapy have a role as well in certain patients. One particular study found that 100% of schwannomas express VEGF and that bevacizumab, a VEGF inhibitor, led to tumor shrinkage and hearing improvement in many though not all patients. This medication may offer hopeful treatment in the future, yet it has its limitations and is not currently standard of care. Many other molecular targeted therapies on VEGF and other pathways, such as VEGF receptor and platelet-derived growth factor receptor, Raf/Mek/Erk pathway (MAP kinase pathway), and mTOR, are currently being under investigation and hold promises as replacing surgery and its morbidity as first line therapy. For those who suffer from severe bilateral sensorineural hearing loss due to vestibular schwannomas, cochlear implants and auditory brain stem implants are available.

Meningiomas and intramedually spinal tumors can typically be monitored without intervention. However, if they become symptomatic, surgery may be warranted. Radiation is rarely used. Eye and skin lesions often are monitored but go untreated, though the different lesions are variably managed (i.e., cataract removal).

SUGGESTED READING

Asthagiri AR, Parry DM, Butman JA, et al. Neurofibromatosis type 2. *Lancet* 2009;373:1974.

Baser EM, Friedman JM, Wallace AJ, et al. Evaluation of clinical diagnostic criteria for neurofibromatosis 2. *Neurology*. 2002;59:1759–1765.

Evans DG. Neurofibromatosis type 2: Genetic and clinical features. *Ear Nose and Throat Journal.* 1999;78(2):97–100.

Kumar, Vinay, Abbas, Abul K. *Fausto, Nelson. Robbins and Cotran Pathologic Basis of Disease*, 7th ed. 2005; 168–169:305.

Plotkin SR, et al. Hearing improvement after bevacizumab in patients with neurofibromatosis type 2. *New Engl J Med.* 2009;361:358–367.

Theodosopoulus PV, Pensak ML. Contemporary management of acoustic neuromas. *The Laryngoscope.* 2011;121(6):1133–1137.

Progressive Weakness and Numbness of the Arms and Legs

Kiril Kiprovski

CHIEF COMPLAINT: **I am weak all over and my arms go to sleep.**

HISTORY OF PRESENT ILLNESS

A 73-year-old, right-handed male presented in the neuromuscular clinic with 6 months history of progressive weakness of the arms and legs and associated numbness. Patient initially started to experience numbness in the ulnar aspect of the right hand. Gradually symptoms progressed, and he started to experience numbness in the left hand as well. Subsequently, he noticed weakness in his arms. He also started to develop some numbness in the right foot, but most significantly, he started to experience weakness in the legs and progressive gait impairment. He developed difficulties using stairs, and he started using a cane. He commented that his hands feel like "sand paper." He was unable to do pushups and curls. There were no chewing or swallowing difficulties or speech impairment. There were no respiratory difficulties or bladder control impairment. His weakness had no diurnal variation. He denied any other constitutional symptoms. He denied any exposure to toxins, tick bite, arthralgias, or skin rash.

PAST MEDICAL HISTORY

Hypertension, BPH.

PAST SURGICAL HISTORY

None.

MEDICATIONS

Aspirin and Terazosin.

ALLERGIES

Penicillin (rash).

FAMILY HISTORY

Is noncontributory.

PHYSICAL EXAMINATION

Patient appears well, and he is in not apparent distress. He is attentive, pleasant, and cooperative gentleman and is able to provide appropriate medical history. He is 5′8″ tall and he weighs 165 pounds. Conjunctivae are pink and sclerae are anicteric. Oropharynx is clear. There are no skin rashes. The blood pressure while sitting is 130/70 mmHg with a heart rate of 80 bpm in regular rhythm.

NEUROLOGICAL EXAMINATION

Higher mental function: Patient has normal cognitive assessment.
CNs II–XII: reveals full eye movements in all directions without nystagmus or diplopia. Visual fields are full on confrontation. Pupils are 3 mm and equally reactive to light.

The face is symmetrical, and he is able to fully close his eyes and pucker his lips. Masticatory muscles are unremarkable. Speech is normal. The tongue protrudes in the midline, and the soft palate elevates bilaterally symmetrical. Sternocleidomastoid and trapezius muscles are with normal bulk and strength.

Motor examination reveals normal bulk and tone in both upper and lower extremities, and there are no involuntary movements. Muscle strength testing reveals proximal and distal weakness in arms and legs graded 4/5 bilaterally.

Sensory examination mildly diminished pin prick in the palms on both sides and mildly diminished pin prick and light touch over the medial aspect of the left foot. There are no skin trophic changes. Vibration sense is mildly decreased to the ankles. Position sense is impaired at the toes. Romberg test is negative.

Muscle stretch reflexes are absent in both upper and lower extremities.

Plantar responses are flexor.

Cerebellar examination is unremarkable. He has to push with both hands in order to stand from a chair. His gait is slow, uncertain, and he needs a cane to ambulate. He is unable to stand on the heel and is able to stand on the toes. He is unable to walk tandem or to squat.

STOP AND THINK QUESTIONS

➢ Is this spinal cord disease?

➢ What is the significance of generalized areflexia?

➢ Which diagnostic tests will be helpful to clarify the diagnosis?

DIAGNOSTIC TEST RESULTS

EMG/NCV showed demyelinating sensorimotor polyneuropathy with conduction block (Figure 47.1). The ulnar nerve motor nerve conduction study shows slowing of the distal conduction velocity of 15 m/s on the right and 17 m/s on the left, and also across the elbow 25 m/s on the right and 17 m/s on the left. There is significant drop in the amplitude and negative area from below the elbow to the wrist of 68% on the right and 75% on the left compatible with conduction block. There is also significant temporal dispersion with proximal stimulation on both sides with 5% increase in duration on the right and 14% on the left. The onset latencies for each individual response are also depicted. CBC, ESR, CRP, PT/PTT, electrolytes, glucose, liver profile, CPK, vitamin B_{12}, folate, thyroid function tests, serum immunoglobulins, serum immunofixation, and RPR are normal or negative; chest X-ray is normal. CSF: total protein, 105 (<60); glucose, 63; cells, 0.

DIAGNOSIS: Chronic inflammatory demyelinating polyneuropathy (CIDP).

DISCUSSION

CIDP is an immune mediated polyneuropathy that in some cases may cause significant disability. As patients with CIDP may improve with immunosuppressant or immunomodulatory treatments, it is important to recognize the disease. The diagnosis is largely based on clinical history, examination, and electrodiagnostic testing. However, there are some patients where it is not possible to establish the diagnosis of CIDP initially. In these cases, additional investigations are needed such as investigating for an associated disorder such

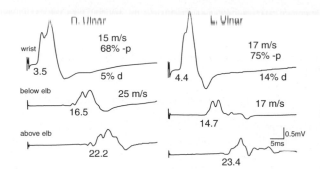

FIGURE 47.1 *Motor nerve conduction studies of right and left ulnar nerves showing slowing of the distal conduction velocity and also across the elbow. There is significant drop in the amplitude from below the elbow to the wrist compatible with conduction block. There is significant temporal dispersion with proximal stimulation on both sides with 5% increase in duration on the right and 14% on the left. The onset latencies for each individual response are also depicted.*

as neoplasm, laboratory studies for associated disease, CSF sampling nerve biopsy, or MRI of plexus or roots.

In the common form of CIDP, the diagnosis must be suspected in patients with progressive symptoms over at least 2 months that involve the upper and lower extremities of predominantly weakness with a proximal and/or distal distribution along with a proprioceptive and/or superficial sensory deficit. Typical CIDP pattern of weakness is characterized by symmetric proximal and distal involvement, but can be purely distal. CIDP is most commonly presents in adults, with a peak incidence at 40 to 60 years of age. Facial and neck flexor muscles can be also involved. Extraocular muscle weakness is rare. Most patients will have some degree of sensory involvement, but the motor symptoms are dominant. The sensory involvement tends to follow a distal to proximal gradient. Sensory involvement of the fingers frequently occurs as early as toes. Sensory symptoms usually consist of numbness and tingling, but painful paresthesias may be present. Many patients have impaired balance due to proprioceptive deficits. Deep tendon reflexes are usually absent or depressed. Autonomic features, sphincter involvement, and respiratory difficulties are infrequent. There is no well-established association between antecedent infections and CIDP. Some patients can progress more rapidly over the first 4 to 8 weeks. The course is slowly progressive in the majority but a relapsing–remitting course is noted in at least one third, more commonly in younger patients. There are various CIDP variants as listed below in Table 47.1.

There are several published recommended criteria for the diagnosis of CIDP. The published criteria are useful for research purposes, but may be too rigid for clinical practice and may exclude many patients with CIDP. Available diagnostic criteria for CIDP need to be viewed as clinical guides and not as firm rules. Various medical illnesses can present with signs and symptoms of CIDP (Table 47.2).

LABORATORY FEATURES

The most important laboratory studies that support the diagnosis of CIDP are the cerebrospinal fluid examination and nerve conduction studies. CSF shows albuminocytologic disassociation. An elevated CSF white blood cell count should lead to consideration of alternate diagnosis such as HIV infection, Lyme disease, neurosarcoidosis, or lymphomatous infiltration of nerve roots. All patients with suspected CIDP should be evaluated for a serum paraprotein. If a paraprotein is present, a search for a lymphoproliferative disorder, such as multiple myeloma or lymphoma, should be undertaken. In some cases, MRI can

TABLE 47.1 *CIDP Variants*

Asymmetric variant of CIDP (Lewis-Sumner syndrome)
Distal acquired demyelinating sensory neuropathy and sensory CIDP
Distal CIDP
Sensory CIDP
Multifocal demyelinating neuropathy with persistent conduction block
Anti-MAG
CIDP with hypertrophic nerves
Subacute demyelinating polyneuropathy
Chronic inflammatory demyelinating neuropathies

TABLE 47.2 *Common Associations with CIDP*

HIV infection: mild lymphocytic pleiocytosis and increased gamma
  globulin
Hodgkin's lymphoma
Paraproteinemias and/or plasma cell dyscrasias
CIDP associated with MGUS: Distal weakness, sensory>motor;
  gammopathy of IgM
Multiple sclerosis
Systemic lupus erythematosus
Chronic active hepatitis (with Hepatitis B or C)
Diabetes mellitus

show enlargement of the spinal roots or increased T2 signal and contrast enhancement in roots of the brachial or lumbosacral plexuses.

HISTOPATHOLOGICAL FINDINGS

In typical cases of CIDP, sural nerve biopsies show demyelination and/or remyelination and, occasional inflammation and decreased density of nerve fibers. Sural nerve biopsy is probably the least useful study compared to CSF and nerve conduction study. In most patients with CIDP, a nerve biopsy is not necessary. A nerve biopsy should be considered if the CSF or nerve conduction studies are not supportive of the diagnosis in a patient who clinically resembles CIDP.

ELECTROPHYSIOLOGICAL FEATURES

Nerve conduction study findings that suggest a demyelinating neuropathy include prolongation of distal motor latency in two or more motor nerves, nonuniform slowing of motor conduction velocity of less than 70% to 80% of the lower limit of normal in two or more motor nerves, delay or absence of F-waves or H-reflex, and the presence of conduction block and/or abnormal temporal dispersion and prolongation of the duration of the compound muscle action potential. Conduction block and temporal dispersion are highly suggestive of an acquired demyelinating process. Sensory responses are usually with decreased amplitude or absent. Somatosensory-evoked potentials can be also useful in some patients.

TREATMENT

CIDP is treated with immunosuppressants. "First line" treatment for CIDP is accepted as steroids, IVIg, or plasma exchange. There are some patients who have CIDP who might have mild disease with minimal impact on function and quality of life. Treatment might not be initiated in these cases. Most patients are impaired significantly, however, by the disorder, and treatment would be indicated.

STEROIDS

Steroids have been widely used in CIDP, and the usefulness of steroids in CIDP has been confirmed. If there is no contraindication to steroids and disability is significant, starting with 1 mg/kg body weight or 60 to 100 mg daily or every other day prednisone or prednisolone for at least 4 weeks is advisable, followed by tapering over months. Continuous oral steroid therapy is the commonest regimen used, but some have proposed pulsed high-dose treatment with dexamethasone or oral methylprednisolone. Steroid treatment seems to be beneficial in 60% to 70% of patients with CIDP, and long-term treatment needs to be individually tailored according to disease course, with careful attention paid to potential side effects.

Pulsed oral methylprednisolone is also efficacious in the long-term treatment of CIDP and is relatively well tolerated. Remission can be induced in most patients. Patients are treated with pulsed oral methylprednisolone, 500 mg once a week, for 3 months, and the dose can be adjusted every 3 months by 50 to 100 mg depending on the clinical status. Intravenous, high-dose methylprednisolone is also an effective treatment for CIDP. One gram of methylprednisolone is administered daily for 3 to 5 consecutive days, followed by one gram weekly for 4 to 8 weeks, and then monthly based on clinical course. Patients treated with intravenous methylprednisolone can have less corticosteroid adverse effects compared with those treated with daily oral prednisone.

Although a minority of patients can eventually be tapered completely off of prednisone, many patients relapse. It is important for both the patient and physician to realize CIDP is a chronic disorder and may require immunosuppressive therapy for many years. Some patients will require a steroid-sparing agent to facilitate the prednisone taper. Azathioprine, mycophenolate mofetil, cyclosporine, and methotrexate can be used.

Blood pressure, blood sugar, and electrolytes need to be monitored with corticosteroid therapy. Before beginning corticosteroids, tuberculin skin testing should be considered. Patients will need regular ophthalmology evaluations for cataracts and glaucoma. Diet program of a low-salt, low-simple sugar, and low-calorie diet to minimize weight gain should be instituted. To help prevent steroid-induced osteoporosis, patients should take 1000 to 1500 mg/d of elemental calcium and 400 to 800 IU of vitamin D per day. Bone densitometry studies can be obtained at baseline and repeated at 6 to 12 month intervals to evaluate for osteoporosis. Consultation with osteoporosis specialist is advisable.

IVIg

IVIg has proven efficacy and is commonly used to treat patient with CIDP. IVIg is usually administered starting with an induction dose of 2 g/kg over 2 to 5 days. Subsequently, maintenance doses of 0.4 g/kg to 1 g/kg are given, usually monthly. Rarely, some patients require infusions every 2 weeks or weekly. If this is the case, smaller infusions can be tried. Optimum frequency and dose of IVIg infusion must be individually adjusted because need varies between patients and the disease course can have spontaneous remission or plateau phases.

The optimal duration of treatment with IVIg in CIDP is unknown, but most of the patient can achieve drug-free remission. If patients continue to require high doses of IVIg for many months, then the addition of steroids or other immunosuppressants might be considered. The IVIg has low side-effect profile. The most common side effects are headache, fever, and hypertension.

Plasma Exchange

PE is effective in patients with CIDP. Most patients can improve with this treatment. Usual protocol is ten courses of PE over 4 weeks. Adverse effects and venous access problems seriously hamper long-term use.

Other Therapies

If treatments other than steroids, IVIg, or PE are considered, the choice of immunosuppressant depends on several factors and must be individualized. These factors include the severity of the disease, which may indicate more aggressive but more risky treatments; the age and gender of patients, which might limit the use of agents that lead to infertility; and coincident medical problems, which may be complicated by certain treatments. Overall, two thirds of CIDP patients respond to one of the three main therapies (prednisone, IVIg, or plasma exchange). If a patient does not respond to one of these first-line therapies, switching to the other is advisable. PE or a combination of steroids and IVIg can be started if neither of these treatments proves effective. Refractory cases might need intensive immunosuppression. Azathioprine, cyclophosphamide, cyclosporine, interferon-α, interferon-β, mycophenolate mofetil, and methotrexate have all been reported to be beneficial in CIDP patients not responsive to initial therapies. Long-term outcome is usually good in patients with CIDP, especially in those with a monophasic or relapsing course. The time from onset to treatment might be determining factor in the prognosis of CIDP.

CONCURRENT ILLNESSES

Several systemic disorders can occur with CIDP such as HIV infection, lymphoma, plasmacytoma, multiple myeloma, POEMS, monoclonal gammopathy of undetermined significance, chronic active hepatitis, hepatitis C, inflammatory bowel disease and connective tissue disease, bone marrow and organ transplants, CNS demyelination, nephrotic syndrome, Lyme disease, diabetes mellitus, hereditary neuropathy, and thyrotoxicosis. These patients should probably be treated no differently from those with idiopathic CIDP.

SUGGESTED READING

Tracy JA, Dyck PJB. Investigations and treatment of chronic inflammatory demyelinating polyradiculoneuropathy and other inflammatory demyelinating polyneuropathies. *Curr Opin Neurol.* 2010;23:242–248.

Vallat JM, Sommer C, Magy L. Chronic inflammatory demyelinating polyradiculoneuropathy: Diagnostic and therapeutic challenges for a treatable condition. *Lancet Neurol.* 2010;9:402–412.

Van den Bergh PY, Hadden RD, Bouche P, et al. European Federation of Neurological Societies/Peripheral Nerve Society guideline on management of chronic inflammatory demyelinating polyradiculoneuropathy: Report of a joint task force of the European Federation of Neurological Societies and the Peripheral Nerve Society—first revision. *Eur J Neurol.* 2010;17(3):356–363.

Vialal K, Maisonobe T, Stojkovic T, et al. A current view of the diagnosis, clinical variants, response to treatment and prognosis of chronic inflammatory demyelinating polyradiculoneuropathy. *Journal of the Peripheral Nervous System.* 2010;15:50–56.

Kimberly Parker Meurer, Chad Carlson, and Anuradha Singh

CHIEF COMPLAINT: **My child has frequent spasms.**

HISTORY OF PRESENT ILLNESS

The patient is a 3-month-old girl referred by her pediatrician for evaluation and treatment of suspected seizures. Her parents describe the events as sudden forward flexion of the head and neck with extension of the arms outward and then inward. Her eyes roll up briefly with each spell. Each episode lasts 2 to 3 seconds, and she has several of these in clusters lasting from 15 to 60 minutes. The eyes do not go one side or the other. In between episodes, she remains quiet with glassy eyes. The episodes do not occur in relation to feeding. These tend to occur as she wakes up from sleep. Parents have not seen any other seizure type.

PAST MEDICAL HISTORY

Product of an uncomplicated, full-term pregnancy and vaginal delivery, birth weight 6 pounds and 4 ounces, Apgars 9/9.

PAST SURGICAL HISTORY

None.

MEDICATIONS

None.

ALLERGIES

NKDA.

PERSONAL HISTORY

Lives at home with parents; she is the only child of her parents.

FAMILY HISTORY

Noncontributory.

PHYSICAL EXAMINATION

Vital signs: Pulse 100/min, regular; respiratory rate, 30/min; blood pressure, 83/59 mm Hg; head circumference, 41.8 cm.

General: Well-nourished interactive 3-month-old female.

HEENT: Normocephalic, anterior and posterior fontannelle patent and soft, tympanic membranes normal, neck supple.

Respiratory: RR 30/min, rate regular, respirations quiet. No nasal flaring, no retractions, or intercostals bulging, chest excursions symmetrical. Trachea midline. Normal breath sounds.

Cardiac: NSR, S1, S2 normal, no murmurs, rubs, gallops, or clicks. +Brachial, radial, pedal pulses.

Abdomen: Soft, flat, and nontender, no hepatosplenomegaly or abdominal pulsatile masses, normoactive bowel sounds, liver edge 1 cm below right costal margin. No groin lymphadenopathy. Femoral pulses full and equal.

Musculoskeletal: Mild decreased tone, strength 5/5 and equal bilaterally, full ROM throughout without observed discomfort.

Skin: Woods lamp examination revealed several 1 to 3 cm elliptical shaped hypopigmented spots located on right thigh, left buttock, and upper and mid back, single leaf-shaped hypopigmented lesion on right arm.

NEUROLOGICAL EXAMINATION

Mental status: Awake and alert, responsive, smiles spontaneously.

CNs II–XII: Normal fundoscopic examination, isocoric pupils, pupils equal and reactive, full EOM, tracks 90 degrees; face symmetric when crying, startles/blink reflex to sharp sound, symmetric soft palate elevation, normal cry, head lag, 45 degrees.

Motor: Normal muscle mass, mild decreased tone, moves all extremities symmetrically, no drift, no fasciculations.

Sensory: Withdrew all extremities equally to tactile stimuli.

Reflexes: Symmetric at 2+ biceps, brachioradialis, triceps, patellar, and Achilles.

Plantars: Bilateral extensors.

Personal/Social: Smiles, regards own hands.

Fine motor/adaptive: Tracks 90 degrees, unable to grasp rattle, does not put hands together.

Language: Ooo/Ahh heard, does not squeal or intentionally laugh.

Gross motor: Holds head 30 degrees while prone, unable to hold head midline with supported sitting.

STOP AND THINK QUESTIONS

➢ How will you classify patient's seizures?

➢ What is the significance of hypopigmented skin lesions?

➢ How are infantile spasms treated?

➢ What are neurophakomatoses?

DIAGNOSTIC TEST RESULTS

MRI brain (Figure 48.1A and 48.1B): Scattered asymmetric patchy areas of abnormal signal within both cerebral hemispheres, predominately involving the gray and subcortical white matter, nodular contour of the bodies of the lateral ventricles.

1st VEEG: Hypsarrhythmia and multifocal spikes.

Echocardiogram: Two small rhabdomyomas in lower ventricular septum of no clinical significance.

Renal ultrasound: Multiple renal cysts and angiomyolipomas bilaterally.

DIAGNOSIS: Tuberous sclerosis complex (TSC) with infantile spasms (IS).

HOSPITAL COURSE

With ACTH, patient's IS resolved and EEG no longer revealed hypsarrhythmia. She was tapered off of ACTH and converted to vigabatrin. After 2 months of seizure freedom, she began to experience seizures with various presentations including moaning, unilateral or

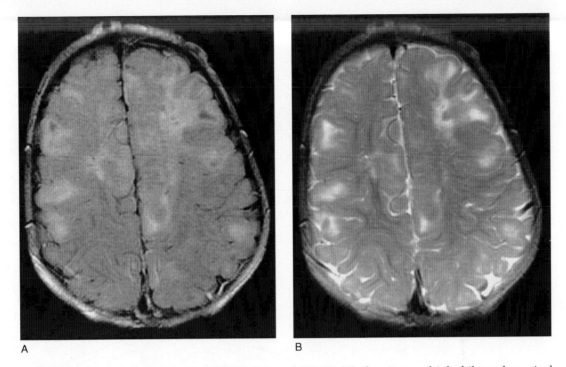

FIGURE 48.1 *Axial MRI brain, FLAIR (A) and T2WI (B) showing multiple bilateral cortical tubers.*

bilateral arm and leg stiffening and jerking, and behavioral arrest. EEG revealed bilateral independent seizure foci as well as multifocal interictal discharges. Despite trials of oxcarbazepine, levetiracetam, topiramate, and lamotrigine, the patient continued to experience frequent seizures and failed to reach developmental milestones. She subsequently underwent a presurgical evaluation to assess candidacy for resective surgery followed by an intracranial EEG monitoring study and resective surgery.

MEG and MSI: Focal hyperexcitability in the right posterior frontal and frontoparietal regions and left frontal region.

Interictal SPECT: Decreased uptake in the left superior and midfrontal regions with decreased perfusion to left anterolateral region of left temporal lobe, decreased perfusion to right temporoparietal region. (Possibility that patient seized during injection.)

Ictal SPECT: Increased perfusion to right superior frontal lobe, stable decreased perfusion to right midfrontal lobe, stable decreased perfusion to left anterolateral temporal lobe and right temporoparietal region. There was perfusion difference in left frontal lobe suggestive of seizure focus when compared with interictal SPECT.

2nd VEEG: Interictal: multifocal spikes, left>right. Ictal: total seizure count 14, 12 from left, 1 right, 1 nonlateralizable.

Intracranial VEEG: 64-point grid, three four-contact strips and one six-contact strip and two eight-contact depth electrodes were placed on the left side (Figure 48.2A). Intracranial ictal EEG onsets were found as shown in Figure 48.2B. Ictal onsets are indicated by red circles.

DISCUSSION

TSC is an autosomal dominant genetic disorder. The mutations causing TSC can be inherited or spontaneous and occur on either of two genes, TSC1 and TSC2, which encode for the

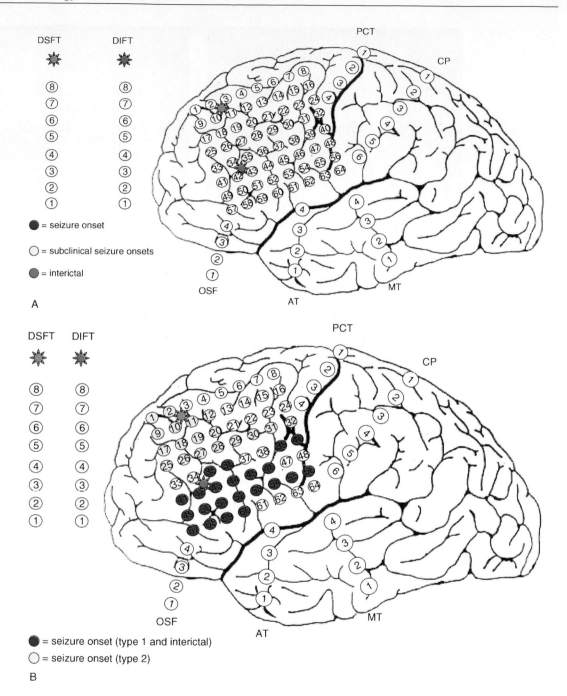

FIGURE 48.2 *Graphic presentation of left hemispheric coverage (A) of the tuber (intracranial 64-point grid, three 4-contact strips and one 6-contact strip and two 8-contact depth electrodes were placed on the left side). Ictal onsets are seen as dark circles (B).*

growth-suppressing proteins, hamartin and tuberin, respectively. TSC2 has been associated with higher tuber burden. Deficient mTOR pathway causes the growth of tumors throughout multiple organs including, but not limited to, the brain, skin, eyes, heart, kidneys, and lungs. mTOR is a central regulator of cell proliferation, angiogenesis, and cell metabolism. The manifestations of the disorder can vary from mild to severe, and neurologically can result in complications such as intractable seizures, developmental delay, and features of autistic spectrum disorder. Once considered rare, the incidence of TSC is currently estimated at 1 in every 6,000 live births, with one million individuals known to be affected worldwide.

Individuals with TSC are often referred to neurological clinics in infancy following the onset of seizures or for the presence of neurocutaneous lesions. Seizures often present in the form of IS, as in the case presented here. Spasms consist of clusters of sudden, briefly sustained movements of the axial musculature and are commonly associated with global developmental delay. The diagnostic and characteristic interictal EEG hallmark in patients with IS is hypsarrhythmia, which involves: (a) multifocal spikes, (b) disorganized high amplitude background, and (c) burst suppression, whereby a burst of brain activity is followed by diminished brain activity. However, during the spasm, electrodecremental pattern is seen at the onset of IS. Although IS resolves by age five, the vast majority of affected individuals go on to develop other types of epilepsy that are often refractory to medication.

Brain imaging findings representative of TSC include: cortical tubers, or benign potato-like growths, that appear along the sulci and gyri, SEN, which line the ventricles and often calcify, and SEGA, which can develop near the foramen of Monro and may result in obstruction of the CSF flow and hydrocephalus. SEN do not enhance on gadolinium while SEGA may enhance.

The skin manifestations of TSC are often recognized in the pediatric or primary care clinic, resulting in neurological referrals. The most common neurocutaneous lesions include hypomelanotic macules, shagreen patch, ungual fibromas, and facial angiofibromas.

Hypomelanotic Macules: Patches of skin lighter than the surrounding skin that vary in size or shape can be in the form of a leaf and called ash leaf spot.

Shagreen Patch: Firm yellowish-red or pink area of nodules slightly elevated above the surrounding skin, texture similar to that of an orange peel.

Periungual Fibromas: Fibrous growths that appear around the fingernails and toenails.

Other non-neurological manifestations of TSC may be present in organs such as the eyes, heart, kidneys, and lungs. Table 48.1 lists all major and minor features. The diagnosis of the TSC requires the presence of either two major features or one major feature and

TABLE 48.1 *Major and Minor Features of Tuberous Sclerosis*

Major Features	Minor Features
Facial angiofibromas or forehead plaque	Multiple randomly distributed pits in dental enamels
Non-traumatic ungual or periungual fibroma	Hamartomatous rectal polyps[c]
Hypomelanotic macules (more than three)	Bone cysts[d]
Shagreen patch	Cerebral white matter migration lines[a,d]
Multiple retinal nodular hamartomas	Gingival fibromas
Cortical tuber[a]	Non-renal hamartoma[c,d]
Subependymal nodule	Retinal achromic patch
Subependymal giant cell astrocytoma	"Confetti" skin lesions
Cardiac rhabdomyoma, single or multiple	Multiple renal cysts[c]
Lymphangiomyomatosis[b]	
Renal angiomyolipoma[b]	

[a]When cerebral cortical dysplasia and cerebral white matter migration tracts occur together, they should be counted as one rather than two features of TSC.
[b]When both lymphangiomyomatosis and renal angiomyolipomas are present, other features of TSC should be present before a definitive diagnosis is made.
[c]Histologic confirmation is suggested.
[d]Radiographic confirmation is sufficient.
Source: Adapted from Roach et al. (1998) *Journal of Child Neurology* 13, 624–628.

TABLE 48.2 *Commonly Used Treatment for Infantile Spasms*

Medication	Dosing	Complications
ACTH	100 u/m² IM, if EEG after one week shows response continue dose, if suboptimal response increase dose to 150 u/m². If no response after 2 weeks consider taper. Consider taper after 2 to 4 weeks of treatment. May elect to continue treatment up to 6 to 8 weeks if good response and acceptable toxicity	Hypotension, sepsis/infection, hypokalemia
Sabril (vigabatrin)	50 to 100 mg per kg divided into 2 doses	Retinal toxicity/visual field defects, drowsiness, fatigue, dizziness, unsteadiness, cognitive difficulties, depression/psychiatric, hyperactivity in children

two minor features. Individuals with one major feature plus one minor feature probably have tuberous sclerosis. Tuberous sclerosis should be suspected in patients who have one major feature or two or more minor features.

TREATMENT

IS are commonly associated with severe delays in development; thus, early recognition of the clinical features and EEG pattern is critical to establishing timely effective treatment (Table 48.2). ACTH has proven to be the most efficacious short-term therapy despite its high risk of adverse effects. Sabril/vigabatrin, the only antiepileptic drug approved in the United States for the treatment of IS, has also been shown to be a beneficial treatment. Additionally, antiepileptic agents such as zonisamide, valproic acid, topiramate, and benzodiazepines, as well as the ketogenic diet, have been utilized in the treatment of IS; however, there is insignificant evidence proving their efficacy. Children with TS can develop other seizure types as they grow. High doses of topamax, depakote (in children older than 2 years), lamictal, levetiracetam, and felbatol are other broad spectrum antiepileptics that are used to treat IS. Trileptal and tegretol can help complex partial seizure types that may originate from the large tubers. Sirolimus (Rapamycin) is an mTOR inhibitor that has been shown to diminish the size of SEGAS and renal angiomyolipomas and improves pulmonary function in lymphangioleiomyomatosis. mTOR inhibitor, Everolimus (Afinitor), has been indicated to reduce SEGA volume. SEGA size may increase after discontinuation of mTor inhibitor therapy and may recur after resective surgery. Due to adverse effects, the chronic use of ACTH or steroids is not advisable. The vagal nerve stimulator has been used in children older than 12 years of age.

SUGGESTED READING

Bollo RJ, Kalhorn SP, Carlson C, Haegeli V, Devinsky O, Weiner HL. Epilepsy surgery and tuberous sclerosis complex: special considerations. *Neurosurg Focus.* 2008 Sep;25(3):E13.

Crino PB. Do we have a cure for Tuberous Sclerosis Complex. *Epilepsy Curr.* 2008 November;8(6):159–162.

Gomez MR, Samson JR, Whittemore VH eds. *Tuberous Sclerosis Complex*, 3rd ed. New York: Oxford University Press; 1999:29–46.

Roach ES, Gomez MR, Northrup H. Tuberous sclerosis complex consensus conference: Revised clinical diagnostic criteria. *J Child Neurol.* 1998 Dec;13(12):624–628.

Amaradha Singh and Minjee Kim

CHIEF COMPLAINT: **Changed mental status.**

HISTORY OF PRESENT ILLNESS

The patient is a 46-year-old, right-handed male with a prior history of TBI due to fall and electrocution in 1987, subsequent cognitive impairment, polysubstance abuse, and recent psychiatric admission for evaluation of acute mental status change. Upon admission, the patient's urine toxicology was positive for cocaine, methadone, and benzodiazepines. Neurology was consulted because a rapid response team was called for a witnessed seizure. Just few minutes before the seizure, he was running around, yelling, screaming, and saying things that were not making sense. Later, while the nurse was changing the patient, the staff witnessed a tonic–clonic seizure. It lasted approximately 1.5 minutes and was associated with fecal incontinence. Patient was seen breathing heavily and did not respond to any tactile stimuli.

Patient was electrocuted in 1987. He suffered from significant traumatic brain injury and remained in a coma for 6 days and was hospitalized for three weeks and received inpatient rehabilitation for another three weeks. He denied any history of febrile seizures, meningitis, or encephalitis of family history of seizures. Two years after the TBI, he started having complex partial seizures with rare secondary generalization and was started on Dilantin. Most of his seizures were either related to noncompliance or the use of recreational drugs.

PAST MEDICAL HISTORY

TBI 1987, subsequent cognitive impairment, polysubstance abuse, psychosis unspecified.

PAST SURGICAL HISTORY

Appendectomy.

ALLERGIES

None.

PERSONAL HISTORY

Smokes one pack of cigarettes per day since 16 years of age, history of alcohol and drug abuse; uses marijuana and cocaine on a regular basis. He is on disability and was not able to work since the fall; he is single and lives in a shelter.

PHYSICAL EXAMINATION

General: The patient was observed lying in bed, looked lethargic, probably postictal.
Vital signs: Blood pressure, 177/51 mm Hg; pulse, 90/min; respiratory rate 18/min; fasting glucose 190 mg/dL.

NEUROLOGICAL EXAMINATION

Higher mental functions: He could tell his name, but could not tell the date, day of the week, or the name of the hospital. He was unable to consolidate information. Speech was nonfluent, and often spoke out of the context with conversation.

CNs II–XII: PERRLA, EOMI, no nystagmus, no facial asymmetry, hearing normal, tongue midline and no atrophy, SCM and trapezii normal.

Motor: Normal bulk and tone. Patient did not comply for good motor examination but was able to move all extremities against gravity.

Sensory: Withdrew all extremities to noxious stimuli.

Reflexes: 2+ and symmetric.

Plantars: Withdraws toes bilaterally.

Gait examination, Romberg, and cerebellar examination: Deferred.

NCHCT: Stable gliosis within the left temporal lobe with mild ex vacuo dilatation of the temporal horn of the lateral ventricle, and inferior left frontal lobe and inferior right parietal lobe hypodensity suggesting old gliosis (see Figure 49.1).

EEG (06/2010): PDR of 7.5 to 8 Hz; mild generalized slowing.

DIAGNOSIS: Status epilepticus (SE).

HOSPITAL COURSE

Patient was given propofol and admitted to the MICU. Initially, he remained stable on Keppra and dilantin only, but when propofol was decreased, he developed nonconvulsive SE and had to be put back on propofol drip.

Video EEG showed left parasagittal slowing and rare sharp transients in the left centroparietal region, maxima in the P3 and C3. Twenty eight subclinical seizures were recorded over 36 hours of monitoring. Seizures were originating from the left parasagittal region, which eventually spreads to the right hemisphere (refer to Figure 49.2).

He was started on high doses of topamax 100 mg bid in addition to Keppra and phenytoin, and on this regimen, seizure activity resolved. At 24 hours seizure free, patient was able to be extubated and maintained on oral 3 drug AED regimen. AEDs at the time of transfer to the floor were Keppra 2000 mg bid, Phenytoin 200 mg bid, and Topiramate 100 mg bid.

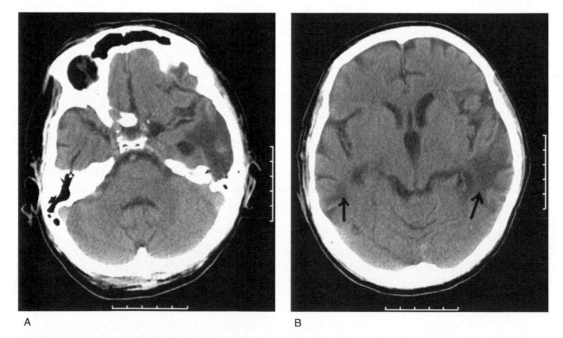

A   B

FIGURE 49.1 *Noncontrast head CT axial images showing left temporal contusion (a); and inferior temporal and posterior parietal areas of gliosis indicated by black arrows (b); left more than right.*

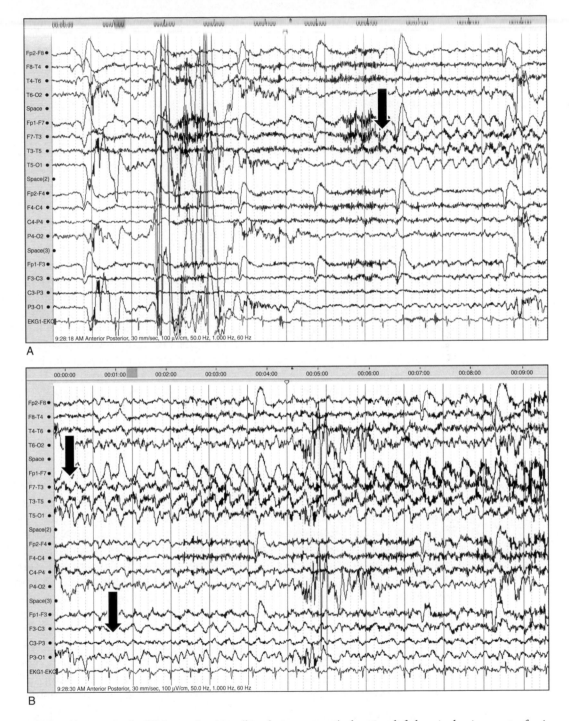

FIGURE 49.2 *Scalp EEG monitorings (bipolar montages) showing left hemispheric onset of seizures (A) and further evolution of ictal rhythms (B).*

Once on the floor, patient's mental status was significant for paranoid ideations, most notably involving delusions that the nurses were tainting his medications; nurses and physicians were stealing his money, and that there were police officers on the unit who were attempting to kill him. Patient also reported on several occasions hearing gunshots, and CMT had to be called on one occasion after patient was found on a different floor of the hospital and refused to go back to his room. Psychiatry recommended starting antipsychotic regimen and patient was placed on Risperidone, titrated up to a dose of 2 mg PO BID.

Patient started refusing medications regularly secondary to concerns that the medication was tainted, on one occasion spitting the pills back out at his nurse, and on numerous other occasions by checking medications. Despite lack of therapeutic levels of AEDs, patient remained seizure free for the remainder of his hospitalization. Repeat vEEG was negative for any epileptiform activity or subclinical seizures. Psychiatry suggested decreasing patient's Keppra dose. Keppra was slowly tapered down, now at a dose of 250 mg PO BID. Phenytoin levels were consistently subtherapeutic, and phenytoin was therefore discontinued. Topomax was increased to 200 mg twice daily; however, last level was 3.9 (8–12 expected range). Patient remained paranoid on the floor, but was in complete behavioral control. Per prior notes in chart, patient appears to have psychosis at baseline; unclear whether this is secondary to multiple TBI or primary psychotic disorder. Postictal psychosis is another possibility after cluster of seizures. Both Topomax and Keppra have been associated with psychosis. Patient was initially determined to be unable to care for himself independently given the extent of his TBI and persisting psychiatric symptoms.

Patient's cognitive function gradually improved over the remainder of his admission. He was evaluated by neuropsychology, who found him to be cognitively impaired especially in the areas of language, immediate and delayed memory, and attention.

DISCHARGE MEDICATIONS

Topamax 200 mg bid; Risperdal 2 mg po bid; Trazodone 100 mg po qhs; Flomax 0.4 mg once daily.

DISCUSSION

Gastaut in 1973 described SE as "seizure that persists for a sufficient length of time or is repeated frequently enough to produce a fixed or enduring epileptic condition." SE refers to a continuous prolonged seizure or rapidly repetitive discrete seizures with impaired consciousness in between seizures. Duration of seizures to qualify as SE is controversial and there is a movement to change the traditional definition of seizures lasting over 30 min. In practical setting, seizures lasting beyond 5 minutes should prompt an emergent use of anticonvulsant therapy. On the contrary, serial seizures can be close together but patient regains consciousness in between. About 12% to 30% of new-onset seizures can present with SE. There are approximately 20 SE cases per 100,000 people in the USA yearly, with higher incidence in early childhood (< 5 years) and in the elderly (> 65 years). SE occurs most commonly in children less than a year of age (135–156 in 100,000/year). Incidence over age 60 years is 3–10 times more common. Incidence is higher in patients with learning disabilities and structural pathology (especially frontal lesions). SE is classified into three main subtypes:

- GCSE
- EPC
- NCSE

Most commonly reported form, ~50% (Knake, 2006) is GCSE. Convulsive SE is clinically obvious initially; however, after 30 to 45 minutes of continuous seizures, clinical signs may become subtle or absent. The only sign may be twitching of eyes or fingers, or autonomic manifestation such as tachycardia, papillary dilatation, or hypertension. In such cases, a continuous EEG would be the only way to monitor seizure activities. GESE can be further classified according to the seizure types, such as partial with secondarily generalized, generalized seizures at onset, absence status, myoclonic status, and febrile status epilepticus.

Focal motor SE, or EPC, is a continuous muscle twitching without generalization, which is frequently seen in a single limb or a side of the face. This subtype is relatively uncommon, and how aggressively one needs to treat EPC largely depends on the clinical context. EPC can be seen with neoplastic lesions such as glioblastoma multiforme or autoimmune inflammatory conditions such as Rasmussen's encephalitis. Simple partial seizures are hardest to treat. Rasmussen's encephalitis presents with intractable seizures, which are medically refractory and often requiring hemispherectomy.

The third subtype, NCSE, represents a heterogeneous group of nonmotor seizures. It includes primary generalized SE (e.g., absence SE), secondary generalized SE, and complex partial SE. Since their clinical presentation varies widely, ranging from somnolent to comatose status, the only way to diagnose NCSE is by doing routine or prolonged EEG. For this reason, NCSE is likely under-recognized, particularly in critically ill patients with impaired mental status. Five to ten percent of comatose patients in the ICU, and up to 34% of neurological ICU patients may be in NCSE if examined by EEG. In patients with severe anoxic-ischemic encephalopathy, NCSE is associated with poor neurological outcome. Nonepileptic SE can be confused with NCSE or GCSE.

ETIOLOGY OF SE

Any factors causing an increase in the glutamate activity can cause prolonged seizures. Prolonged seizures themselves can desensitize GABA receptors causing more excitotoxicity leading on to apoptosis by sustained high influx of calcium ions into neurons. Neuronal injury caused by prolonged seizures gets worse if there are co-existing conditions, such as hyperthermia, hypoxia, and hypotension. The most common risk factor of SE is a prior history of epilepsy (22%–26%). However, more than half of SE occurs in patients without prior seizures. In adults, most common causes of SE are cerebrovascular accidents (25%); change in medications (18%–20%), alcohol/substance withdrawal (10%–13%), and less frequent causes include anoxia, metabolic derangement, infection, trauma, and tumor, in a descending order. In contrast, one third of pediatric SE cases are due to infections followed by low antiepileptic drug levels. Other causes of SE are listed in Table 49.1.

Etiology and age are two main determinants of prognosis in SE, and there is an intricate relationship between them, as discussed below. The prognosis of SE is greatly dependent on age, etiology, promptness of treatments, and complications that occur in its course. Short-term mortality, measured as death rate during hospitalization for SE or within 30 days of

TABLE 49.1 *Causes of SE*

Acute	Chronic
CNS infections (meningitis or encephalitis)	Known seizure disorder
Stroke	Alcohol/drug withdrawal
Neoplasms	Remote CNS insult
Head trauma	
Drug toxicity	
Hypoxia	
Metabolic encephalopathy: Abnormal lytes, renal failure	

SE, ranges from 8% to 22% across all age groups. Most of these early deaths occur in those with acute symptomatic etiology. Although long-term mortality of SE is not as well studied as short-term outcomes, a population-based cohort study showed that among survivors of the initial 30 days after their first SE, over 40% died in the next 10 years. This is approximately three-fold higher mortality compared to general population. Mirroring risk factors for short-term mortality, acute symptomatic etiology (vs. idiopathic/cryptogenic etiology; relative risk [RR] =2.2), myoclonic SE (vs. GCSE; RR= 4.0), and SE duration > 24 hours (vs. < 2 h; RR =2.3) were associated with increased 10-year mortality. Interestingly, patients with idiopathic SE appear to have no significant increase in long-term mortality compared to general population, suggesting that SE alone does not modify long-term mortality. The means by which SE affects mortality remains to be elucidated. However, serious medical complications during the hospitalization, irreversible neurological damage, and functional deterioration on discharge likely contribute to the long-term outcome. Children have a much lower mortality rate (3%–15%) than adults (15%–22%), which is probably due both to their physiologic resilience and to the nature of etiology in this age group. For example, prolonged febrile seizures carry a low mortality rate, rarely last longer than 2 hours, and are generally more responsive to treatments than GCSEs of other etiologies. Etiologies that cause severe persistent systemic disturbances such as anoxia are less common in children yet carries similar mortality as when it occurs in adults.

Prolonged seizures morbidity and mortality rates of SE appear to have crude correlation to its etiology. In the past, NCSE has been thought to be a benign condition. However, recent studies indicate that even NCSE is associated with significant complications. Unremitting seizure activities result in cardiorespiratory, autonomic, and metabolic complications as well as irreversible neuronal injury. Prolonged convulsive seizures may lead to hypothermia, acidosis, rhabdomyolysis, renal failure, trauma, and pulmonary aspiration. It is believed that in the Phase I of the SE (0–30 minutes), the compensatory mechanisms are still intact. In the Phase 2 of SE (>30 minutes), compensatory mechanisms start failing (see Table 49.2).

Prolonged seizure activities lasting as little as 30 to 60 minutes may result in irreversible neuronal damage secondary to excitotoxicity, apoptosis, synaptic reorganization, and impaired protein and DNA synthesis. Seizures lasting longer than 1 hour are predictive of poor outcome. Certain regions of the brain are more likely to be affected by SE than others. They include hippocampal complex, amygdala, thalamus, and cerebellar pyramidal cells, all of which have abundant receptors for excitatory neurotransmitters and are therefore more prone to excitotoxicity and other mechanisms of insult. Some victims of SE suffer from irreversible dysfunction in memory, balance, affect, and cognition. Prolonged febrile convulsions, considered benign in the past, are thought to result in acute hippocampal injury and MTS, later leading to development of temporal epilepsy. A causal association, however, is still being argued, since genetic predisposition is an important cause both for

TABLE 49.2 *Phases of SE*

Phase I (0–30 min)	Phase II (>30 min)
Adrenaline and noradrenaline release	Failure of cerebral autoregulation
Increased cerebral blood flow and metabolism	Cerebral edema
Hypertension and hyperpyrexia	Respiratory depression
Hyperventilation and tachycardia	Cardiac arrhythmias
Lactic acidosis	Hypotension
	Hypoglycemia
	Hyponatremia
	Renal failure rhabdomyolysis, hyperthermia
	Disseminated intravascular coagulation

febrile seizures and MTS. Since SE often requires an intensive level of care and prolonged hospitalization, there are additional complications associated with treatment. Adverse effects of anticonvulsant drugs, drug–drug interactions, ventilator-associated pneumonia, and other nosocomial infections are just a few examples.

Treatment: SE is a true neurological and medical emergency, requiring prompt recognition and initiation of treatments. Many old and newer anticonvulsant drugs have been studied for their effectiveness in SE. Out-of-hospital options include rectal Diazepam, buccal and intranasal Midazolam, and Klonopin ODT wafers.

Management includes:

- ABCs
- Start pharmacotherapy (Table 49.3)
- Vitals monitoring, oxygen, IV access; intubation to protect airway as needed, avoid long-acting neuromuscular blockers (they can mask seizure acitivity)
- Passive cooling for hyperthermia
- Draw ABG, electrolytes and AED levels

Most commonly used agents are summarized in Table 49.3. Ideal agent would be something that is easy to administer, 100% effective, has prompt onset of action and long duration of action.

In general, IV benzodiazepines are the first line agents for GCSE in adults. Lorazepam is a preferred agent to diazepam and midazolam because of its better water solubility and

TABLE 49.3 *Treatment of SE*

I/V Lorazepam	0.1 mg/kg (4 mg to 8 mg loading dose)
I/V Phenytoin	*Loading dose:* 20 mg/kg IV
	Maximum infusion rate: 50 mg/min
I/V Fosphenytoin	*Loading dose:* 20 mg/kg IV
	Maximum infusion rate: 150 mg/min
I/V Valproate	*Loading dose:* 20 mg/kg IV, higher doses 30–60 mg/kg can be used.
	Infusion rate: 5 mg/kg/min
I/V Phenobarbital	*Loading dose:* 15 mg/kg to 20 mg/kg
	Maximum rate: 50–100 mg/min
Midazolam (Versed) I/M, nasal, buccal	0.2 mg/kg (nasal/buccal faster than IM)
Continuous IV Midazolam Infusion*	*Bolus dose:* 0.2 mg/kg, repeat boluses of 0.2–0.4 mg/kg every 5 min until seizures stop, up *to maximum total loading dose* of 2 mg/kg
	Initial infusion rate: 0.1 mg/kg/h
	Maintenance: 0.05 mg/kg/h–2.9 mg/kg/h
	(Continuous IV rate should be increased by 20%)
Continuous IV Propofol infusion*	*Bolus dose:* 1 mg/kg
	Repeat 1 mg/kg to 2 mg/kg boluses q 3–5 min until seizures stop, up to 10 mg/kg
	Initial infusion rate: 2 mg/kg/h
	Continuous infusion rate: 1 mg/kg/h to 15 mg/kg/h
	Do not exceed >5 mg/kg/h for >48 h
Continuous IV Pentobarbital Infusion*	*Loading dose:* 5 mg/kg, repeat 5 mg/kg boluses until seizures stop. Maximum bolus rate: 25 mg/min to 50 mg/min (based on BP)
	Initial infusion rate: 1 mg/kg/h
	Maintenance rate: 0.5 mg/kg/h to 10.0 mg/kg/h

*All continuous infusions should be kept on a steady dose for 12 to 24 hours and slow withdrawal of infusions is recommended over 24 h. If seizures return, try even slower withdrawal.

TABLE 49.4 *AEDs as precipitants of SE*

Drugs	Types of SE
Benzodiazepines	Tonic SE
Carbamazepine	Absence, myoclonic, ESES
Oxcarbmazapine	Myoclonic and absence SE
Lamotrigine	Myoclonic SE
Tiagabine	Nonconvulsive SE (partial and absence)
Vigabatrin	Nonconvulsive SE (partial and absence)

hence a longer serum half-life (4–6 hours). Sixty-five percent of GCSE can be terminated with the initial benzodiazepine therapy. If seizures stop and the cause of SE are promptly corrected, additional emergency agents may not be necessary. If seizures continue after the administration of lorazepam, IV phenytoin or fosphenytoin is the next choice of agent (Table 49.3). Although not as widely available, fosphenytoin has advantages over phenytoin in that it can be infused three times faster, can be administered intramuscularly, and has a better side-effect profile. Following a loading dose, an additional smaller dose (i.e. 25%–50% of the initial dose) of phenytoin or fosphenytoin can be given. For continuing seizures, a loading dose of IV phenobarbital may be administered, followed by a second dose (i.e. 25%–50% of the initial dose). Alternatively, newer agents with broad spectrum, such as IV valproic acid or levetiracetam, can be used at this point, depending on past experiences, drug availability, and personal preferences. At any point during the treatment, an emergency intubation may be necessary, especially if the patient develops emesis, because loss of protective airway reflexes is common with repeated or prolonged seizures, increasing the risk of pulmonary aspiration. If the patient has seizures continuing over an hour on presentation, has severe systemic derangement, or develops SE while in the intensive care unit, the treating physician can immediately proceed with continuous infusion of general anesthetic agents such as propofol, midazolam, or pentobarbital (see Table 49.3).

If patients with known epilepsy develop status epilepticus, it is often due to a low serum level of their antiepileptic drugs, and the administration of their home medications may be necessary unless one is absolutely sure of their compliance. For absence SE, first-line agents sodium valproate, ethosuximide, and benzodiazepines are effective. On the other hand, benzodiazepines, phenytoin, carbamazepine, lamotrigine, oxcarbmazepine, vigabatrin, and tiagabine can paradoxically cause SE (see Table 49.4).

The key to the management of SE is early recognition and early intervention by pharmacotherapy and avoiding complications.

SUGGESTED READING

DeLorenzo RJ, Pellock JM, Towne AR, Boggs JG. Epidemiology of status epilepticus. *J Clin Neurophysiol.* 1995;12(4):316–325.

Hirsch LJ. Levitating Levetiracetam's status for status epilepticus. *Epilepsy Curr.* 2008;8(5):125–126.

Lowenstein, DH. Status epilepticus, *N Engl J Med.* 1998;338:970–976.

Shorvon S. Definition, classification and frequency of status epilepticus. In: Shorvon S, ed. *Epilepticus: Its Clinical Features and Treatment in Children and Adults.* Cambridge: Cambridge University Press; 1994:21–33.

Treiman DM. Generalized convulsive, nonconvulsive, and focal status epilepticus. In: Feldman E, ed. *Current Diagnosis in Neurology.* St. Louis: Mosby-Year Book;1994:11–18.

Treiman DM, Meyers PD, Walton NY, et al. A comparison of four treatments for generalized convulsive status epilepticus. Veterans Affairs Status Epilepticus Cooperative Study Group. *N Engl J Med.* 17 Sep 1998;339(12):792–798.

Left-Arm Weakness in a Patient With Lung Cancer

Jonathan H. Howard

CHIEF COMPLAINT: **Weakness in left arm for the last few days.**

HISTORY OF PRESENT ILLNESS

The patient is a 76-year-old, right-handed man who was admitted with a one-day history of pain in his left leg and three-day weakness of his left arm. His history and work-up since admission were reviewed. His ER examination revealed that his left lower extremity was cold, pale, and peripheral pulses could not be palpated. On review of symptoms, the patient also complained of hemoptysis and dyspnea. Further history revealed that the patient had been a heavy smoker for many years. A chest radiograph revealed a large right pleural effusion. A bronchoscopy with biopsy of a subcarinal lymph node was performed, and pathological examination revealed the diagnosis of nonsmall cell lung cancer. An angiogram of his leg revealed an arterial thrombus, and the patient had his leg amputated below his knee.

On postoperative day 6, he informed the primary team that he was having trouble moving his left arm and neurology was consulted. The onset of this weakness had been gradual over the past several days. He also said that he felt his hands were clumsy, and he had difficulty buttoning his shirt and eating his food. He also reported a dull, diffuse headache of several days duration. The patient denied visual complaints, sensory complaints, or difficulty speaking.

PAST MEDICAL HISTORY

Hypertension and HLD.

PAST SURGICAL HISTORY

Cholecystectomy.

MEDICATIONS

Norvasc and Crestor once daily (did not recall the dosages).

ALLERGIES

None.

PERSONAL HISTORY

He has 30 years of smoking history but denied any history of alcohol or drug abuse.

PHYSICAL EXAMINATION

Vital signs: Blood pressure, 120/88 mm Hg; pulse, 78/min; respiratory rate, 16/min; afebrile.

General physical examination was significant for decreased movements of the chest on the right side, stony dullness to percussion and diminished breath sounds with decreased vocal resonance and pleural friction rub. Patient had below-knee amputation of the left lower extremity.

NEUROLOGICAL EXAMINATION

Higher mental functions: The patient was awake and alert. He knew the name of the hospital and the year though he was unsure of month. His memory was 1/3. His spontaneous speech was fluent and he was able to name objects appropriately. He had difficulty following complex commands and was unable to sustain attention for tasks such as naming the months of the year backwards or serial 7s.

CNs II–XII: Unremarkable except left UMN facial.

Motor: Left upper extremity strength was 3–4/5. He was able to lift his left thigh off the bed and the remainder of his left leg had been amputated. Strength on the right side was 5/5.

Sensory: Intact to all modalities of sensation.

Reflexes: Symmetrical except slight left hyperreflexia in the upper extremity.

Cerebellar: Bilateral dysmetria and difficulty with rapid-alternating movements.

Gait examination was deferred.

STOP AND THINK QUESTIONS

➢ Where could the lesion be in this patient?

➢ Does the relatively gradual onset of the patient's symptoms help determine the nature of the lesion? How could the same pathological process explain his mental status abnormalities and ataxia?

➢ What treatment options are available in this case?

DIAGNOSTIC TEST RESULTS

An MRI scan of the brain with gadolinium was obtained (Figure 50.1A–50.1C). This revealed numerous, round lesions scattered throughout the brain, brain stem, and cerebellum. The lesions displayed ring-like enhancement on post-gad T1 sequences (Figure 50.1A–50.1C). Most of the brain lesions were located at the gray–white junctions. A large lesion was seen in the subcortical white matter in the right frontal lobe accounting for his weakness of the left arm (Figure 50.1C). All of the lesions were associated with a variable degree of vasogenic edema and mass effect upon adjacent brain parenchyma. There was mild compression of the fourth ventricle on the right, imposed by an adjacent metastatic lesion; however, the ventricle remained patent on the left. Ventriculomegaly disproportionate to the degree of age-related sulcal enlargement suggested mild obstructive hydrocephalus.

Due to the number of brain lesions, our patient was treated with WBR, though he unfortunately expired several weeks after the radiation.

DIAGNOSIS: Metastatic small-cell lung cancer with intracranial metastases (ICM).

DISCUSSION

ICM are amongst the most dreaded and unfortunately common complications in patients with cancer. Approximately 170,000 cancer patients develop ICM every year in the United States, compared with approximately 20,000 primary brain tumors. ICM are seen in about 10% to 30% of adult patients with cancer and 5% to 10% of children with cancer. ICM can be classified based on the location of the tumor with the skull, dura, leptomeninges, and brain parenchyma all being sites of possible spread. About 80% of ICM localize to the brain or leptomeninges.

The most common primary tumor in patients with ICM is lung carcinoma, which accounts for almost half of all brain metastases. Other primary tumors that metastasize to the brain

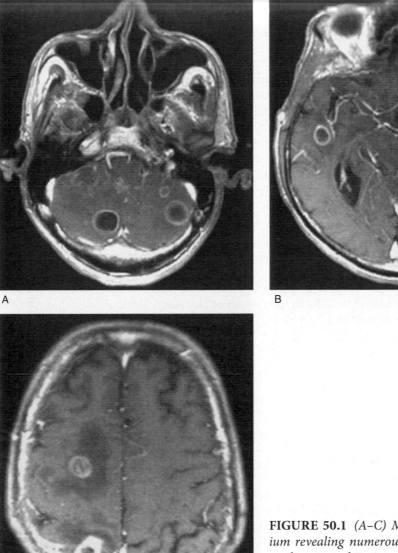

FIGURE 50.1 *(A–C) MRI brain with gadolinium revealing numerous, round lesions located at the gray–white junctions scattered throughout the brain, brain stem, and cerebellum. The lesions display ring-like enhancement on postgad T1 sequences.*

include breast, melanoma, sarcomas, thyroid, renal, and colon cancers. Hemorrhage into malignant neoplasms accounts for approximately 10% of all spontaneous intracranial hematomas. Significant hemorrhage can occur in 3% to 14% of brain metastases. Intracerebral metastases most prone to hemorrhage include bronchogenic carcinoma, malignant melanoma, choriocarcinoma, renal cell carcinoma, and thyroid malignancy. Rarely colorectal malignancy and malignant fibrous histiocytoma can also present as brain metastases with hemorrhage.

Tumor cells most commonly reach the brain by hematogenous spread. Therefore, metastases are frequently located at the junction of the gray matter and white matter where blood vessels narrow. The distribution of metastases to the CNS is proportional to the amount of blood flow to various regions. About 80% are located in the cerebral hemispheres, 15% are located in the cerebellum, and 5% are located in the brain stem.

As with primary brain tumors, ICM can produce a wide range of neurological signs and symptoms depending on the location of the tumor and its rate of growth. Neurological dysfunction is the presenting symptom of an underlying cancer in about 10% to 20% of cases.

Headache is probably the most frequent complaint in patients with ICM and is present in about half of such patients. Such headaches are typically insidious in onset and may resemble tension-type headaches. The classic picture of a headache on awakening in the morning is certainly a worrisome feature of any headache, but actually not a common feature of patients with ICM.

ICM commonly produce focal neurological deficits such as weakness, numbness, seizures, visual field abnormalities, aphasias, or ataxia. Usually, such symptoms are subacute in onset, though occasionally patients may have a presentation that mimics a stroke. Often times, this occurs when a patient has had a hemorrhage into a tumor. The patient may present with lethargy, personality change, or memory impairment. Such patients typically have tumors located in the frontal or temporal lobes. Additionally, patients with blockage of the ventricular system may develop nausea and vomiting in addition to headache due to obstructive hydrocephalus.

In patients in whom ICM are suspected, an MRI with gadolinium is the diagnostic study of choice, although in the emergency department, a CT with contrast may be more feasible. ICM are usually multiple, round lesions that are seen at the gray–white junction, with mass effect and surrounding vasogenic edema. With the administration of gadolinium, a ring-like pattern of enhancement is characteristic, reflecting breakage of the blood–brain barrier. Biopsy should be reserved for patients without a clear diagnosis of ICM. This includes patients with an isolated lesion, or patients with multiple brain lesions in whom no underlying, systemic cancer can be found despite a meticulous search.

In patients with suspected ICM but without a known primary tumor, an investigation for an underlying cancer should be performed. The site of the underlying cancer may be obvious from history and physical examination alone. In patients for whom this is not the case, the initial evaluation should consist of a chest radiograph and a CT chest given the high incidence of lung cancer. Other frequent primary, yet occult tumors include breast cancer, colon cancer, renal cancer, and melanoma. If imaging of the chest is unremarkable, a CT of the abdomen and pelvis should be performed to search for these cancers. Mammogram in females and colonoscopy in both sexes should be considered in the right clinical context. In about 25% of cases, no primary tumor can be identified.

TREATMENT

Once the diagnosis is made, high-dose steroids are usually started to relieve vasogenic edema and lower the intracranial pressure. This often has a rapid and dramatic improvement in the patient's symptoms and can be life-saving in certain patients. Our patient was started on high-dose steroids (Decadron 10 mg IV every 6 h). The following day, he was able to lift his left arm above his head. Further treatment consists of neurosurgical resection, radiotherapy, or a combination of the two treatments. Radiotherapy, in turn, consists of stereotactic radiosurgery and WBR.

The exact combination of these treatments must be individualized on a case-by-case basis. For most patients, the goal of treatment is relief of symptoms rather than increased survival. Factors that influence further treatment include the size, number, and location of the metastases, as well as the overall prognosis of the patient. Three prognostic classes have been identified based on the age of the patient, their performance status, and the extent of extracranial disease. Indications of a favorable prognosis include age less than 65, a Karnofsky performance score of greater than 70, and a well-controlled primary tumor. For patients with a favorable prognosis, a more aggressive treatment approach using surgery or stereotactic radiosurgery can be justified.

Surgeries combined with WBR can double the life expectancy for patients with a single metastasis. Surgical interventions are being increasingly used in patients with multiple metastatic lesions. The primary indication for surgery in patients with multiple metastases is relief of focal symptoms due to mass effect from large lesions. In other cases, tissue may be needed for pathological diagnosis. Surgery is usually followed by WBR. In one randomized trial, postsurgical patients who received WBR had a lower incidence of tumor recurrence in the brain and were less likely to die of neurological causes, though overall mortality and function were not improved. WBR alone is used in patients with a poor prognosis and in those with numerous brain metastases. It has been shown to decrease the amount of tumor edema as well as improve neurologic function. The survival usually depends on the degree of extracranial disease. WBR has been shown to increase survival from 1 to 2 months to 3 to 6 months. Patients who receive WBR should be pretreated with steroids to minimize the risk of worsening cerebral edema.

Stereotactic radiosurgery is a technique using multiple convergent beams of radiation to specifically target a discrete area of pathology while sparing the surrounding, unaffected brain tissue. Though there have been no trials directly comparing SR with surgical resection, based on observational studies, SR is comparable to surgery in certain patients. The size of the tumor is the primary factor in deciding whether surgery or SR is preferable. For lesions greater than 3 cm, surgery offers more immediate debulking of the lesion and minimizes the risk of radiation necrosis of normal tissue associated with SR. Adding WBR to SR has been shown to improve local tumor control, but does not prolong overall survival. SR has been shown to be effective in sarcomas, melanomas, and renal cancers, which are traditionally thought of as radio resistant.

In addition to focal neurological deficits due to mass effect, patients with ICM are at risk for seizures. Postsurgical patients are often temporarily placed on prophylactic anticonvulsants, but there is little evidence to support their prolonged use. In patients who suffer from seizures, however, lifelong antiepileptic treatment is indicated.

SUGGESTED READING

Suh JH, Vogelbaum MA, Barnett GH. Update of stereotactic radiosurgery for brain tumors. [Review] [33 refs] [Journal Article. Review] *Curr Opin Neurol*. Dec 2004;17(6):681–686.

Wen PY, Loeffler JS. Management of brain metastases. *Oncology (Huntingt)* Jul 1999;13(7):941–954, 957–961; discussion 961–962, 969.

Note: Page references followed by "*f*" and "*t*" denote figures and tables, respectively.